Zoology
NCERT
Pointers and Practice

DR. LAXMI KANT GUPTA

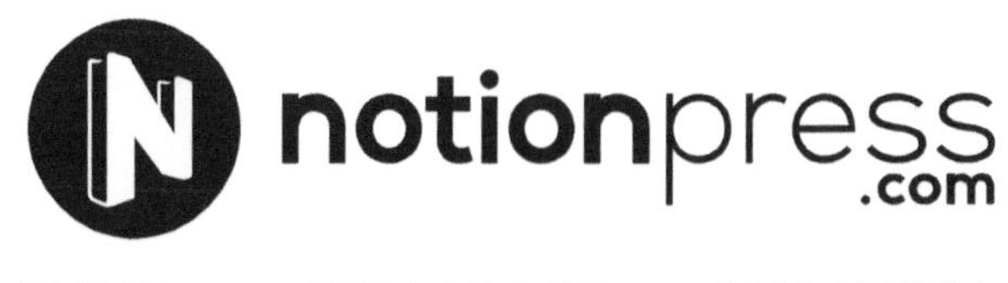

ISBN 979-8-89446-068-0

Contents

PREFACE

NCERT – Pointers and Practice for NEET-Zoology and other Medical Entrance Examinations is a comprehensive practice material for students aspiring to get admission into prestigious medical colleges. The contents of this book have been carefully created to help students master the latest trends in questions from across key medical entrance examinations. This book can also be used as a resource to prepare for class XI and XII board examinations—**100% based on NCERT**.

HIGHLIGHTS OF THE BOOK:

- Framed as per class XI and XII syllabus of NCERT.
- Content designed to help maximise scores in NEET.
- Assertion and Reason questions to help critical analysis.
- Latest pattern based LIST 1/ LIST 2 type questions in every chapter.
- Well designed Exclusively NCERT based Statement based questions in every chapter.
- Questions in end of each chapter and test papers for student's self-practice.

STUDENTS NOTE:

As an experienced teacher/mentor, I would suggest a student should meticulously scan the theory and diagrams of **NCERT –Pointer and Practice** minimum three times. In my opinion, the book will prove to be an asset and will serve to fulfill the requirement of the medical aspirants.

Dr. Laxmi Kant Gupta

Ph.D., CSIR-NET

Former CSIR-SRF

About the Author

Dr Laxmi Kant Gupta has completed his Ph.D. form IIPR, Kanpur and qualified CSIR-NET. After This he was appointed as Lecturer/Assistant Professor In **D.A.V. College**, Kanpur.

Qualifications

- **PH.D** - Genetics & Plant Breeding
- **CSIR-NET** - Life Sciences
- **Former CSIR-SRF**

Experience

1. **Research Experience:-**

   3 Year Research Experience as CSIR-SRF in **Indian Institute of Pulses Research** Kanpur.

2. **Teaching Experience in College:-**

   5 year Teaching Experience as Lecturer/Assistant Professor in **D.A.V. College**, Kanpur.

3. **Teaching Experience in Coachings:-**

   23 Year+ In Various Prestigeous Institute Of India.

Administrative Experience

- Worked as **HOD** Science & Technology Department of **Spectra Coaching Centre**.
- Worked as Member of Libarary Advisory Committee in **D.A.V. College**, Kanpur.

Acknowledgment

This book is a result of the enormous support given by **Aashish Arora sir** who always there to support me. I believe that the blessings of my parents (Late **Dr. Raj Kumar Gupta** and Late **Smt. Pushplata Gupta**) and my grandparents always helped me. My wife **Neetu Gupta** and son **Abhishek Varshney** always played a prime role in making me more focused and determined towards my goal. All other family members inspired me throughout the preparation of this book. My sincere thanks to the team of **Notion Press** for providing me the platform to serve students. I appreciate their efforts in bringing out this book in such an excellent manner. Careful attempts have been made in making the book error free; however, corrections, suggestions, queries, and criticism will be highly appreciated and are welcome. Once again special thanks to my wife **Neetu Gupta** and son **Abhishek Varshney** for always being there with me and helping me in ensuring high quality throughout the book.

Dr. Laxmi Kant Gupta

Ph.D., CSIR-NET

Former CSIR-SRF

ANIMAL KINGDOM

1.1 Basis of Classification

1.2 Classification ofAnimals

- Over **a million species of animals have been discovered till now** so the need for classification becomes all the more important.

- The classification helps in assigning a systematic position to newly find species.

1.1 BASIS OF CLASSIFICATION

- With respect to differences in structure and form of different animals, there are fundamental features common to various individuals in relation to the arrangement of cells, body symmetry, nature of coelom, patterns of digestive, circulatory or reproductive systems.

- These above features are used as the basis of animal classification.

1.1.1 Levels of Organisation

- According to **RH whittaker** all members of Animalia are multicellular, all of them do not exhibit the same pattern of organisation of cells.

- **In sponges,** the cells are arranged as loose cell aggregates, i.e., they exhibit **cellular level** of organisation.

- **Some division of labour (activities) occur among the cells in sponges.**

- **In coelenterates,** the arrangement of cells is more complex.

- The cells performing the same function are arranged into tissues, hence is called **tissue level** of organisation.

- **Organ level** is exhibited by members of **Platyhelminthes.**

- In other higher phyla where tissues are grouped together to form organs, each specialized for a particular function. In animals like **Annelids, Arthropods, Molluscs,**

- **Echinoderms and Chordates**, organs have associated to form functional systems, each system concerned with a specific physiological function which is called **organ system** level of organisation.

- Organ systems in different groups of animals exhibit various patterns of complexities.

- The digestive system **in Platyhelminthes has only a single opening** to the outside of the body that serves as both mouth and anus, hence **called incomplete.**

- **A complete digestive system** has two openings, mouth and anus. Similarly, the circulatory system may be of two types:

- (i) **open type** in which the blood is pumped out of the heart and the cells and tissues are directly bathed in it. Examples **Arthropoda, Non cephalopod Mollusca, Tunicata, Hemichordata, Echinodermata, Leech**

- (ii) **closed type** in which the blood is circulated through a series of vessels of varying diameters (arteries, veins and capillaries). Examples **Most of Annelida, Chordata Except Urochodata**

1.1.2 Symmetry

- Animals can be classified on the basis of their symmetry.

a. Asymmetry

- Sponges are mostly **asymmetrical,** i.e., any plane that passes through the center does not divide them into equal halves. Example **most of sponges, Gastropod Mollusca**

- **In Gastropoda mollusca due to torsion Asymmetry found.**

b. Radial symmetry

- When any plane passing through the central axis of the body divides the organism into two identical halves, it is called **radial symmetry.**

- Coelenterates, ctenophores and adult echinoderms shows radial symmetry.

c. Bilateral symmetry

- **Bilateral symmetry found** in Animals like Flatworm, Round worm, annelids, arthropods to chordates except adult Echinodermata and Gastropod mollusca.

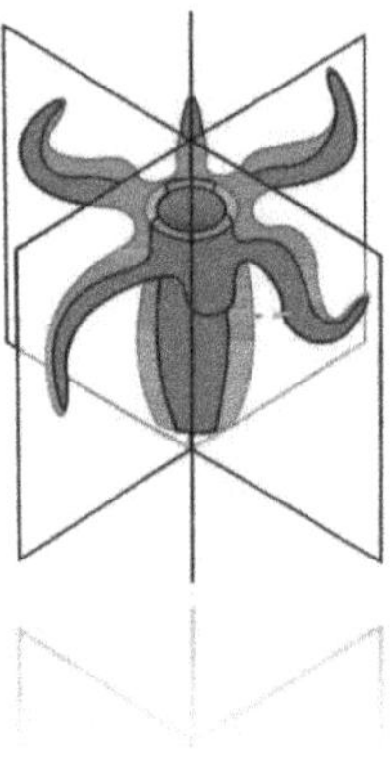
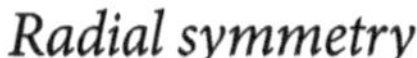

Radial symmetry

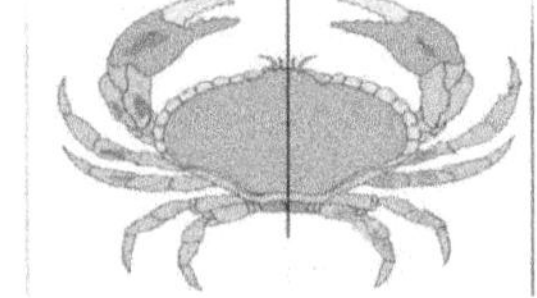

Bilateral symmetry

1.1.3 Diploblastic and Triploblastic Organisation

Diploblastic animals

- Animals in which the cells are arranged in two embryonic layers, an external **ectoderm** and an internal **endoderm,** are called **diploblastic** animals, e.g., coelenterates.

- An undifferentiated layer, mesoglea, is present in between the ectoderm and the endoderm example **cnidarians.**

Triploblastic animals

- **Triploblastic:** Those animals in which the developing embryo has a third germinal layer– Mesoderm in between the ectoderm and endoderm e.g. Platyhelminthes to chordates.

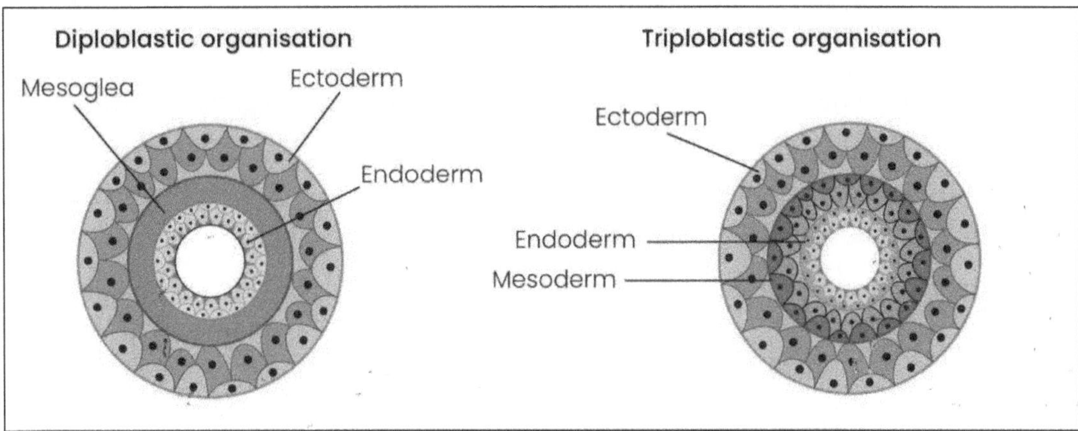

1.1.4 Coelom

- **Presence or absence of a cavity** between the body wall and the gut wall is very important in classification.
- The body cavity, which is lined by mesoderm is called **coelom**.

Coelomates

- Animals possessing coelom are called **coelomates,** e.g., annelids, molluscs, arthropods, echinoderms, hemichordates and chordates.

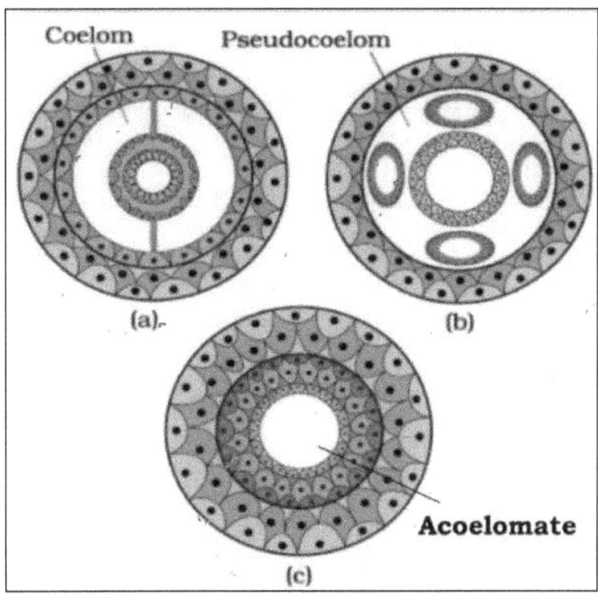

Pseudocoelomates

- The body cavity in which the mesoderm is present as scattered pouches in between the ectoderm and endoderm is called pseudocoelom and the animals possessing them are called **pseudocoelomates,** e.g., Roundworms.

Acoelomates

- The animals in which the body cavity is absent are called **acoelomates,** e.g., Flatworms.
- In **acoelomates body cavity absent** because mesodermal parenchymatous cell densely present.
- The animals in which the developing embryo has a third germinal layer, **mesoderm**, in between the ectoderm and endoderm, are called **triploblastic** animals e.g. platyhelminthes to chordates.

1.1.5 Segmentation

- In some animals, the body is **externally** and **internally** divided into segments with a serial repetition of at least some organs.
- In earthworm, the body shows **metameric segmentation** and the phenomenon is known as **metamerism.** Example - **Annelida, Arthropoda, Chordata**
- **Pseudometamerism** found in *Taenia.*

1.1.6 Notochord

- Notochord is a **mesodermal** in origin.
- **Rod-like structure.**
- Notochord formed on the dorsal side during embryonic development in chordates.
- Animals with notochord are called chordates and those animals which do not form this structure are called non-chordates, e.g., porifera to echinoderms.
- In Urochordata notochord is present in the tail of larva only.
- In Hemichordata stomochord presen

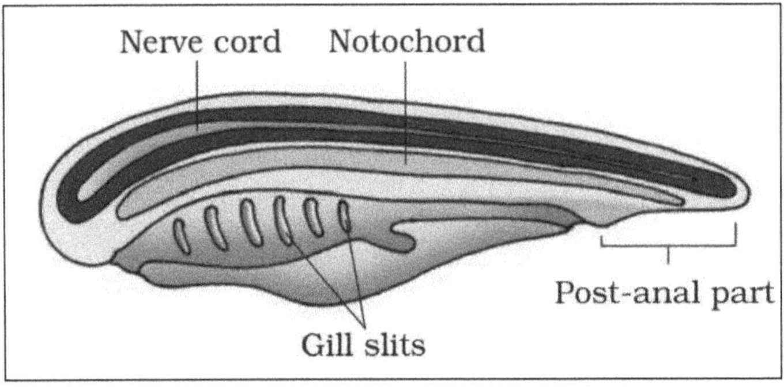

Figure shows position of Notochord

1.1.7 Embroyonic Development

On the basis of fate of blastopore, animals can be divided into two categories:

(a) **Protostomiates:** Animals in which Blastopore firstly forms mouth. e.g. Platyhelminthes to Mollusca

(b) **Deuterostomiates:** Animals in which Blastopore firstly forms anus.e.g. Echinoderms, Hemichordates and Chordates

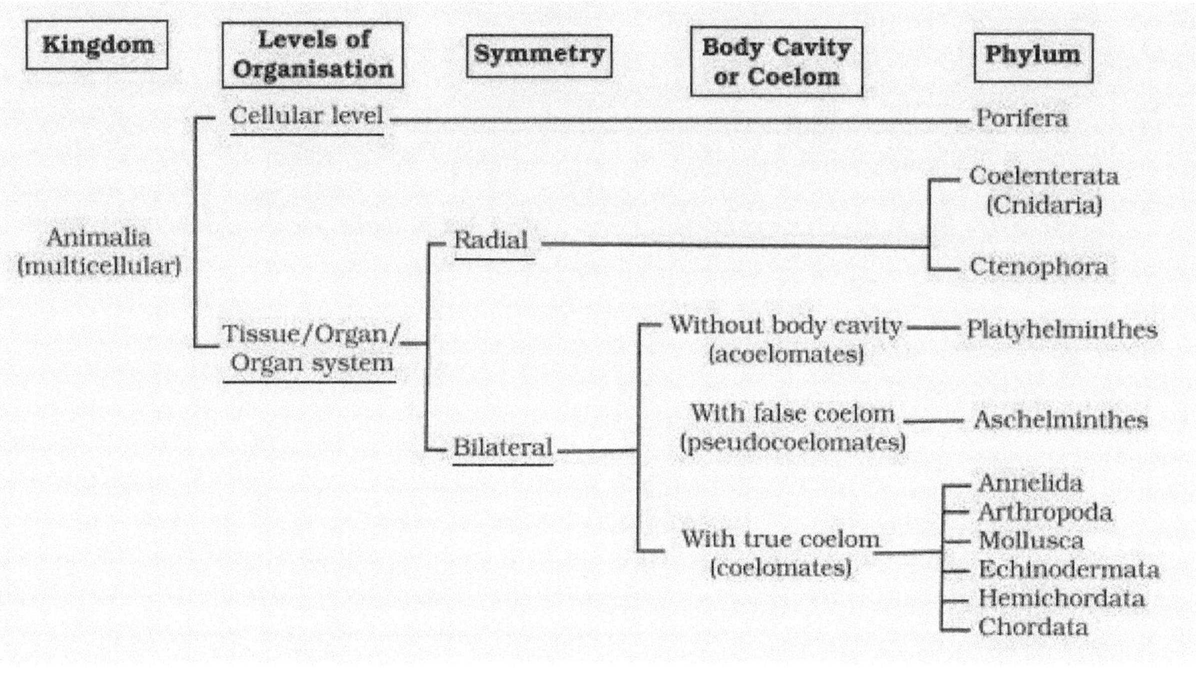

Kingdom
Levels of Organisation
Symmetry
Body Cavity or Coelom
Phylum
Animalia (multicellular)
Cellular level
Porifera
Tissue/Organ/ Organ system
Radial
Coelenterata (Cnidaria)
Ctenophora
Bilateral
Without body cavity (acoelomates)
Platyhelminthes
With false coelom (pseudocoelomates)
Aschelminthes
With true coelom (coelomates)
Annelida
Arthropoda
Mollusca
Echinodermata
Hemichordata
Chordata

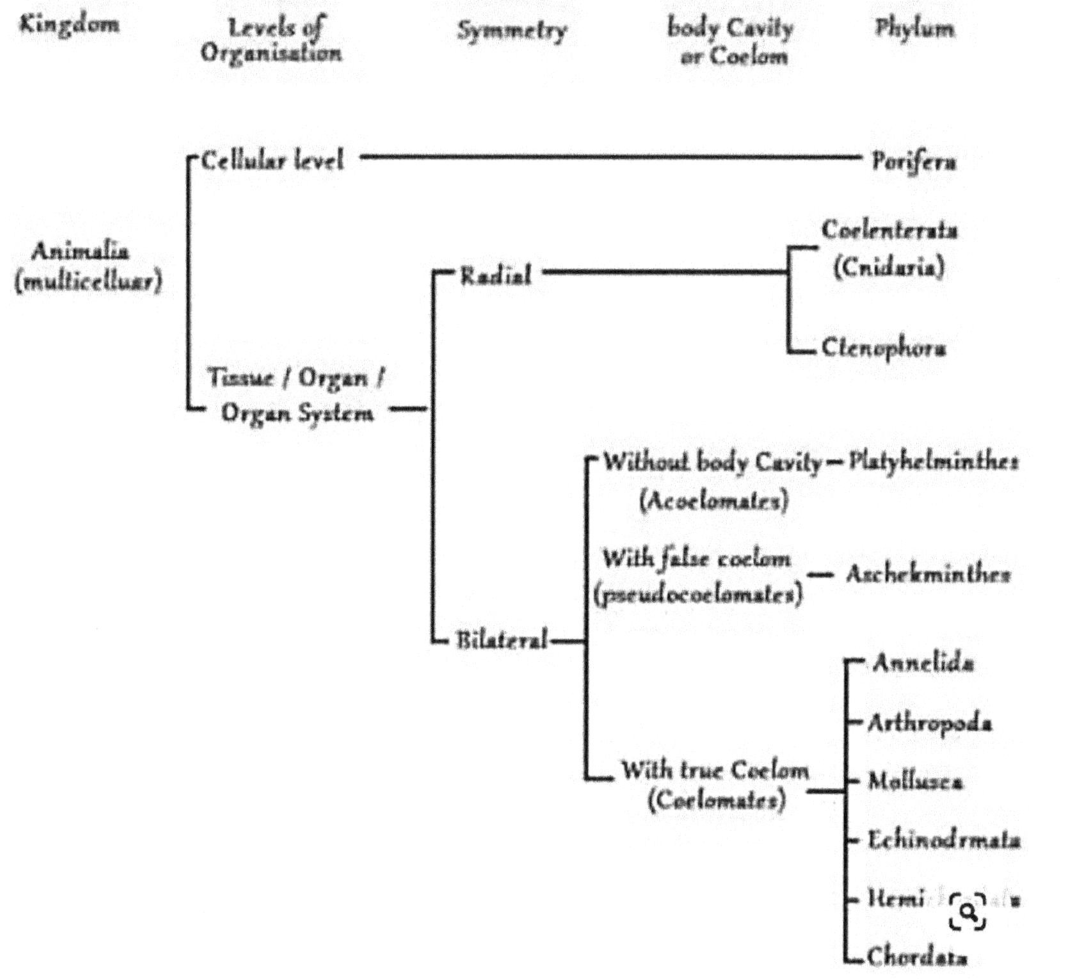

Kingdom
Levels of Organisation
Symmetry
body Cavity or Coelom
Phylum
Animalia (multicellular)
Cellular level
Porifera
Tissue / Organ / Organ System
Radial
Coelenterata (Cnidaria)
Ctenophora
Bilateral
Without body Cavity (Acoelomates)
Platyhelminthes
With false coelom (pseudocoelomates)
Aschekminthes
With true Coelom (Coelomates)
Annelida
Arthropoda
Mollusca
Echinodrmata
Hemi
Chordata

Salient Features of Different Phyla in the Animal Kingdom

Phylum	Level of Organisation	Symmetry	Coelom	Segmentation	Digestive System	Circulatory System	Respiratory System	Distinctive Features
Porifera	Cellular	Many	Absent	Absent	Absent	Absent	Absent	Body with pores and canals in walls.
Coelenterata (Cnidaria)	Tissue	Radial	Absent	Absent	Incomplete	Absent	Absent	Cnidoblasts present.
Ctenophora	Tissue	Radial	Absent	Absent	Incomplete	Absent	Absent	Comb plates for locomotion.
Platyhelminthes	Organ & Organ-system	Bilateral	Absent	Absent	Incomplete	Absent	Absent	Flat body, suckers.
Aschelminthes	Organ-system	Bilateral	Pseudo coelomate	Absent	Complete	Absent	Absent	Often worm-shaped, elongated.
Annelida	Organ-system	Bilateral	Coelomate	Present	Complete	Present	Present	Body segmentation like rings.
Arthropoda	Organ-system	Bilateral	Coelomate	Present	Complete	Present	Present	Exoskeleton of cuticle, jointed appendages.
Mollusca	Organ-system	Bilateral	Coelomate	Absent	Complete	Present	Present	External skeleton shell usually present.
Echinodermata	Organ-system	Radial	Coelomate	Absent	Complete	Present	Present	Water vascular system, radial symmetry.
Hemichordata	Organ-system	Bilateral	Coelomate	Absent	Complete	Present	Present	Worm-like with proboscis, collar and trunk.
Chordata	Organ-system	Bilateral	Coelomate	Present	Complete	Present	Present	Notochord, dorsal hollow nerve cord, gill slits with limbs or fins.

1.2 CLASSIFICATION OF ANIMALS

1.2.1 Phylum – Porifera (pore bearing animals)

- Members of this phylum are commonly known as sponges.
- They are generally marine.
- Mostly asymmetrical animals.
- *Spongilla* is a fresh water sponges.
- These are primitive multicellular animals
- They have cellular level of organisation.
- Sponges have a water transport or canal system.
- Water enters through minute pores (**ostia**) in the body wall into a central cavity, **spongocoel**, from where it goes out through the **osculum**.

- The canal system is helpful in food gathering, respiratory exchange and removal of waste.
- The **Choanocytes** or collar cells line the spongocoel and the canals.
- Digestion is intracellular.
- The body is supported by a skeleton made up of **spicules** or **sponging fibres**.
- Sexes are not separate (**hermaphrodite**), i.e., eggs and sperms are produced by the same Individual.
- Sponges reproduce asexually by fragmentation and sexually by formation of gametes.
- Fragmentation and Budding present.
- Fertilisation is internal
- The larval stage present.
- Larva is morphologically distinct from the adult.
- Examples: *Sycon* (Scypha), *Euspongia* (Bath sponge) **and** *Spongilla* (Fresh water sponge)

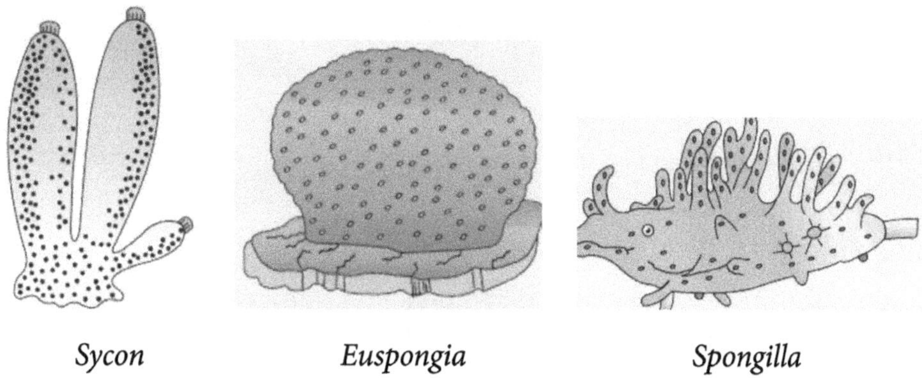

Sycon   *Euspongia*   *Spongilla*

1.2.2 Phylum – Coelenterata (Cnidaria)

- Cnidarias are aquatic, mostly marine.
- *Hydra is a fresh water polyp.*
- They are sessile or free-swimmer
- Radially symmetrical animals.
- The name cnidaria is derived from the **cnidoblasts or cnidocytes** (which contain the stinging capsules or nematocytes) present on the tentacles and the body.

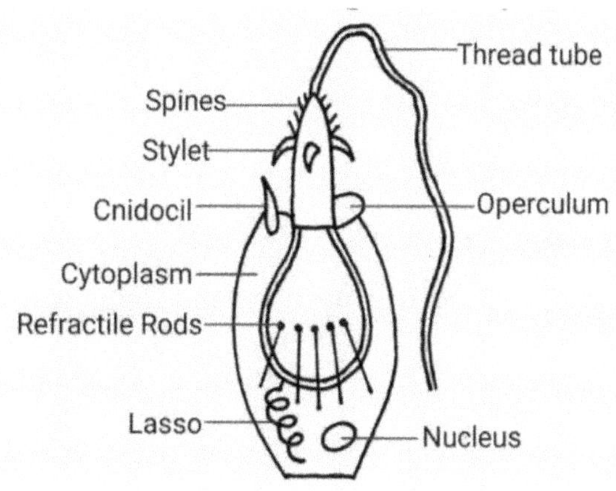

- **Cnidoblasts**/Nematoblast cells are used for anchorage, defense and for the capture of prey.
- Cnidarians exhibit tissue level of organization.
- Cnidarians are **diploblastic**.
- They have a central gastro-vascular cavity with a single opening
- **Hypostome** present below mouth.
- Digestion is extracellular and intracellular.
- Some of the cnidarians, e.g., **corals** have a skeleton composed of calcium carbonate.
- Cnidarians exhibit two basic body forms called **polyp** and **medusa**.
- The polyp is a sessile and cylindrical form like *Hydra, Adamsia*, etc.
- The medusa is umbrella-shaped and free-swimming like *Aurelia* **or jelly fish.**

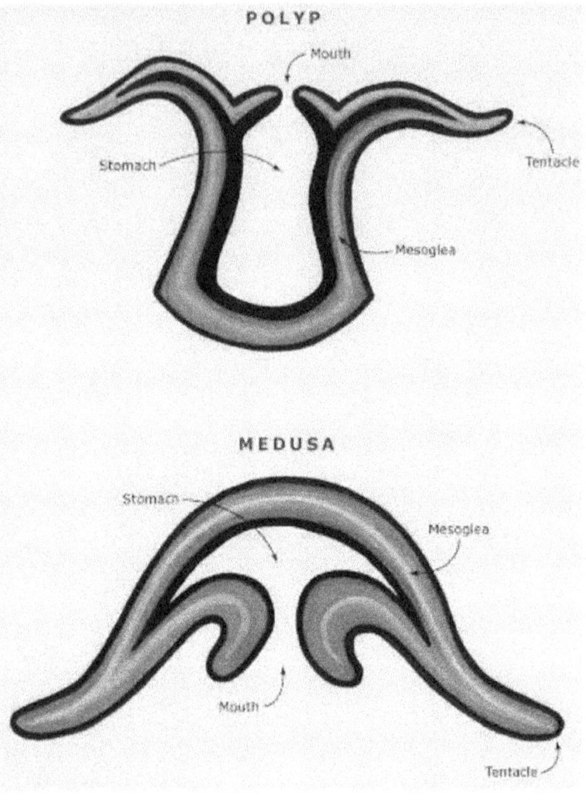

- Those cnidarians which exist in both polyp and medusa forms and exhibit alternation of generation, which is also known as **Metagenesis.**
- The polyps produce medusae by asexual reproduction and medusae form the polyps by sexual reproduction (e.g., *Obelia*).
- Larva mostly present.
- Examples: *Physalia* **(Portuguese man-of-war)**, *Adamsia* **(Sea anemone)**, *Pennatula* **(Sea-pen)**, *Gorgonia* **(Sea-fan) and** *Meandrina* **(Brain coral)**.

1.2.3 Phylum – Ctenophora

- Ctenophores, commonly known as **sea walnuts** or **comb jellies.**
- They are exclusively marine.
- **They shows radial symmetry.**
- They diploblastic organisms.
- Tissue level of organization present.
- The body bears eight external rows of ciliated **comb plates**, which help in locomotion.
- Digestion is both extracellular and intracellular.
- **Bioluminescence** (the property of a living organism to emit light) is well-marked in ctenophores.
- Bisexual.

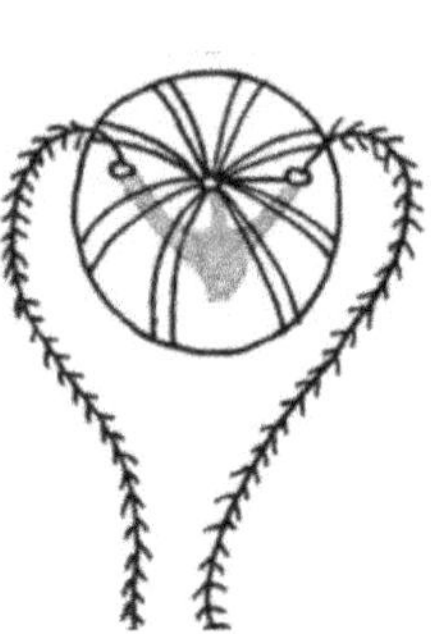

Pleurobrachia

- Only **sexual reproduction** present.
- Fertilisation is external.
- **Larva** present.

Examples: ***Pleurobrachia* and *Ctenoplana.***

1.2.4 Phylum – Platyhelminthes

- They have dorso-ventrally flattened body, hence are called **flatworms.**
- These are mostly endoparasites found in animals including human.
- ***Planaria* is free living.**
- Flatworms are **bilaterally symmetrical.**
- Triploblastic and acoelomate animals with organ level of organisation.
- Hooks and suckers are present in the parasitic forms.
- In ***Taenia* mouth is absent.**
- Some of them absorb nutrients from the host dire
- ctly through their body surface.
- Specialised cells called flame cells help in osmoregulation and excretion.
- Bisexual(mostly) but ***Schistosoma(blood fluke)*** is unisexual.
- Fertilisation is internal
- Larva present.
- Some members like ***Planaria (Dugesia)* possess high regeneration capacity.**

Examples: ***Taenia* (Tapeworm), *Fasciola* (Liver fluke).**

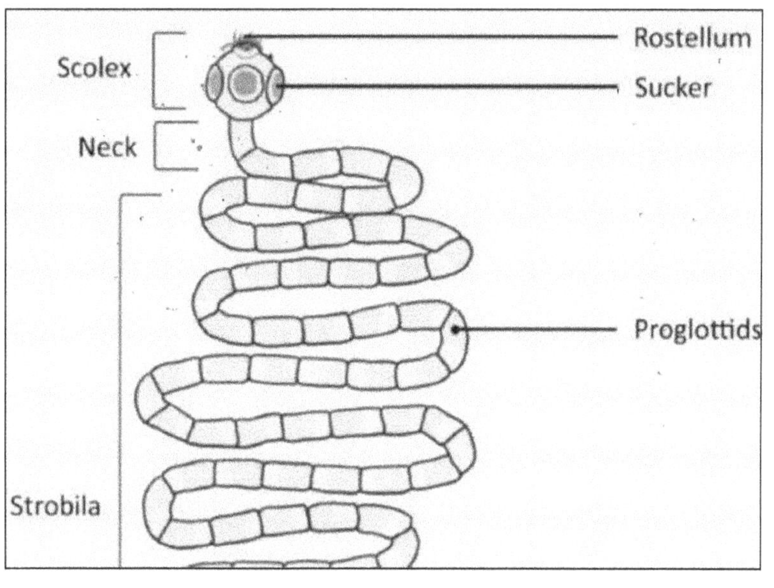

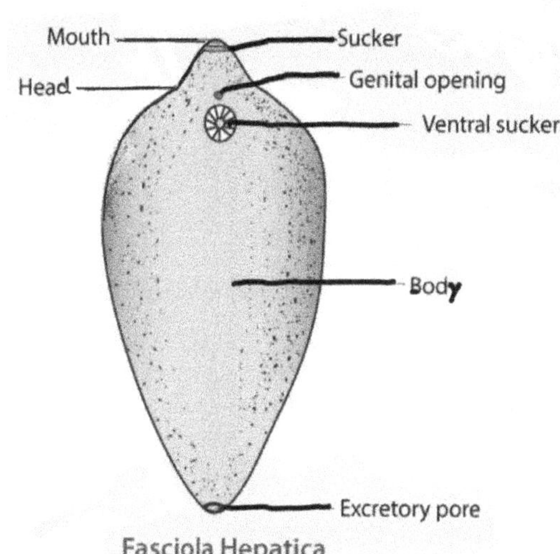

Fasciola Hepatica

1.2.5 Phylum – Aschelminthes

- The body of the aschelminthes is circular in cross-section, hence, the name **roundworms**.
- They may be freeliving, aquatic and terrestrial or parasitic in plants and animals.
- Roundworms have organ-system level of body organisation.
- They are bilaterally symmetrical, triploblastic and pseudocoelomate animals.
- Alimentary canal is complete with a well developed **muscular pharynx.**
- An excretory tube removes body wastes from the body cavity through the excretory pore.
- Sexes are separate(**dioecious**), i.e., males and females are distinct.
- Often females are longer than males.
- Fertilisation is internal and development may be direct (the young ones resemble the adult) or indirect.

Examples: *Ascaris* **(Round Worm)**, *Wuchereria* **(Filaria worm)**, *Ancylostoma* **(Hookworm)**

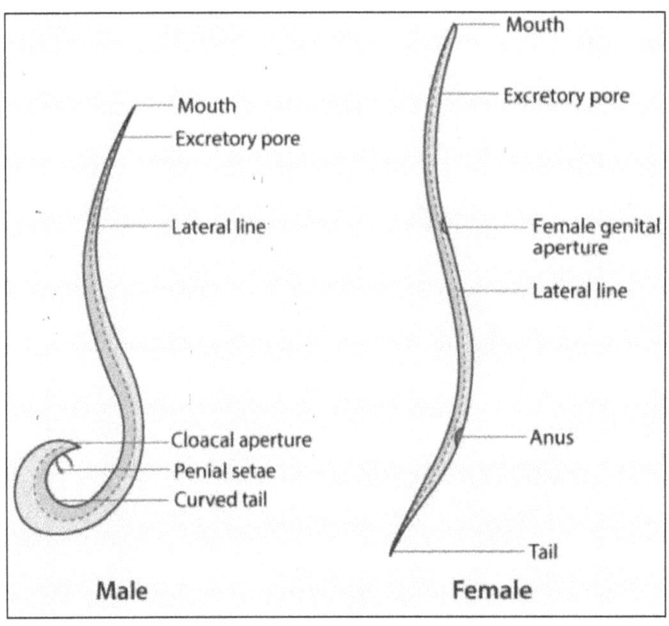

Ascaris

1.2.6 Phylum – Annelida

- They may be aquatic (marine and fresh water) or terrestrial; free-living, and sometimes parasitic
- They **exhibit organ-system level of body organisation**
- Bilateral symmetry
- They are triploblastic,
- **Metamerically** segmented
- Coelomate animals.
- Their body surface is distinctly marked out into **segments** or **metameres** (Latin, *annulus*: little ring) and, hence, the phylum name Annelida.
- They possess longitudinal and circular muscles which help in locomotion.

- Aquatic annelids like *Nereis* possess lateral appendages, **parapodia**, which help in swimming.
- A closed circulatory system is present.
- **Nephridia** (sing. nephridium) help in osmoregulation and excretion.
- Neural system consists of paired ganglia (sing. ganglion) connected by lateral nerves to a double ventral nerve cord.
- ***Nereis,* an aquatic form, is unisexual.**
- The earthworms and leeches are bisexual.
- Reproduction is sexual.
- In earthworm larva absent.
- Larva present in ***Nereis.***

Examples: ***Nereis, Pheretima* (Earthworm) and *Hirudinaria* (Blood sucking leech).**

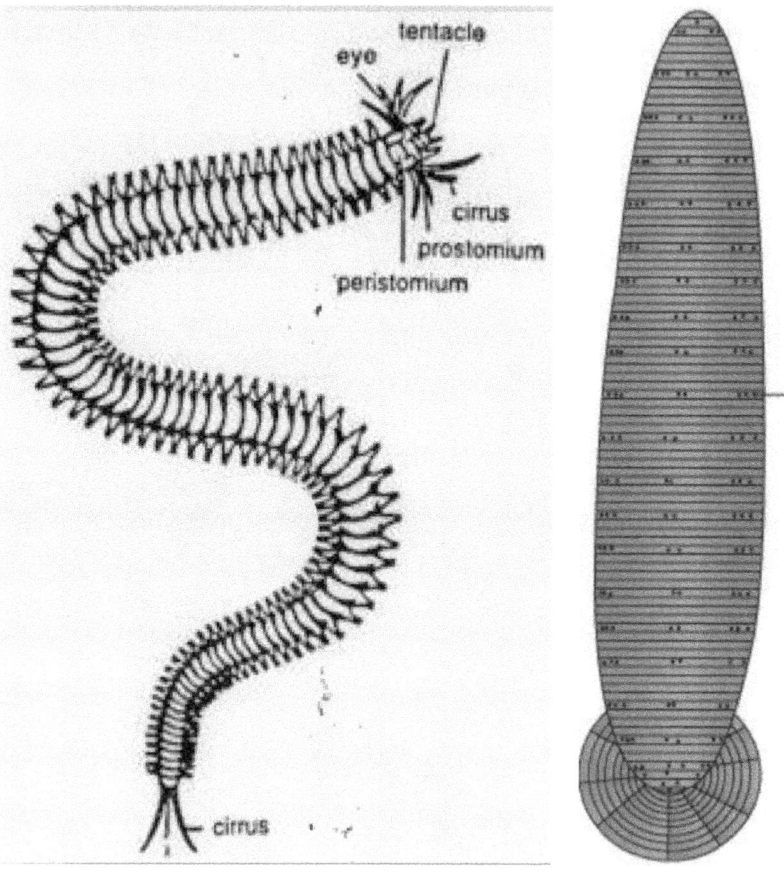

Nereis   Hirudinaria

1.2.7 Phylum – Arthropoda

- This is the **largest phylum** of Animalia which includes insects.
- Over two-thirds of all named species on earth are arthropods.
- They have organ-system level of organisation.
- **They are bilaterally symmetrical**

- Triploblastic animals.
- **Segmented animals.**
- Coelomate animals.
- The body of arthropods is covered by chitinous exoskeleton.
- The body consists of **head, thorax** and **abdomen.**
- They have **jointed appendages**(arthros-joint, poda-appendages).
- Respiratory organs are gills, book gills, book lungs or tracheal system.
- Trachea present in Insects.
- Book lungs Present in **Scorpians.**
- Book gills present in *Limulus*
- Circulatory system is of **open type.**
- Sensory organs like antennae, eyes (compound and simple), statocysts or balance organs are present.
- Excretion takes place through **malpighian tubules.**
- They are mostly unisexual.
- Fertilisation is usually internal.
- They are mostly oviparous.

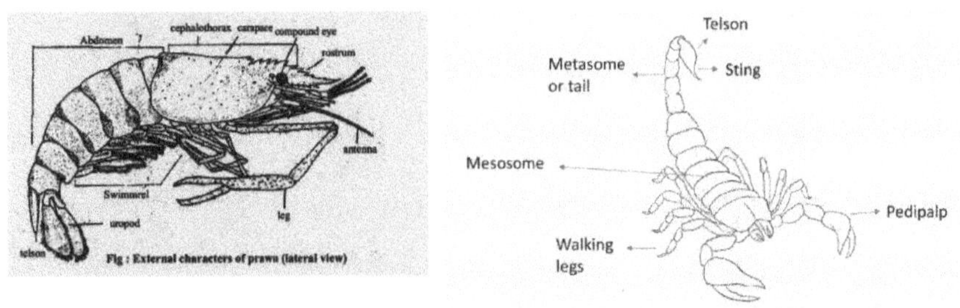

Prawn   *Scorpian*

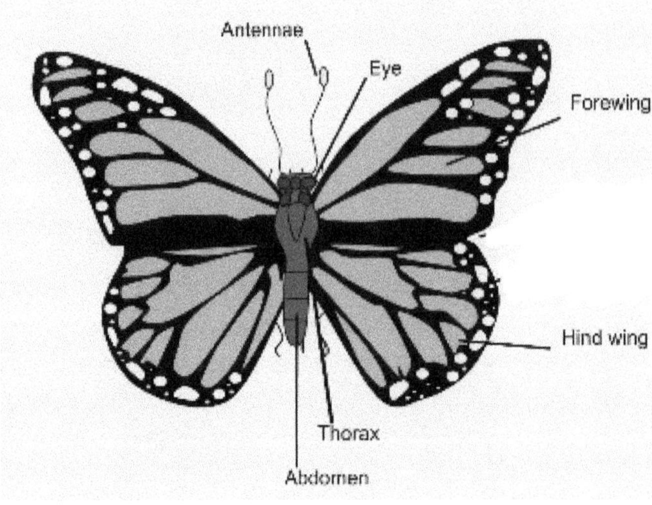

Butterfly   *Locusta*

- Development may be direct or indirect.
- Examples: **Economically important insects** – *Apis* (Honey bee), *Bombyx* (Silkworm), *Laccifer* (Lac insect)
- **Vectors** – *Anopheles, Culex* and *Aedes* (Mosquitoes)
- **Gregarious pest** – *Locusta* (Locust)
- **Living fossil** – *Limulus* (King crab).

1.2.8 Phylum – Mollusca

- Mollusca is the **second largest** animal phylum.
- Molluscs are terrestrial or aquatic (marine or fresh water) having an organ-system level of organisation.
- They are bilaterally symmetrical
- Triploblastic and coelomate animals.
- Body is covered by a calcareous shell and is unsegmented with a distinct **head, muscular foot** and **visceral hump.**
- **Muscular foot helps in locomotion.**
- A soft and spongy layer of skin forms a mantle over the visceral hump.
- The space between the hump and the mantle is called the mantle cavity in which feather like gills are present.
- Feather like gills called as ctenidia.
- **Gills** have respiratory and excretory functions.
- The anterior **head** region has sensory tentacles.
- The mouth contains a file-like rasping organ for feeding, called **radula.**
- They are usually **dioecious**
- **Oviparous**
- Indirect development.

Examples: *Pila* (Apple snail), *Pinctada* (Pearl oyster), *Sepia* (Cuttlefish), *Loligo* (Squid), *Octopus* (Devil fish), *Aplysia* (Seahare), *Dentalium* (Tusk shell) and *Chaetopleura* (Chiton).

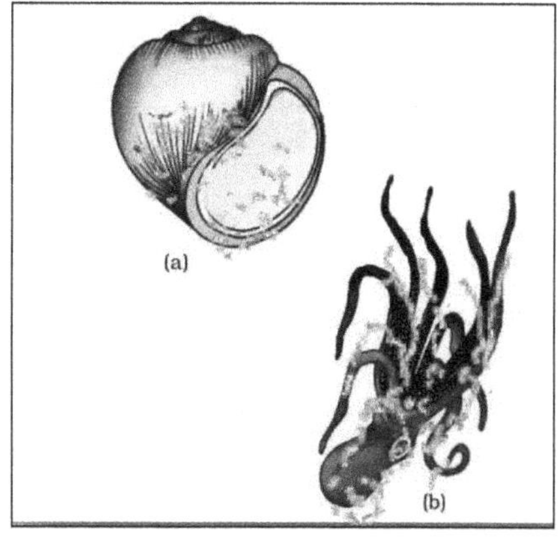

a. Pila   b. Octopus

1.2.9 Phylum – Echinodermata

- These animals have an **endoskeleton of calcareous ossicles** and, so, the name Echinodermata (Spiny bodied animals).
- **All are marine** with organ-system level of organisation.
- The adult echinoderms are radially symmetrical but larvae are bilaterally symmetrical.
- They are **triploblastic** and coelomate animals.
- Digestive system is complete
- They have **mouth on the lower (ventral) side** and anus on the upper (dorsal) side.
- The most distinctive feature of echinoderms is the presence of **water vascular system/ Amulacral system** which helps in locomotion, capture and transport of food and respiration.
- Tube feet are component of **water vascular system and helps in locomotion.**
- **Open circulation present.**
- An excretory system is absent.
- **Unisexual.**
- Reproduction is sexual.
- Fertilisation is usually external.
- Development is indirect with free-swimming larva.

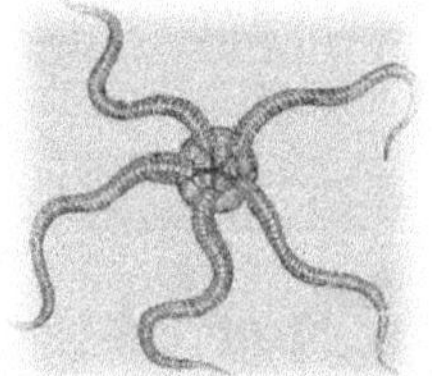
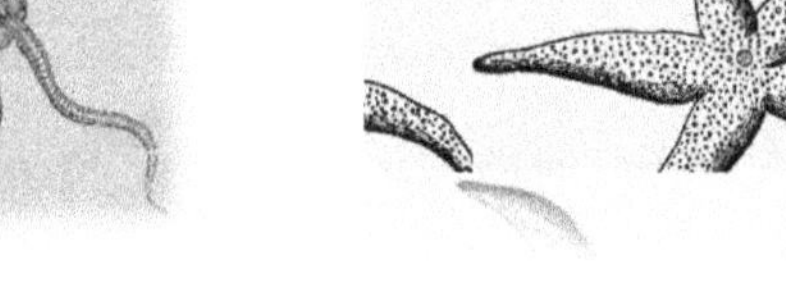

Ophiura   *Asterias*

Examples: ***Asterias* (Star fish), *Echinus* (Sea urchin), *Antedon* (Sea lily), *Cucumaria* (Sea cucumber) and *Ophiura* (Brittle star)**

1.2.10 Phylum – Hemichordata

- Hemichordata was earlier considered as a sub-phylum under phylum Chordata.
- Also known as half chordata.
- Notochord absent, so placed as a separate phylum under non-chordata.
- Stomochord present, which is endodermal, rudimentary structure, extends up to Collar region.
- This phylum consists of a small group of **worm-like** marine animals with organ-system level of organisation.
- They are bilaterally symmetrical.
- Triploblastic and coelomate animals.
- The body is cylindrical.
- The body is composed of an anterior **proboscis**, a **collar** and a long **trunk.**
- Circulatory system is of **open type.**
- Respiration takes place through gills.
- Excretory organ is **proboscis gland.**
- Unisexual.

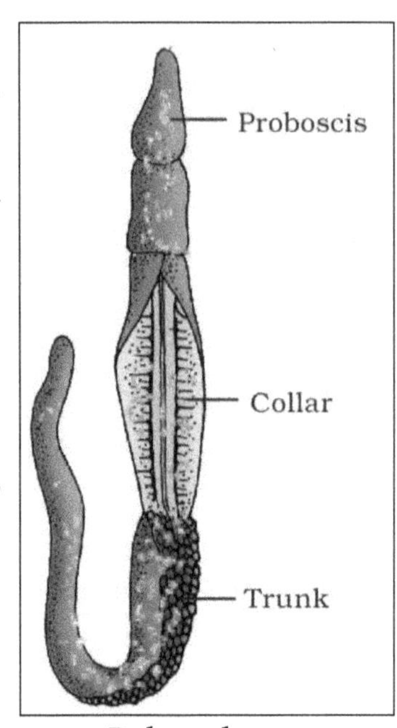

Balanoglossus

- Fertilisation is external.
- Development is indirect.

Examples: *Balanoglossus* and *Saccoglossus.*

1.2.11 Phylum – Chordata

- Chordates are fundamentally characterised by the presence of a **notochord**, a **dorsal hollow nerve cord** and **paired pharyngeal gill slits.**
- These are bilaterally symmetrical
- Triploblastic
- Coelomate
- Organ-system level of organisation.
- Chordates possess a post anal tail and a closed circulatory system.
- The comparison of salient features of chordates and non-chordates-

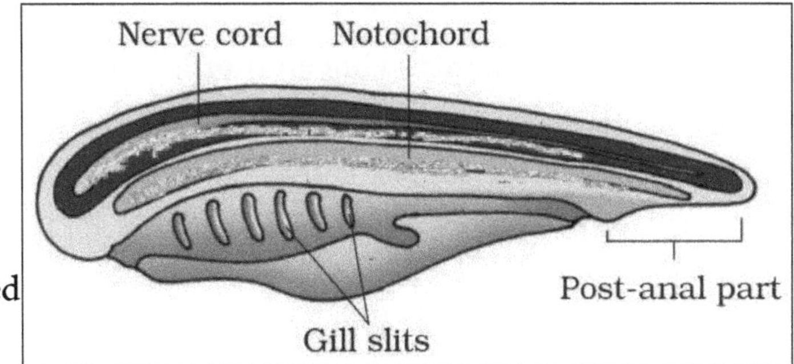

Figure Showing Fundamental Features of Chordata

Chordata	Non Chordata
1. Notochord present	Absent
2. CNS dorsal, hollow, single	CNS ventral, solid, double
3. Post anal tail present	Post anal tail absent
4. Heart is ventral	Heart is dorsal
5. Pharynx perforated by gill slits	Pharynx not perforated by gill slits

- Phylum Chordata is divided into 3 subphyla: 1.**Urochordata /Tunicata**, 2.**Cephalochordata** and 3.**Vertebrata.**

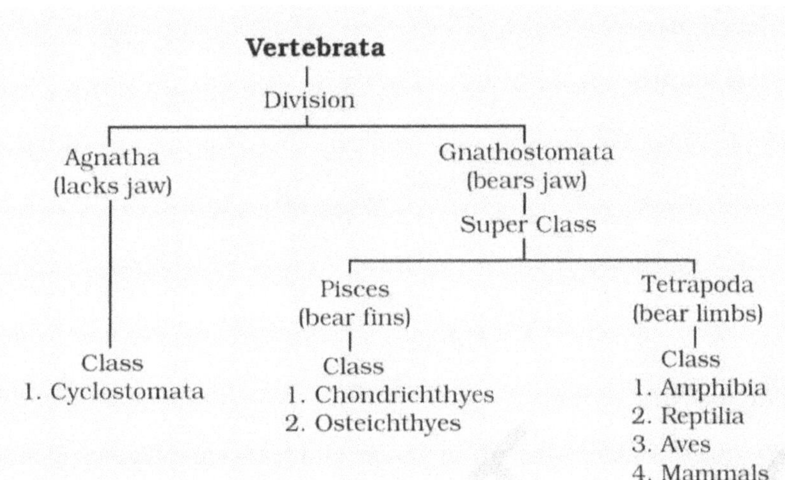

- Subphyla **Urochordata and Cephalochordata** are often referred to as **protochordates** and are exclusively marine.

- In **Urochordata**, notochord is present only in larval tail Examples of **Urochordata** – *Ascidia, Salpa, Doliolum*
- In **Cephalochordata**, notochord extends from head to tail region and is persistent throughout their life.

Example of **Cephalochordata** - *Branchiostoma* (**Amphioxus or Lancelet**).

The members of subphylum **Vertebrata** possess notochord during the embryonic period.

The notochord is replaced by a cartilaginous or bony **vertebral column** in the adult.

All vertebrates are chordates but all chordates are not vertebrates.

Besides the basic chordate characters, vertebrates have a ventral muscular heart with two, three or four chambers, kidneys for excretion and osmoregulation and paired appendages which may be fins or limbs.

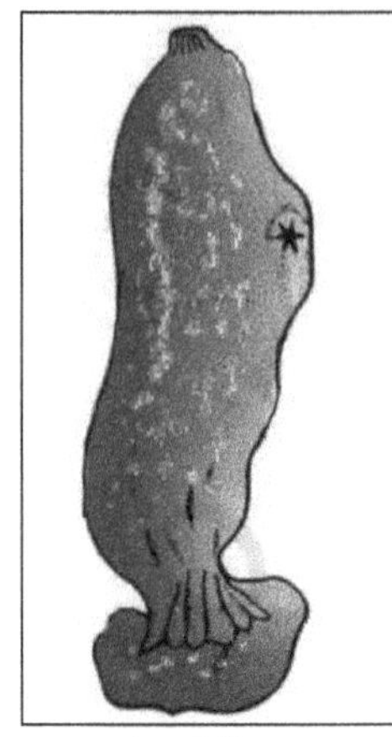

Ascidia

1.2.11.1 Class – Cyclostomata

- All living members of the class **Cyclostomata are ectoparasites** on some fishes.
- Elongated body bearing 6-15 pairs of **gill slits** for respiration.
- Cyclostomes have a **sucking and circular mouth** without jaws.
- On body **scales and paired fins absent.**
- Cranium and vertebral column are made by cartilage.
- Circulation is of closed type.
- Cyclostomes are marine but migrate for spawning to fresh water this is an example of Anadromous migration.
- After spawning, within a few days, they die.
- Their larvae, after metamorphosis, return to the ocean this is an example of Catadromous migration.
- In hagfish larva is absent.
- *In Petromyzon larva present.*

Examples: *Petromyzon* (**Lamprey**) **and** *Myxine* (**Hagfish**).

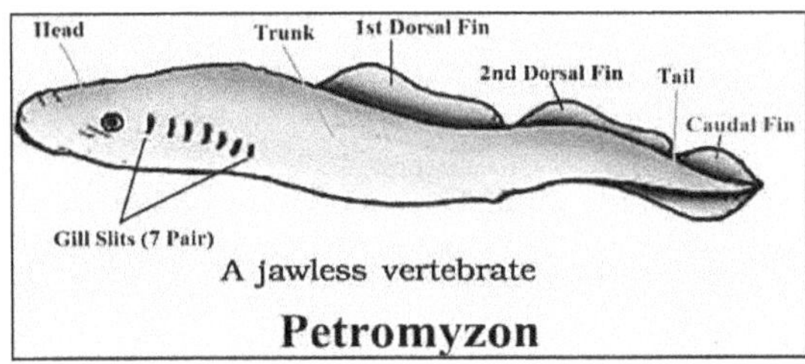

A jawless vertebrate

Petromyzon

1.2.11.2 Class – Chondrichthyes

- They are **marine animals with streamlined body** and have **cartilaginous endoskeleton.**
- Mouth is **located ventrally.**
- **Notochord** is **persistent** throughout life.
- Gill slits are separate and without **operculum** (gill cover).

- The skin is tough, containing minute **placoid scales.**
- Placoid scales are **Ecto-mesodermal** in origin like teeth.
- Teeth are modified **placoid scales** which are backwardly directed.
- Jaws are very powerful.
- These animals are predaceous.
- Due to the absence of air bladder, they have to swim constantly to avoid sinking.
- Heart is two-chambered (one auricle and one ventricle).
- Some of them have **electric organs** (e.g., *Torpedo*) and some possess **poison sting** (e.g., *Trygon*).
- They are cold-blooded (**poikilothermous**) animals, i.e., they lack the capacity to regulate their body temperature.
- Sexes are separate.
- In males **pelvic fins** bear claspers.
- They have internal fertilisation and many of them are viviparous.

Examples: *Scoliodon* **(Dog fish),** *Pristis* **(Saw fish),** *Carcharodon* **(Great white shark),** *Trygon* **(Sting ray).**

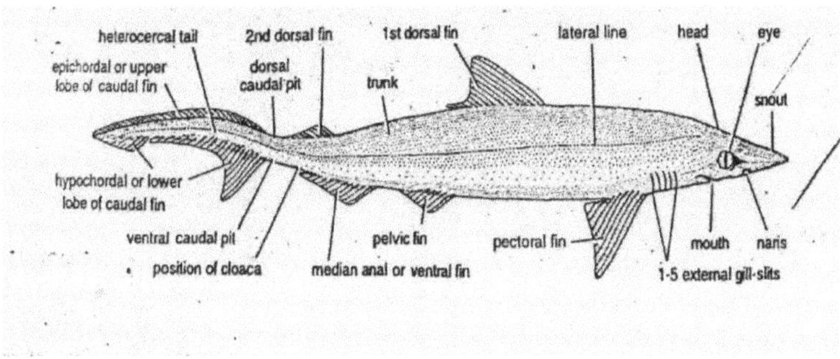

Dog fish

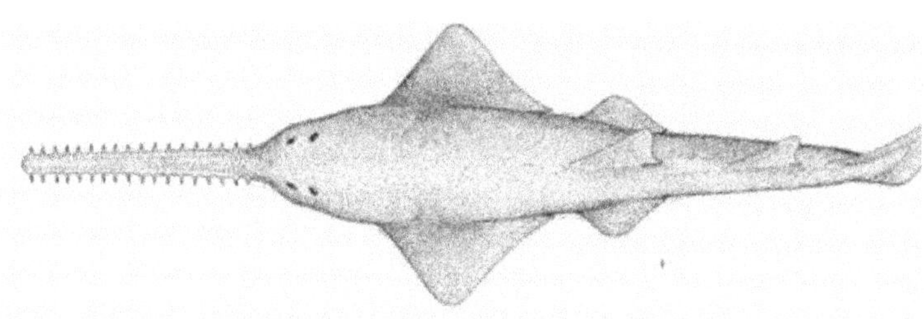

Saw fish

1.2.11.3 Class – Osteichthyes

- It includes **both marine and fresh water fishes** with bony endoskeleton.
- Their body is **streamlined.**
- Mouth is **mostly terminal.**
- They have four pairs of gills which are covered by an **operculum** on each side.

- Skin is covered with **cycloid/ctenoid scales.**
- **Air bladder** is present which regulates buoyancy.
- Heart is two chambered (one auricle and one ventricle).
- They are cold-blooded animals.
- Unisexual.
- Fertilisation is usually external.
- They are mostly oviparous and development is direct.

Examples: **Marine –** *Exocoetus* **(Flying fish),** *Hippocampus* **(Sea horse); Freshwater –** *Labeo* **(Rohu),** *Catla* **(Katla),** *Clarias* **(Magur); Aquarium –** *Betta* **(Fighting fish),** *Pterophyllum* **(Angel fish).**

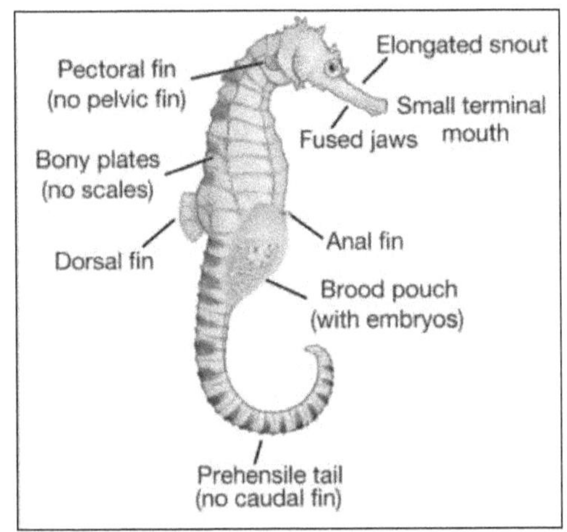

Sea Horse

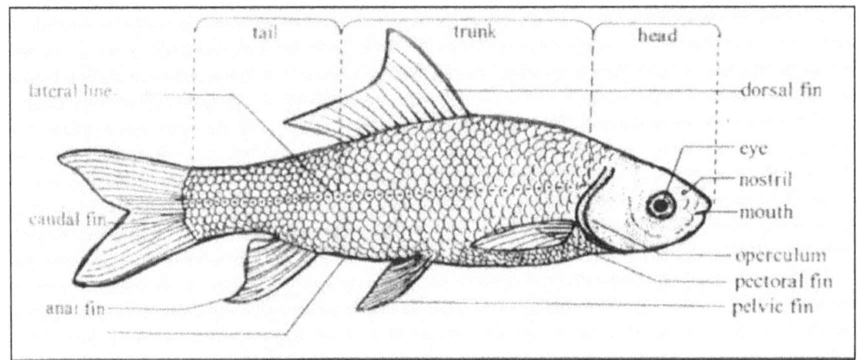

Rohu

1.2.11.4 Class – Amphibia

- Amphibia is a Greek name indicates (*Amphi:* dual, *bios,* life), amphibians can live in aquatic as well as terrestrial habitats.
- The amphibians have adapted to live both on land and water.
- Most of them have two pairs of limbs.
- Body is divisible into **head** and **trunk.**
- Tail may be present in some like Salamander.
- The amphibian skin is moist (without scales).
- But scales present in *Ichthyophis.*
- The eyes have eyelids.
- A **tympanum** represents the ear from outside.
- Alimentary canal, urinary and reproductive tracts open into a common chamber called **cloaca** which opens to the exterior.
- Respiration is by gills, lungs and through skin.
- The heart is three chambered (two auricles and one ventricle).

- These are cold-blooded animals.
- Unisexual.
- Fertilisation is external.
- They are oviparous and development is direct or indirect.

Examples: ***Bufo*** **(Toad),** ***Rana*** **(Frog),** ***Hyla*** **(Tree frog),** ***Salamandra*** **(Salamander),** ***Ichthyophis*** **(Limbless amphibia).**

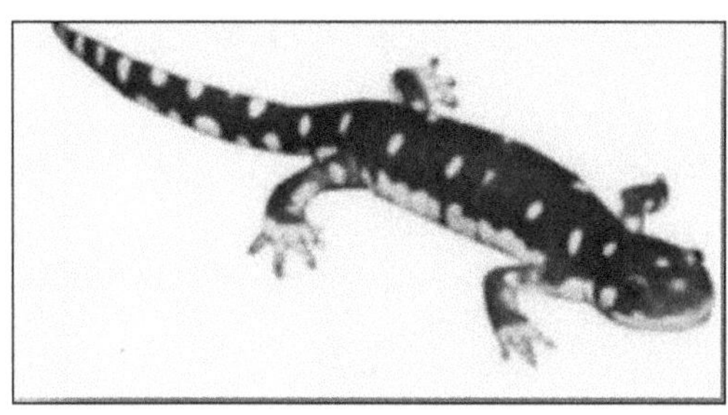

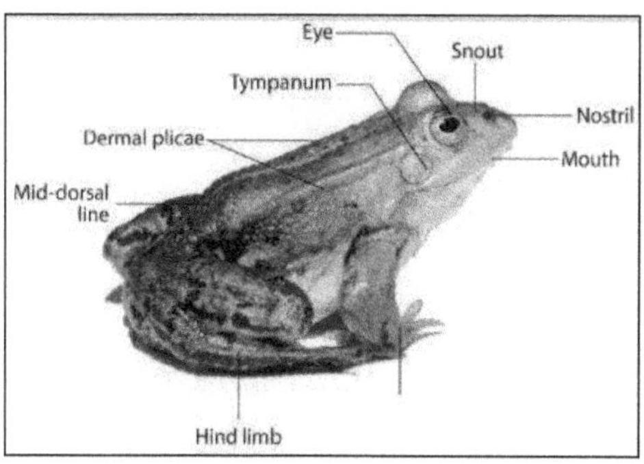

a. Salamandra   *b. Rana*

1.2.11.5 Class – Reptilia

- The class name refers to their creeping or crawling mode of locomotion (*Latin, repere* or *reptum,* to creep or crawl).
- They are mostly terrestrial animals and their body is covered by dry and cornified skin, epidermal **scales** or **scutes.**
- They do not have external ear openings.
- Tympanum represents ear.
- Limbs, when present, are two pairs.
- Limbs are absent in snakes.
- Heart is usually three-chambered, but four-chambered in crocodiles.
- Reptiles are poikilotherms.
- Snakes and lizards shed their scales as skin cast.
- Sexes are separate.
- Fertilisation is internal.
- They are oviparous and development is direct.

Examples: ***Chelone*** **(Turtle),** ***Testudo*** **(Tortoise),** ***Chameleon*** **(Tree lizard),** ***Calotes*** **(Garden lizard),** ***Crocodilus*** **(Crocodile),** ***Alligator*** **(Alligator).** ***Hemidactylus*** **(Wall lizard), Poisonous snakes –** ***Naja*** **(Cobra),** ***Bangarus*** **(Krait),** ***Vipera*** **(Vipra).**

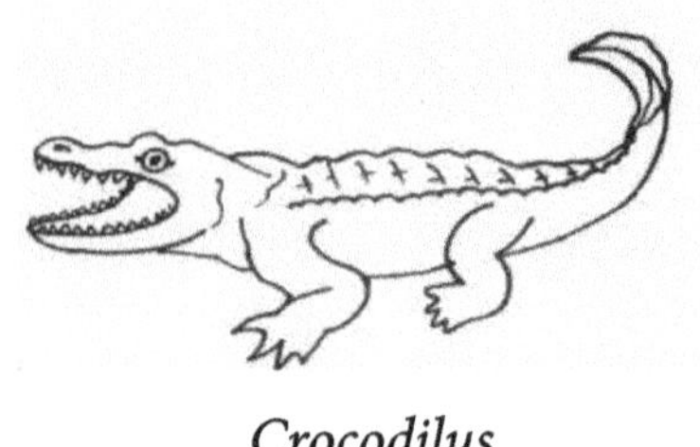

Crocodilus

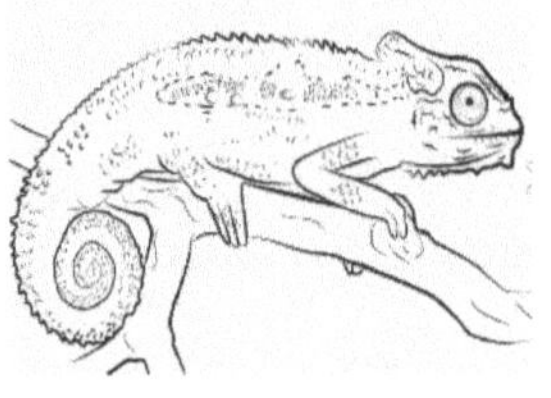

Chameleon

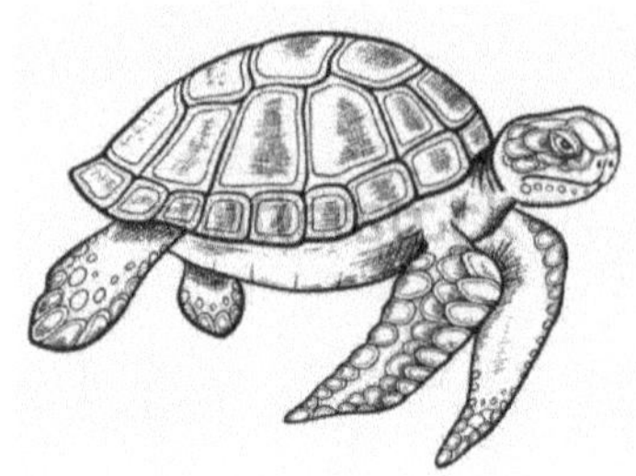

Chelone

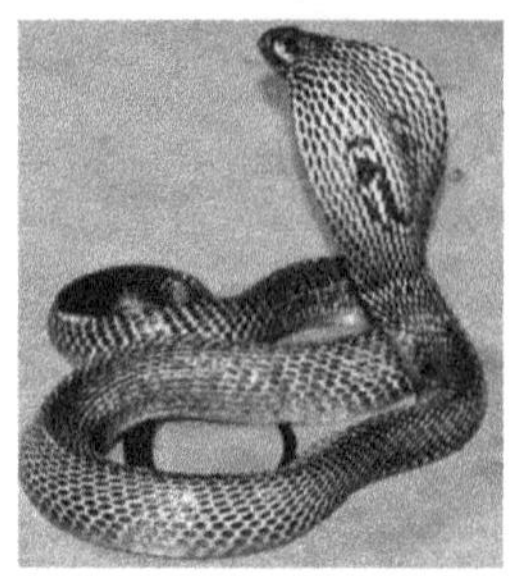

Naja

1.2.11.6 Class – Aves

- The characteristic features of Aves (birds) are the presence of **feathers**
- Most of them can fly except flightless birds (e.g., Ostrich).
- They possess **beak.**
- The forelimbs are modified into **wings**.
- The hind limbs generally have **scales.**
- The hind limbs **are modified for walking, swimming or clasping the tree branches.**
- Skin is dry without glands except the **Oil gland/Preen glands** at the base of the tail.
- Endoskeleton is fully ossified (bony) and the long bones are hollow with **air cavities** (pneumatic).
- The digestive tract of birds has additional chambers, **the crop and gizzard.**
- Heart is completely four chambered.
- Complete double circulation present.
- They are warm-blooded (**homeothermous**) animals, i.e., they are able to maintain a constant body temperature.
- Respiration is by Lungs.
- Air sacs connected to lungs for supplement respiration.
- Unisexual.
- Fertilisation is internal.
- They are oviparous
- The development is direct means larva absent.

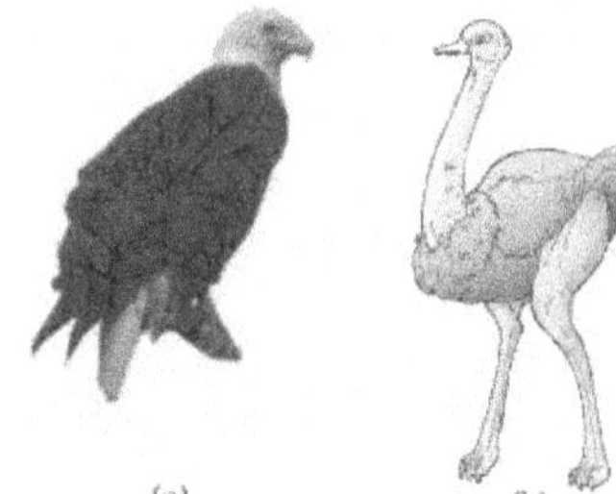

a. Neophron   *b. Struthio*

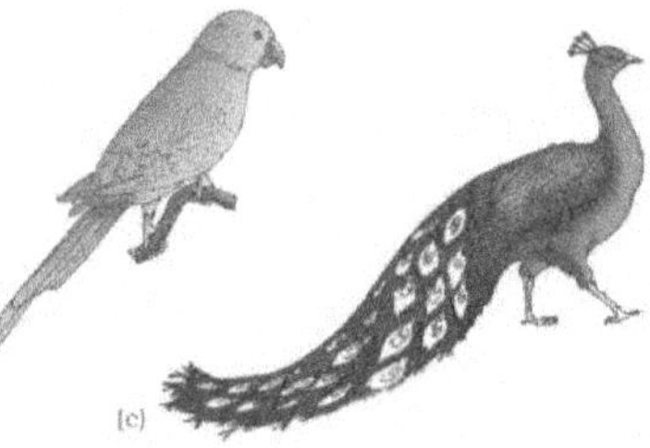

c. Psittacula   *d. Pavo*

Examples: *Corvus* (**Crow**), *Columba* (**Pigeon**), *Psittacula* (**Parrot**), *Struthio* (**Ostrich**), *Pavo* (**Peacock**), *Aptenodytes* (**Penguin**), *Neophron* (**Vulture**).

1.2.11.7 Class – Mammalia

- The most unique mammalian characteristic is the presence of milk producing glands (**mammary glands**) by which the young ones are nourished.
- On skin sweat and oil gland present.

- They are found in a variety of habitats – polar region, deserts, mountains, forests, grasslands and dark caves.
- Some of them have adapted to **fly (Bats) or live in water(Whale)**
- They have two pairs of limbs.
- The limbs adapted for walking, running, climbing, burrowing, swimming or flying.
- The skin of Mammals is unique in possessing **hair**.
- In External ears, **pinnae** are present.
- Different types of teeth(**Heteordont) are present in the jaw socket(thecodont).**
- Heart is four chambered (two auricle and two ventricle)
- They are **homoiothermous.**
- **Respiration** is by lungs.
- Sexes are separate and fertilisation is internal.
- They are viviparous with few exceptions and development is direct.
- They commonly **exhibit viviparity.**
- River dolphin is the national aquatic animal of india.
- *Panthera tigris* (**tiger)** is the national animal of india.
- **Perissodactyla** is the order of horse.

Examples:

Oviparous mammals-*Ornithorhynchus* (Platypus);

Viviparous mammals - *Macropus* (Kangaroo), *Pteropus* (Flying fox), *Camelus* (Camel), *Macaca* (Monkey), *Rattus* (Rat), *Canis* (Dog), *Felis* (Cat), *Elephas* (Elephant), *Equus* (Horse), *Delphinus* (Common dolphin), *Balaenoptera* (Blue whale), *Panthera tigris* (Tiger), *Panthera leo* (Lion).

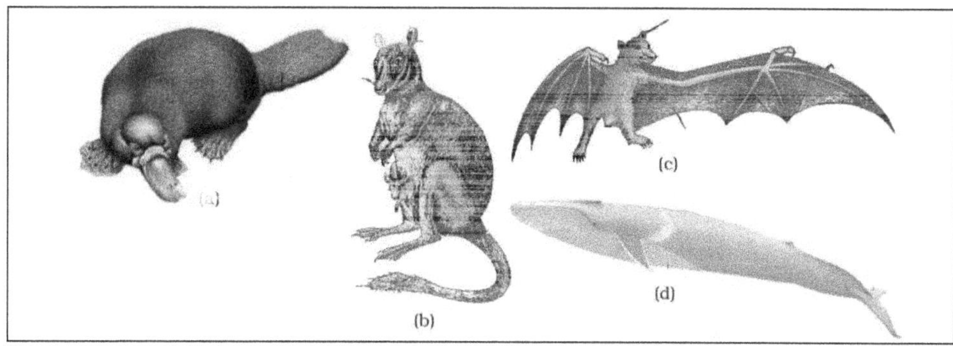

a. *Ornithorhynchus*   b. *Macropus*   c. *Pteropus*   d. *Balaenoptera*

1. **Consider the following matchings and find out the incorrect with respect to Arthropoda-**

    A. Vectors – *Culex*

    B. Gregarious pest – *Locusta* (Locust)

    C. Living fossil – *Limulus*

    D. Economically important insects – *Cockroach and ticks*

    1. A,C

    2. B,D

    3. D

    4. A,B,C,D

2. **Match the list 1 and 2-**

    List1 List2

a.	*Aedes*	j. cnidoblasts
b.	*Pila*	k. jointed appendages
c.	*Hydra*	l. visceral hump
d.	*Asterias*	m. water vascular system

    Find out the correct option –

    1. a.k, b.j, c.l, d.m

    2. a.k,b.l,c.j,d.m

    3. a.l,b.j,c.k,d.m

    4. a.l,b.j,c.m,d.k

3. **Consider the following features-**

    a) The presence of water canal system.

    b) The space between the hump and the mantle is called the mantle cavity in which feather like gills are present.

    c) The anterior head region has sensory tentacles.

    d) The mouth contains a file-like rasping organ for feeding, called radula.

    e) Larva never present

Which above features are found in phylum Mollusca-

1. a,b

2. only e and c

3. b,c,d

4. a,b,c,d,e

4. **Read the following statement carefully with respect to Reptilia -**

   I.   They do not have external ear openings.

   II. Tympanum represents ear.

   III. Limbs, when present, are one pairs.

   IV. Heart is usually three-chambered, but four-chambered in crocodiles.

   V.   Reptiles are poikilotherms.

   VI. Snakes and lizards shed their scales as skin cast.

   VII. Bisexual.

   How many of them are correct-

   1. three

   2. four

   3. five

   4. six

5. **Consider the following statements and find out the correct option-**

   STATEMENT 1. Animals like annelids, arthropods the body can be divided into identical left and right halves in only one plane, exhibit bilateral symmetry

   STATEMENT 2. When any plane passing through the central axis of the body divides the organism into two identical halves, it is called radial symmetry.

   1. Both are wrong statements

   2. Only Statement 1 correct

   3. Both are correct statements

   4. Only statement 2 correct

6. **Go through the following statements-**

   ASSERTION(A). In earthworm, the body shows metameric segmentation.

   REASON(R). The body is externally and internally divided into segments with a serial repetition of at least some organs.

   1. A correct and R is correct explanation of A

   2. A correct and R is also correct but R is not correct explanation of A

   3. A correct but R incorrect

   4. A and R both are incorrect

7. **Find out the incorrect statement-**

   1. Notochord is a mesodermally derived rod-like structure formed on the dorsal side during embryonic development in some animals.

   2. Animals with notochord are called chordates and those animals which do not form this structure are called non-chordates, e.g., porifera to echinoderms.

   3. Sponges have a water vascular system.

   4. In sponges water enters through minute pores (ostia) in the body wall into a central cavity called spongocoel.

8. **Go through the following statements-**

   a) Choanocytes or collar cells line the spongocoel and the canals.

   b) Digestion is intracellular.

   c) The body is supported by a skeleton made up of spicules or sponging fibres.

   d) Sexes are not separate (hermaphrodite), i.e., eggs and sperms are produced by the same Individual.

   e) Sponges reproduce asexually by fragmentation and sexually by formation of gametes.

   f) Fertilisation is internal and development is indirect having a larval stage which is morphologically distinct from the adult.

   Find out the correct statements and choose the suitable option for sponges-

   1. a,b only

   2. a,b,c,d only

   3. b,c,a only

   4. a,b,c,d,e,f

9. **Match the list 1 and 2-**

   List1 List2

a. *Physalia*	J. Sea-pen
b. *Adamsia*	k.. Portuguese man-of-war
c. *Pennatula*	l. Sea anemone
d. *Gorgonia*	m. Sea-fan

   Find out the correct option –

   1. a.k, b.j, c.l, d.m

   2. a.k,b.l,c.j,d.m

   3. a.l,b.j,c.k,d.m

   4. a.l,b.j,c.m,d.k

10. **Consider the following statements and find out the correct option-**

    STATEMENT 1. Ctenophores, commonly known as sea walnuts or comb jellies.

    STATEMENT 2. The body bears eight intenral rows of ciliated comb plates, which help in locomotion.

    1. Both are wrong statements

    2. Only Statement 1 correct

    3. Both are correct statements

    4. Only statement 2 correct

11. **Read the following statements very carefully and find out the incorrect with respect to Cnidaria-**

    1. They are aquatic, mostly marine, sessile or free-swimming, radially symmetrical animals.

    2. The name cnidaria is derived from the cnidoblasts or cnidocytes (which contain the stinging capsules or nematocytes) present on the tentacles and the body.

    3. Cnidoblasts are used for anchorage, defense and for the capture of prey.

    4. Cnidarians exhibit tissue level of organisation and are triploblastic.

12. **Go through the following statement-**

    ASSERTION(A). Cnidarians exhibit two basic body forms called polyp and medusa.

    REASON(R). Those cnidarians which exist in both forms exhibit alternation of generation (Metagenesis), i.e., polyps produce medusae asexually and medusae form the polyps sexually (e.g., *Obelia*).

    1. A correct and R is correct explanation of A

    2. A correct and R is also correct but R is not correct explanation of A

    3. A. correct but R incorrect

    4. A and R both are incorrect

13. **Go through the following statements-**

    a) Ctenophores, commonly known as sea walnuts or comb jellies are exclusively marine, radially symmetrical, diploblastic organisms with tissue level of organisation.

    b) The body bears eight internal rows of ciliated comb plates, which help in locomotion.

    c) Digestion is both extracellular and intracellular.

    d) Bioluminescence (the property of a living organism to emit light) is well-marked in ctenophores.

    e) Sexes are not separate.

    Find out the correct statements and choose the suitable option for Ctenophora-

    1. a,b only

    2. a, only

    3. b,c,a only

    4. a,c,d,e

14. **Read the following statements and find out correct option-**

    a) Organ-system level of body organisation.

    b) They are bilaterally symmetrical, triploblastic and pseudocoelomate animals.

    c) Alimentary canal is complete with a well developed muscular pharynx.

    d) An excretory tube removes body wastes from the body cavity through the excretory pore.

    How many of them are correct for roundworm-

    1. three

    2. four

    3. two

    4. one

15. Consider the following statements and find out the correct option with respect to Mollusca-

STATEMENT 1. Body is covered by a calcareous shell and is unsegmented with a distinct head, muscular foot and visceral hump.

STATEMENT 2. The space between the hump and the mantle is called the mantle cavity in which feather like gills are not present.

1. Both are wrong statements

2. Only Statement 1 correct

3. Both are correct statements

4. Only statement 2 correct

16. Find out the incorrect statement for hemichordate-

1. Hemichordata was earlier considered as a sub-phylum under phylum Chordata.

2. Hemichordata now placed as a separate phylum under chordata.

3. Hemichordata consists of a small group of worm-like marine animals with organ-system level of organisation.

4. Hemichordata are bilaterally symmetrical, triploblastic and coelomate animals.

17. Consider the following statements-

a) The members of subphylum Vertebrata possess notochord during the embryonic period.

b) The notochord is replaced by a cartilaginous or bony vertebral column in the adult.

c) All vertebrates are chordates but all chordates are not vertebrates.

d) Besides the basic chordate characters, vertebrates have a ventral muscular heart with two, three or four chambers, kidneys for excretion and osmoregulation and paired appendages which may be fins or limbs.

Which above statement are correct for vertebrates-

1. a and c only

2. a,b,c only

3. b,c,d only

4. a,b,c,d

18. Match the list 1 and 2-

List 1   List 2

a. *Ophiura*	Brittle star
b. *Echinus*	Sea urchin
c. *Antedon*	Sea lily

Find out the correct option –

1. only a

2. only a,b

3. only c, b

4. a,b,c

19. Consider the following statements and find out the incorrect one-

1) Urochordata and Cephalochordata are often referred to as protochordates and are exclusively fresh water.

2) In Urochordata, notochord is present only in larval tail, while in Cephalochordata, it extends from head to tail region and is persistent throughout their life.

3) Examples of Urochordata are *Ascidia, Salpa and Doliolum*

4) Example of Cephalochordata is *Branchiostoma*

20. Find out the odd one out with respect to flatworm-

1. *Planaria*

2. *Taenia*

3. *Fasciola*

4. *Ctenoplana*

21. Consider the following statements and find out the correct option

STATEMENT 1. The body of the Aschelminthes is circular in cross-section, hence, the name roundworms.

STATEMENT 2. Roundworms have tissue level of body organisation.

1. Both are wrong statements

2. Only Statement 1 correct

3. Both are correct statements

4. Only statement 2 correct

22. Go through the following statement and find out the correct option-

ASSERTION(A). Annelids like *Nereis* possess lateral appendages, parapodia,which help in swimming.

REASON(R). *Nereis,* an aquatic form, is dioecious.

1. A correct and R is correct explanation of A

2. A correct and R is also correct but R is not correct explanation of A

3. A correct but R incorrect

4. A and R both are incorrect

23. Go through the following statement and find out the correct option-

A. Circulatory system is of open type.

B. Sensory organs like antennae, eyes (compound and simple), statocysts or balance organs are present.

C. Excretion takes place only through Trachea.

D. They are mostly dioecious.

E. Fertilisation is usually internal.

Which above statement are correct for Arthropods?

1. A and C only

2. C and E only

3. A,B,D,E only

4. All are correct

24. Molluscs are terrestrial or aquatic (marine or fresh water) having-

   A.   organ-system level of organisation.

   B.   bilaterally symmetrical.

   C.   triploblastic and coelomate animals.

   D.   Body is covered by a calcareous shell.

   Which above statement are correct ?

   1. B,C, D only

   2. A and C only

   3. D and A only

   4. All are correct

25. Which statement is incorrect for Echinodermata-

   1.   An excretory system is well developed.

   2.   Reproduction is sexual.

   3. Sexes are separate.

   4. Fertilisation is usually external.

26. Consider the following statements for Cyclostomata-

   I.   Cyclostomes have a sucking and circular mouth without jaws.

   II.   Their body is devoid of scales and paired fins.

   III.   Cranium and vertebral column are cartilaginous. Circulation is of closed type.

   IV.   Cyclostomes are marine but migrate for spawning to fresh water.

   V.   After spawning, within a few days, they die.

   How many of them are correct-

   1. five

   2. two

   3. three

   4. four

27. Match the list 1 and 2-

   List 1   List 2

a. *Scoliodon*	j. Magur
b. *Clarias*	k. sting ray
c. *Betta*	l. Dog fish
d. *Trygon*	m. Fighting fish

   Find out the correct option –

   1. a.k, b.j, c.l, d.m

   2. a.k,b.l,c.j,d.m

   3. a.l,b.m,c.k,d.j

   4. a.l,b.j,c.m,d.k

28. Consider the following statements and find out the correct with respect to *Osteichthyes* -

a)   Mouth is mostly terminal.

b)   They have four pairs of gills which are covered by an operculum on each side.

c)   Skin is covered with placoid scales.

d)   Air bladder is present which regulates buoyancy.

How many of them are correct-

1. one

2. two

3. three

4. four

29. Find out the incorrect one for Cyclostomata-

1.   Cyclostomes have a sucking and circular mouth without jaws.

2.   Their body covered by scales and paired fins.

3.   Cranium and vertebral column are cartilaginous.

4.   Circulation is of closed type.

30. Read the following statements -

a)   Most of them have two pairs of limbs.

b)   Body is divisible into head and trunk.

c)   Tail may be present in some.

d)   The amphibian skin is moist (without scales).

e)   The eyes have eyelids.

How many of them are correct for Amphibians –

1. five

2. two

3. three

4. four

31. Read the following statements and find out the correct option-

STATEMENT 1. *Reptilia* name refers to their creeping or crawling mode of locomotion (*Latin, repere* or *reptum*, to creep or crawl).

STATEMENT 2. They are mostly terrestrial animals and their body is covered by dry and cornified skin, epidermal scales or scutes

1. Both are wrong statements

2. Both are correct statements

3. Only statement 1 correct

4. Only statement 2 correct

32. Go through the following statement and find out the correct option-

ASSERTION(A). *Amphibia* name indicates (*Gr., Amphi:* dual, *bios,* life), amphibians can live in aquatic as well as terrestrial habitats.

REASON(R). Alimentary canal, urinary and reproductive tracts open into a common chamber called cloaca which opens to the exterior.

1. A correct and R is correct explanation of A

2. A correct and R is also correct but R is not correct explanation of A

3. A correct but R incorrect

4. A and R both are incorrect

33. Read the following statements-

a) Notochord is persistent throughout life.

b) Gill slits are separate and without operculum (gill cover).

c) The skin is tough, containing minute placoid scales.

d) Teeth are modified placoid scales which are backwardly directed.

e) Their jaws are very powerful.

f) These animals are predaceous.

How many of them are correct for *Chondrichthyes* –

1. five

2. six

3. three

4. four

34. Read the following pairs -

a) *Bufo* - Toad

b) *Rana* - Frog

c) *Hyla* - Tree frog

d) *Salamandra* - Salamander

e) *Ichthyophis* - Limbless amphibia

How many of above are correctly matched-

1. three

2. four

3. five

4. two

35. Which of the following is incorrect with respect to Hemichordata-

1. Circulatory system is of closed type.

2. Respiration takes place through gills.

3. Excretory organ is proboscis gland.

4. Sexes are separate.

36. Find out the incorrect statement-

1. The ctenophores are marine animals with comb plates.

2. The platyhelminthes have flat body and exhibit bilateral symmetry.

3. Aschelminthes are pseudocoelomates and include parasitic as well as non-parasitic round worms.

4. Annelids are metamerically segmented animals with a pseudocoelom.

37. Read the following statements-

i. Heart is four chambered.

ii. They are homoiothermous.

iii. Respiration is by lungs.

iv. Sexes are separate and fertilisation is internal.

v. They are viviparous with few exceptions and development is direct.

Which above statements are correct for Mammals-

1. i and ii only

2. iii And ii only

3. iv and iii only

4. all are correct

38. Consider the following statements –

a) Phylum Chordata includes animals which possess a notochord either throughout or during early embryonic life.

b) Other common features observed in the chordates are the dorsal, hollow nerve cord and paired pharyngeal gill slits.

c) Some of the vertebrates do not possess jaws (Agnatha) whereas most of them possess jaws (Gnathostomata).

d) Agnatha is represented by the class, Cyclostomata.

e) Cyclostomata are ectoparasites on fishes.

Which of above are correct-

1. a and b only

2. b and c only

3. a,b,c,d,e

4. d only

39. Find out the correct statements-

   a) The amphibians have adapted to live both on land and water.

   b) Reptiles are characterised by the presence of dry and cornified skin.

   c) Limbs are absent in snakes.

   d) Fishes, amphibians and reptiles are poikilothermous (coldblooded).

   e) Aves are warm-blooded animals with feathers on their bodies and forelimbs modified into wings for flying.

   Which of the following are correct-

   1. a and d only

   2. a,b and e only

   3. b and d only

   4. All are correct

40. Read the following animals-

   a) *Rattus*

   b) *Canis*

   c) *Columba*

   d) *Psittacula*

   e) *Struthio*

   f) *Pavo*

   g) *Aptenodytes*

   Which of them are mammals-

   1. a and b only

   2. b and c only

   3. c and d only

   4. d only

41. Read the following for birds and find out the incorrect for Birds-

   1) The hindlimbs are modified into wings.

   2) The hind limbs generally have scales and are modified for walking, swimming or clasping the tree branches.

   3) Skin is dry without glands except the oil gland at the base of the tail.

   4) Endoskeleton is fully ossified (bony) and the long bones are hollow with air cavities (pneumatic).

42. Consider the following statements-

   a) They have organ-system level of organisation.

   b) They are bilaterally symmetrical, triploblastic,segmented and coelomate animals.

   c) The body of arthropods is covered by chitinous exoskeleton.

d) The body of insects normally consists of head, thorax and abdomen.

e) They have jointed appendages(arthros-joint, poda-appendages).

f) Respiratory organs are gills, book gills, book lungs or tracheal system.

Which of the following are correct for Arthropoda-

1. a and b only

2. b and e only

3. a,b,c,d,e

4. All are correct

43. Read the following statements with respect to Flatworm-

a) Specialised cells called flame cells help in osmoregulation and excretion.

b) Sexes are not separate.

c) Fertilisation is internal and development is through many larval stages.

d) Some members like *Planaria* possess high regeneration capacity.

How many of them are correct-

1. one

2. two

3. three

4. four

44. Find out the incorrect for roundworms-

1) Alimentary canal is complete with a well developed muscular pharynx.

2) An excretory tube removes body wastes from the body cavity through the excretory pore.

3) Sexes are separate(dioecious), i.e., males and females are distinct.

4) The males are longer than females.

45. Consider the following and find out the incorrect one-

1) The name cnidaria is derived from the cnidoblasts or cnidocytes (which contain the stinging capsules or nematocytes) present on the tentacles and the body.

2) Cnidoblasts are used for anchorage, defense and for the capture of prey.

3) Cnidarians exhibit tissue level of organisation and are diploblastic.

4) Digestion is extracellular only.

46. Read the following statements and find out the correct option

STATEMENT 1. The body of arthropods is covered by chitinous exoskeleton.

STATEMENT 2. This is the largest phylum of Animalia which includes insects.

1. Both are correct statements

2. Both are wrong statements

3. Only statement 1 correct

4. Only statement 2 correct

47. Go through the following statement and find out the correct option-

ASSERTION(A). When any plane passing through the central axis of the body divides the organism into two identical halves, it is called radial symmetry.

REASON(R). Sponges exhibit bilateral symmetry.

1. A correct and R is correct explanation of A

2. A correct and R is also correct but R is not correct explanation of A

3. A correct but R incorrect

4. A and R both are incorrect

48. Read the following statements -

a) They are cold-blooded (poikilothermous) animals, i.e., they lack the capacity to regulate their body temperature.

b) Sexes are separate.

c) In males pelvic fins bear claspers.

d) They have internal fertilisation and many of them are viviparous

e) These animals are predaceous.

f) Due to the absence of air bladder, they have to swim constantly to avoid sinking.

How many of above are correct for cartilaginous fishes-

1. three

2. six

3. five

4. two

49. Consider the following statements -

A. Animals in which the cells are arranged in two embryonic layers, an external ectoderm and an internal endoderm, are called diploblastic animals, e.g., coelenterates.

B. An undifferentiated layer, mesoglea, is present in between the ectoderm and the endoderm.

C. Animals possessing coelom are called coelomates, e.g., annelids, molluscs, arthropods, echinoderms, hemichordates and chordates.

D. Those animals in which the developing embryo has a third germinal layer, mesoderm, in between the ectoderm and endoderm, are called triploblastic animals (platyhelminthes to chordates)

Which above statements are correct-

1. A and C only	2. A,B,D only
3. B and D only	4. All are correct

50. Consider the following statements and find out the incorrect for Mammals-

1. External ears or pinnae are present.	2. Heart is four chambered.
2. They are homoiothermous.	4. Sexes are separate and fertilisation is external.

2

STRUCTURAL ORGANISATION OF ANIMALS

- In **unicellular** organisms, all functions like digestion, respiration and reproduction are performed by a single cell.

- In the complex body of **multicellular** animals the same basic functions are carried out by different groups of cells in a well organised manner.

- The body of a simple **organism** like **Hydra** is made of different types of cells and the number of cells in each type can be in thousands.

- The **human body comprises billions of cells** performing a variety of functions. In multicellular entities, a group of similar cells, along with intercellular substances, perform a particular function, which **is termed a tissue.**

- In other words a **tissue is a group of cells** usually have a common origin and function to carry out specialized activities.

2.1.1 Epithelial Tissue/Covering tissue

- **An epithelial tissue has a free surface,** which faces either a body fluid or the outside environment and thus provides a covering or a lining for some part of the body.

- We commonly refer to an epithelial tissue as **epithelium (pl.: epithelia).**

- Origin From all three germ layers.

- The cells in epithelial tissue are compactly packed with little intercellular matrix.

- There are two types of epithelial tissues namely **simple epithelium** and **compound epithelium.**

- Simple epithelium is composed of a single layer of cells and functions as a lining for body cavities, ducts, and tubes.

- The compound epithelium consists of two or more cell layers and has protective function as it does in our skin.

SIMPLE EPITHELIUM

- On the basis of structural modification of the cells, simple epithelium is further divided into following types. These are **(A) Squamous, (B) Cuboidal, (C) Columnar (D) Ciliated (E) Glandular.**

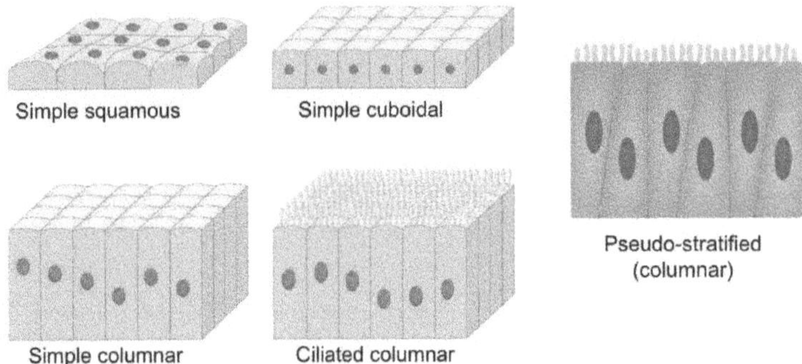

A. Simple squamous epithelium/Pavement epithelium

- The **squamous epithelium** is made of a single thin layer of flattened cells with irregular boundaries.
- Nucleus of cells centrally located.
- They are found in the walls of blood vessels and air sacs of lungs and are involved in a functions like forming a diffusion boundary.

B. Simple cuboidal epithelium

- The **cuboidal epithelium** is composed of a single layer of cube-like cells.
- Nucleus of cells centrally located.
- This is commonly found in ducts of glands and tubular parts of nephrons in kidneys and its main functions are secretion and absorption.
- The epithelium of proximal convoluted tubule (PCT) of nephron in the kidney has microvilli.
- The **cuboidal epithelium also found in gonads.**

C. Simple columnar epithelium

- The **columnar epithelium** is composed of a single layer of tall and slender cells.
- Their nuclei are located at the base.
- Free surface may have microvilli.
- They are found in the **lining of stomach and intestine.**
- **Simple columnar epithelium** helps in secretion and absorption.

D. Ciliated epithelium

- If the columnar or cuboidal cells bear cilia on their free surface they are called **ciliated epithelium.**
- Their function is to move particles or mucus in a specific direction over the epithelium.
- They are mainly present in the inner surface of hollow organs like bronchioles and fallopian tubes.

E. Glandular epithelium

- Some of the columnar or cuboidal cells get specialised for secretion and are called **glandular epithelium.**

- They are mainly of two types: unicellular, **consisting** of isolated glandular cells (goblet cells and goblet cells of the alimentary canal), and multicellular, consisting of cluster of cells (salivary gland).

- On the basis of the mode of pouring of their **secretions**, glands are divided into two categories namely **exocrine** and **endocrine** glands.

- Exocrine glands secrete **mucus, saliva, earwax, oil, milk, digestive enzymes** etc. These products are release through ducts or tubes.

- In **endocrine** glands do not have ducts so also called ductless gland.

- The product of endocrine glands called **hormones** are secreted directly into the fluid bathing the gland.

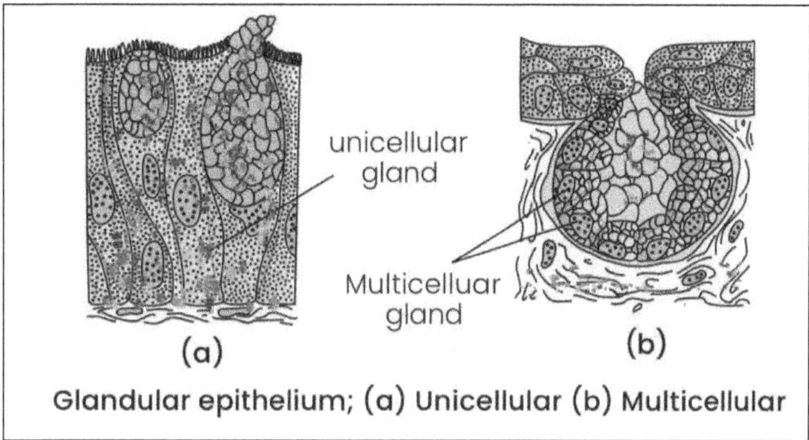

Glandular epithelium; (a) Unicellular (b) Multicellular

COMPOUND EPITHELIUM

- **Compound epithelium** is made of more than one layer (multi-layered) of cells and thus has a limited role in secretion and absorption.

- Their main function is to provide **protection** against chemical and mechanical stresses. They cover the dry surface of the skin, the **moist** surface of buccal cavity, pharynx, inner lining of ducts of salivary glands and of **pancreatic** ducts.

- In skin stratified squamous keratinized epithelium present.

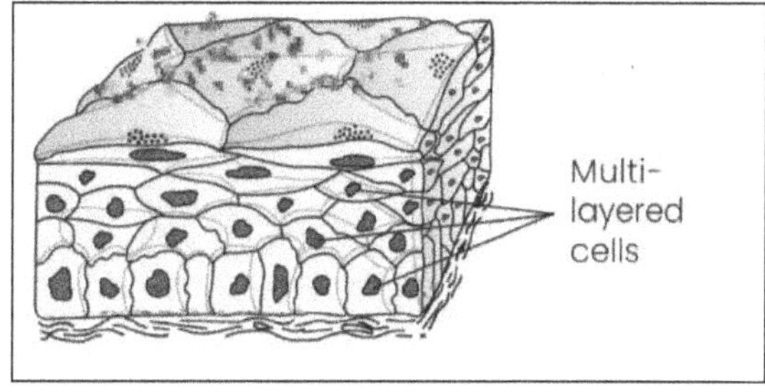

Figure showing stratified Epithelium

CELL JUNCTIONS

- All cells in epithelium are held together with little intercellular material.

- In nearly all animal tissues, specialised junctions provide both structural and functional links between its individual cells.

- Three types of cell junctions are found in the epithelium and other tissues.
- These are called as tight, adhering and gap junctions.

   a. Tight junctions/Zonula occludens help to stop substances from leaking across a tissue.

   b. Adhering junctions/ Zonula adherens perform cementing to keep neighbouring cells together.

   c. Gap junctions facilitate the cells to communicate with each other by connecting the cytoplasm of adjoining cells, for rapid transfer of ions, small molecules and sometimes big molecules.

2.1.2 Connective Tissue

- **Connective tissues** are most abundant and widely distributed in the body of complex animals.
- **Connective tissues** mesodermal in origin.
- They are named **connective** tissues because of their special function of linking and supporting other tissues/organs of the body.
- They range from soft connective tissues to specialised types, which include **cartilage, bone, adipose, and blood.**
- In all connective tissues except blood, the cells secrete fibres of structural proteins called collagen or elastin.
- The fibres forming cells called **Fibrolasts.**
- The fibres provide strength, elasticity and flexibility to the tissue.
- These cells also secrete modified **polysaccharides**, which accumulate between cells and fibres and act as matrix(ground substance).
- Mast cells also found.

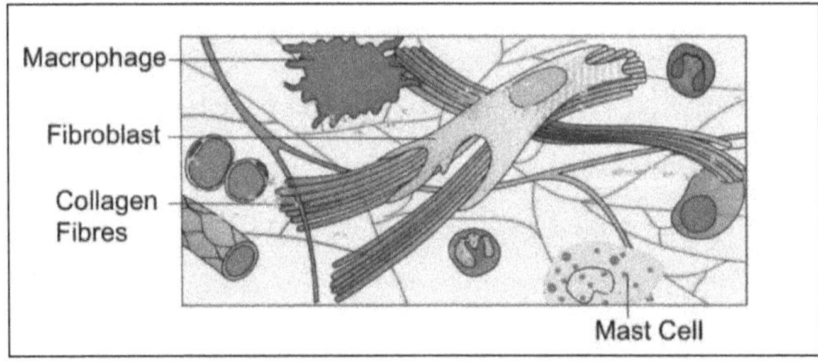

Figure showing component of connective tissue

- Connective tissues are classified into three types:

   (i) **Loose connective tissue**   (ii) **Dense connective tissue**

   (iii) **Specialised connective tissue.**

- **Loose connective tissue also form packing material.**
- **Loose connective tissue** has cells and fibres loosely arranged in a semi-fluid ground substance, for example, **areolar tissue** present beneath the skin.
- **Areolar tissue** it serves as a support framework for epithelium.
- It contains fibroblasts (cells that produce and secrete fibres), macrophages and mast cells.

- **Adipose tissue** is another type of loose connective tissue located mainly beneath the skin.
- The cells of this tissue are specialised to store fats.
- The excess of nutrients which are not used immediately are converted into fats and are stored in this tissue.
- **Adipose tissue helps in heat loss and act as shock absorber.**

(ii) **Dense connective tissue**

- Fibres and fibroblasts are compactly packed in the **dense connective tissues**.
- The orientation of fibres show a regular or irregular pattern and are called **dense regular** and **dense irregular tissues.**
- In the dense **regular connective tissues**, the collagen fibres are present in rows between many parallel bundles of fibres.
- Example of dense **regular connective tissues are Tendon and Ligament.**
- Tendons, which attach skeletal muscles to bones and ligaments which attach one bone to another are examples of this tissue.
- Dense irregular connective tissue has **fibroblasts** and many fibres (mostly collagen) that are oriented differently.
- Dense irregular **connective** tissue is found in the skin.

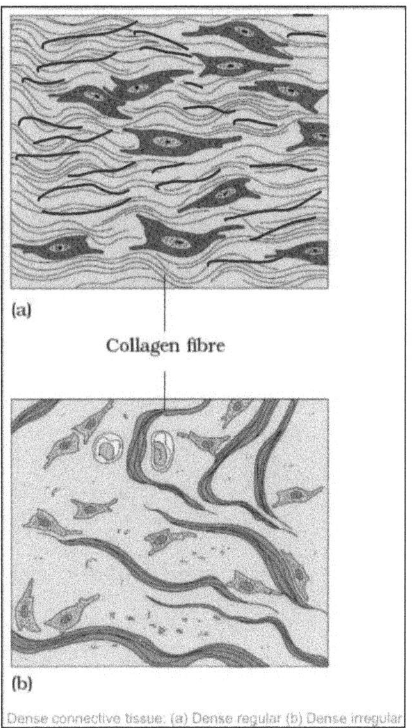

Dense connective tissue: (a) Dense regular (b) Dense irregular

Specialised connective tissues.

- Cartilage, bones and blood are various types of **specialised connective tissues.**

Cartilage

- The intercellular material of **cartilage** is solid and pliable and resists compression.

- Cells of **cartilage called as** chondrocytes.
- Chondrocytes are enclosed in small cavities within the **matrix** secreted by them.
- Most of the cartilages in **vertebrate** embryos are replaced by bones in adults.
- Cartilage is present in the tip of nose, outer ear joints, between adjacent bones of the vertebral column, limbs and hands in **adults**.

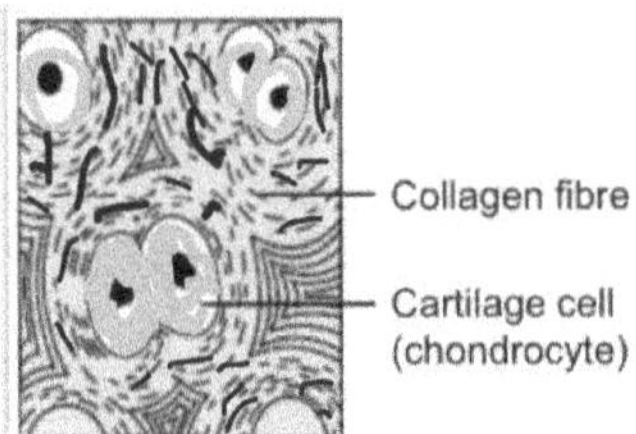

T.S. of Cartilage

Bones

- **Bones** have a **hard** and **non-pliable.**
- **The** ground substance of bone rich in calcium salts and collagen fibres.
- **Calcium salts and collagen fibres** gives strength to bone.
- It is the main tissue that provides **structural** frame to the body.
- Bones support and protect softer **tissues** and organs.
- The bone cells (**osteocytes**) are present in the spaces called lacunae.
- One lacuna contain one **osteocyte**.
- Limb bones, such as the long **bones** of the legs, serve weight-bearing functions.
- They also interact with **skeletal** muscles attached to them to bring about movements.
- The bone marrow in some bones is the site of **production** of blood cells.
- Haversian system is found in **mammalian** bone.

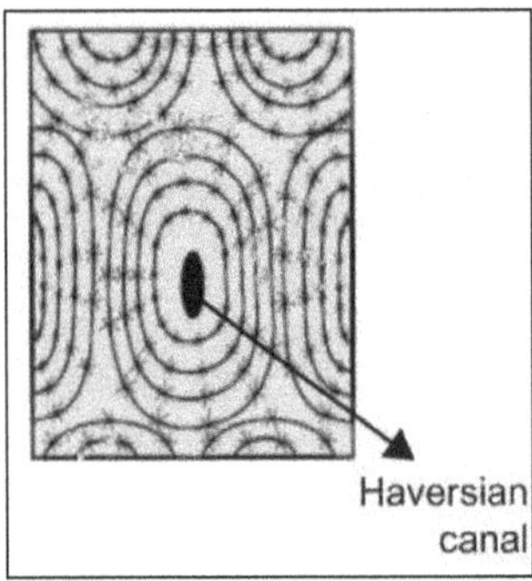

T.S. of Bone

Blood

Blood is a fluid connective tissue containing plasma, red blood cells (RBC), white blood cells (WBC) and platelets.

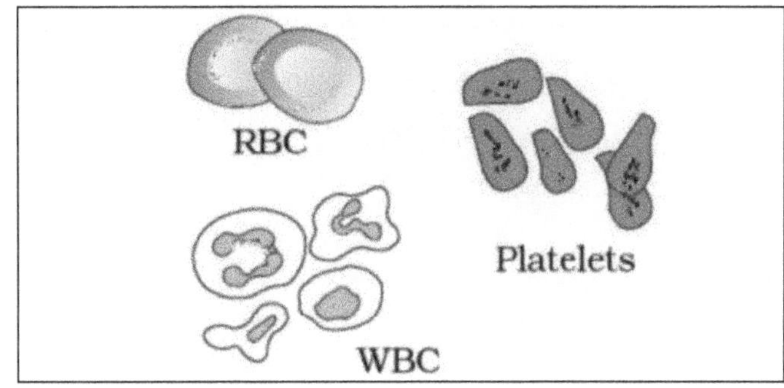

2.1.3 MUSCLE TISSUE

- Each muscle is made of many long, cylindrical fibres arranged in parallel arrays.
- Muscle fibres are composed of numerous fine fibrils, called myofibrils.
- Muscle fibres contract (shorten) in response to stimulation, then relax (lengthen) and return to their uncontracted state in a coordinated fashion.
- Their **action** moves the body to adjust to the changes in the environment and to maintain the positions of the various parts of the body.
- **Muscles** play an active role in all the movements of the body.
- Muscles mostly **mesodermal** in origin.
- Muscles are of three types, skeletal, smooth, and cardiac.

a. Skeletal muscle

- **Skeletal muscle** tissue is closely attached to skeletal bones.
- In a typical muscle such as the biceps, striated (striped) skeletal muscle fibres are bundled together in a parallel fashion.
- A and I band present.
- A sheath of tough connective tissue encloses several bundles of muscle fibres.

b. Smooth muscle

- The **smooth muscle** fibres taper at both ends (fusiform) and do not show striations.
- Cell junctions hold them together and they are bundled together in a connective tissue sheath.
- The wall of **internal** organs such as the blood vessels, stomach and intestine contains this type of muscle tissue.
- A and I band absent.
- Smooth muscles are 'involuntary' as their functioning cannot be directly controlled. We usually are not able to make it contract merely by thinking about it as we can do with skeletal muscles.

c. Cardiac muscle

- **Cardiac muscle tissue** is a contractile tissue present only in the heart.
- **Cell junctions** fuse the plasma membranes of cardiac muscle cells and make them stick together.
- A and I band **present** but not distinct.

- Communication junctions (**intercalated discs**) present.
- **Communication junctions** (intercalated discs) at some fusion points allow the cells to contract as a unit, i.e., when one cell receives a signal to contract, its neighbours are also stimulated to contract.

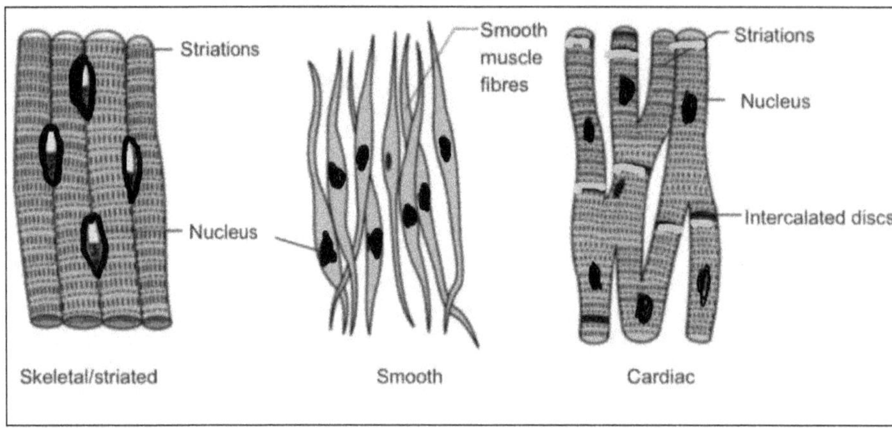

2.1.4 NEURAL TISSUE

- **Neural tissue** exerts the greatest control over the body's responsiveness to changing conditions.
- Neural tissue has two component - **Neuron** and **Neuroglial** cells.
- Neuron is a **structural and functional unit** of nervous system.
- Neurons, the unit of **neural system are excitable cells.**
- The neuroglial cell **which constitute the rest** of the neural **system** protect and support neurons. **Neuroglia make** up more than one half the volume of neural tissue in our body.
- When a neuron is **suitably** stimulated, an electrical disturbance is generated which swiftly travels along its plasma membrane Arrival of the disturbance at the neuron's endings, or output zone, triggers events that may cause **stimulation** or inhibition of adjacent neurons and other cells.

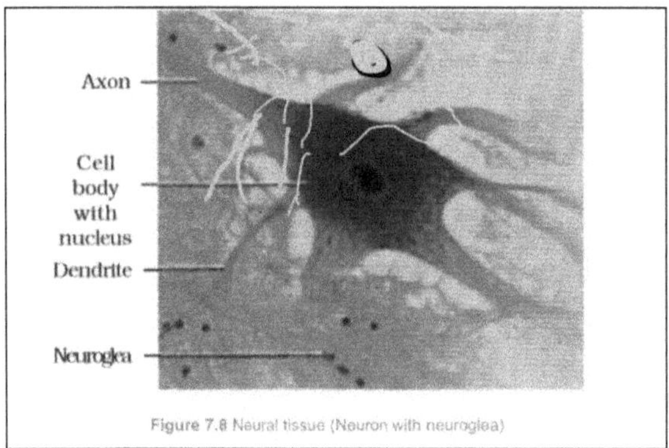

Figure 7.8 Neural tissue (Neuron with neuroglea)

2.2 ORGAN AND ORGAN SYSTEM

- The basic tissues organise to form organs which in turn **associate** to form organ systems in the multicellular organisms.
- Such an **organisation** is essential for more efficient and better coordinated activities of millions of cells constituting an organism.

- Each organ in our body is made of one or more type of tissues.
- Our heart consists of all the four types of tissues, i.e., epithelial, connective, muscular and neural.
- Morphology refers to study of form or **externally** visible features.
- In case of animals this refers to the external **appearance** of the organs or parts of the body.
- The word **anatomy** is used for the study of morphology of internal organs in the animals.

2.3 Cockroach

- Cockroaches are **brown or black bodied animals**
- Cockroaches are included in class **Insecta of Phylum Arthropoda.**
- Cockroaches are **bright yellow, red and green coloured.**
- Cockroaches have also been reported in tropical regions.
- Their size ranges from ¼ inches to 3 inches (0.6-7.6 cm) and have long antenna, legs and flat extension of the upper body wall that conceals head.
- Cockroaches are **nocturnal, omnivores** that live in damp places throughout the world.
- Some Cockroaches shows **cannibalism.**
- They have become residents of human homes and thus are serious pests and vectors of several diseases.

2.3.1 Morphology

- The adults of the common species of cockroach,
- *Periplaneta americana* are about 34-53 mm long with wings *that extend beyond the tip of the abdomen in males.*

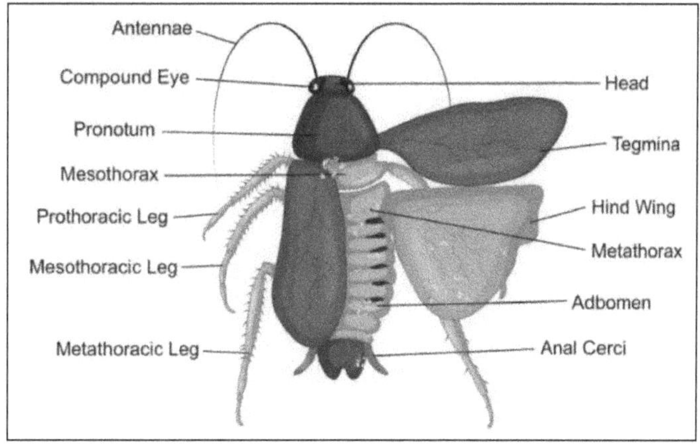

Morphology of Cockroach

- The body of the **cockroach** is segmented and divisible into three distinct regions – head, thorax and abdomen.
- The entire body is covered by a hard **chitinous** exoskeleton (brown in colour).

- In each segment, exoskeleton has hardened plates called **sclerites**(**tergites** dorsally, **pleurite** laterally and **sternites** ventrally) that are joined to each other by a thin and flexible articular membrane (arthrodial membrane).

Head

- Head is **triangular** in shape and lies anteriorly at right angles to the longitudinal body axis.
- It is formed by the fusion of **six segments.**
- Head shows **great mobility in all directions** due to flexible neck.
- Neck is a **modification of Thorax.**
- **The head capsule bears** a pair of compound eyes.
- A pair of thread like antennae arise from membranous sockets lying in front of eyes.
- **Antennae** have sensory receptors that help in monitoring the environment.
- **Anterior** end of the head bears appendages forming biting and chewing type of mouth parts.
- The mouth parts consisting of a labrum (act as upper lip), a pair of mandibles, a pair of maxillae and a labium (act as lower lip).
- A **median** flexible lobe, acting as tongue (hypopharynx), lies within the cavity enclosed by the mouthparts.
- **Common** salivary duct open at the base of hypopharynx.

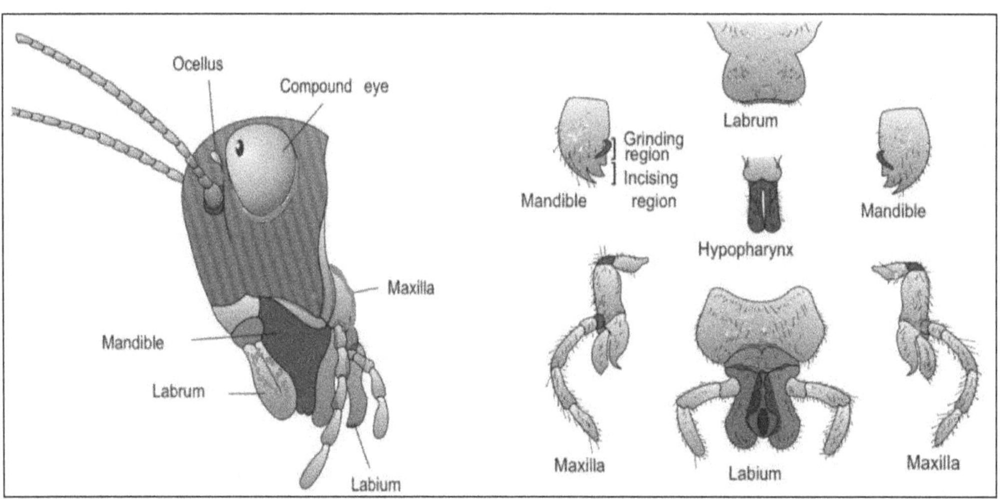

Mouth parts of Cockroach

Thorax

- Thorax consists of three parts – **prothorax, mesothorax and metathorax**.
- The head is connected with **thorax by a short extension of the prothorax known as the neck.**
- **Each thoracic segment bears** a pair of walking legs.

Wings

- **The first pair of wings arises from mesothorax** and the second pair from metathorax.
- Forewings (mesothoracic) called **Tegmina/Elytra** are opaque dark and leathery and cover the hind wings when at rest.

- The hind wings are **transparent, membranous** and are used in flight.

Abdomen

- The abdomen in both males and females consists of 10 segments.
- In females, the **7th sternum** is boat shaped.
- **10th Tergum** Bowl shaped.
- Together with the **8th and 9th sterna** forms a brood or genital pouch whose anterior part contains female gonopore, spermathecal pores and collateral glands.
- In males, genital pouch or chamber lies at the hind end of abdomen bounded dorsally by 9th and 10th terga and ventrally by the **9th sternum.**
- Genital pouch or chamber contains on dorsal side anus and on ventral side male genital pore and gonapophysis present.
- **Ventrally** on **9th segment Males** bear a pair of short, thread like anal styles which are absent in females.
- In both sexes, **dorsally 10th segment** bears a pair of jointed filamentous structures called anal cerci.

7.3.2 ANATOMY

Digestive system

- The alimentary canal present in the body cavity is divided into three regions: **foregut, midgut and hindgut.**
- The mouth opens into a **short tubular pharynx.**
- Mouth open in to a narrow tubular passage called **oesophagus**.
- Oesophagus opens into a sac like structure called crop used for storing of food.
- The crop is followed by **gizzard** or **proventriculus.**
- It has an outer layer of thick circular muscles and thick inner cuticle forming six highly chitinous plate called teeth.
- **Gizzard helps** in grinding the food particles.
- The entire **foregut and hindgut** is lined by cuticle.
- A ring of 6-8 blind tubules called **hepatic or gastric caecae** is present at the junction of **foregut and midgut**, which secrete digestive juice.
- At the junction of midgut and hindgut is present another ring of 100-150 yellow coloured thin filamentous **Malphigian tubules**.
- They help in removal of excretory products from **haemolymph.**

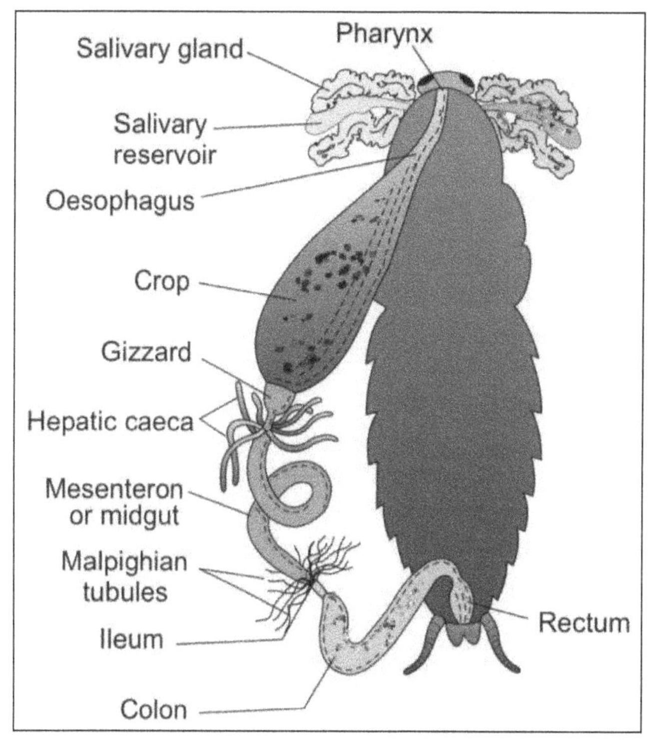

- The hindgut is broader than midgut and is differentiated into ileum, colon and rectum.
- The rectum opens in to anus.

Blood vascular system

- Blood vascular system of cockroach is an **open type/Lacunar type.**
- Blood vessels are **poorly developed** and open into space (haemocoel).

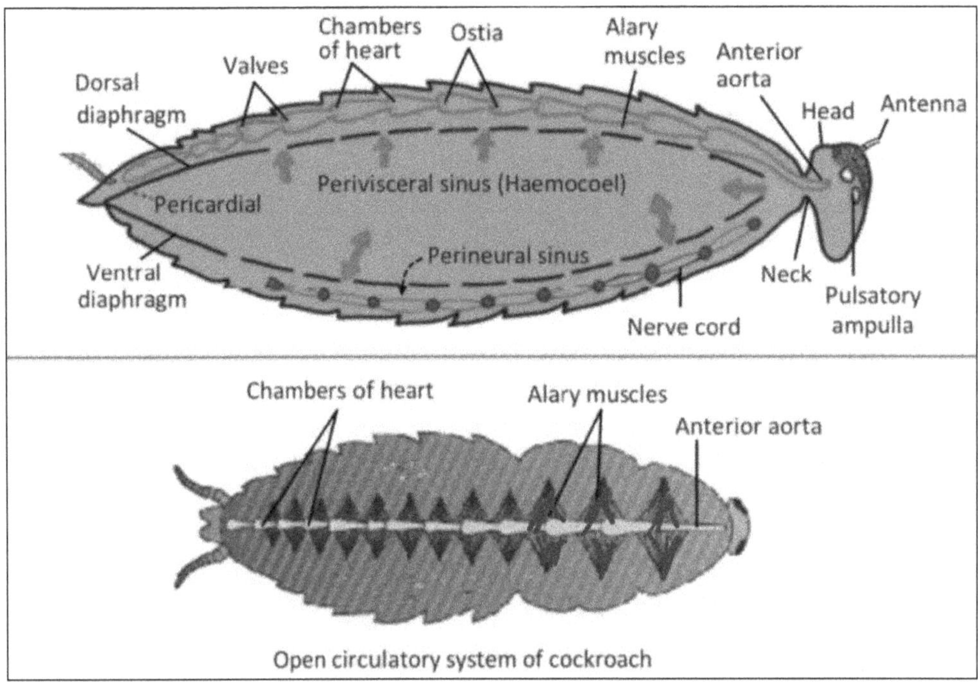

Open circulatory system of cockroach

- **Visceral organs** located in the haemocoel are bathed in blood (haemolymph).
- **The haemolymph** is composed of **colourless plasma** and haemocytes.
- **Heart of cockroach** consists of elongated muscular tube lying along mid dorsal line of thorax and abdomen.
- It is differentiated into **funnel shaped chambers** with ostia on either side.
- Blood from sinuses enter heart through **ostia** and is pumped anteriorly to sinuses again.

Respiratory system

- The respiratory system consists of a network of **trachea,** that open through **10 pairs of small holes called spiracles** present on the lateral side of the body.
- **Thin branching tubes (tracheal tubes subdivided into tracheoles)** carry oxygen from the air to all the parts.
- The opening of the spiracles is **regulated by the sphincters.**
- Exchange of gases take place at the tracheoles by diffusion.

Execratory system

- Excretion is performed by **Malpighian tubules.**
- 100-150 **Malpighian tubules found at the junction of foregut and hind gut.**

- Each tubule is lined by glandular and ciliated cells.
- They absorb nitrogenous waste products and convert them into uric acid which is excreted out through the hindgut.
- Therefore, this insect is called **uricotelic**.
- In addition, the **fat body, nephrocytes and urecose** glands also help in excretion.

Nervous system

- Mid ventral in postion.
- The nervous system of cockroach consists of a series of fused, segmentally arranged ganglia joined by **paired** longitudinal **connectives** on the ventral side.

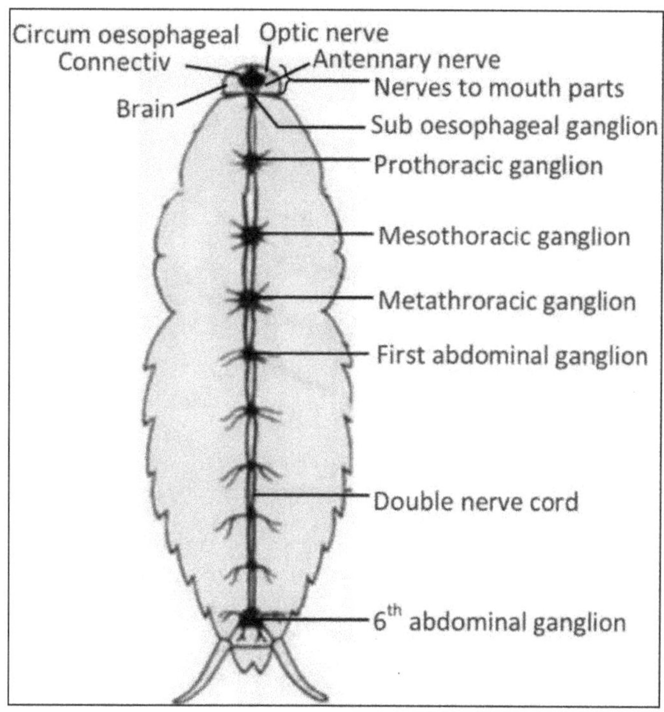

Nervous System of Cockroach

- Three **ganglia** found in the thorax, and **six** in the abdomen.
- The nervous system of cockroach is spread throughout the body.
- The head holds a **bit** of a nervous system while the rest is **situated** along the ventral (belly-side) part of its body.
- So if the head of a cockroach is cut off, it will still live for as long as one week.

Receptors

- In the head region, the brain is represented by **supra-oesophageal ganglion** which supplies nerves to antennae and compound eyes.
- In cockroach, the sense organs are **antennae, eyes, maxillary palps, labial palps, anal cerci**, etc.
- Anal cerci helps to **detect** vibration.
- **Antennae act as Thigmoreceptor.**

Compound eyes

- For vision **compound** eyes are situated at the dorsal surface of the head.
- Each eye consists of about **2000 hexagonal ommatidia (sing.: *ommatidium*)**.
- With the help of several **ommatidia**, a cockroach can receive several images of an object.
- The above type of vision is known as **mosaic** vision with more sensitivity but less resolution, being common **during** night (hence called nocturnal vision).

Reproductive system

- Cockroaches are dioecious and both sexes have well developed **reproductive** organs.

Male reproductive system

- **Male reproductive system** consists of a pair of testes lying one on each lateral side in the 4th–6th abdominal segments.
- From each testis arises a thin **vas** deferens, which opens into ejaculatory duct through seminal vesicle.
- The ejaculatory duct opens into male **gonopore** situated ventral to anus.
- A characteristic mushroom shaped gland is present in the 6th-7th abdominal segments which functions as an accessory reproductive gland.
- Mushroom gland also Known as Utricular glands.
- Phallic/Conglobate gland also found in male cockroach.

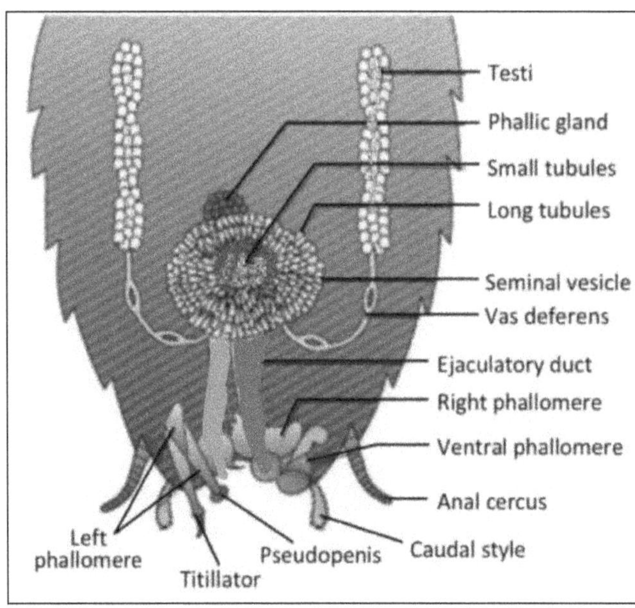

- The external genitalia are represented by male **gonapophysis** or **phallomere** (chitinous **asymmetrical** structures, surrounding the male gonopore).
- **Phallomeres** are three types - Right, Left and ventral.
- **Titillator** and **pseudopenis** are part of left phallomere.
- The sperms are stored in the **seminal vesicles** and are glued together in the form of bundles called spermatophores which are discharged during copulation.

Female reproductive system

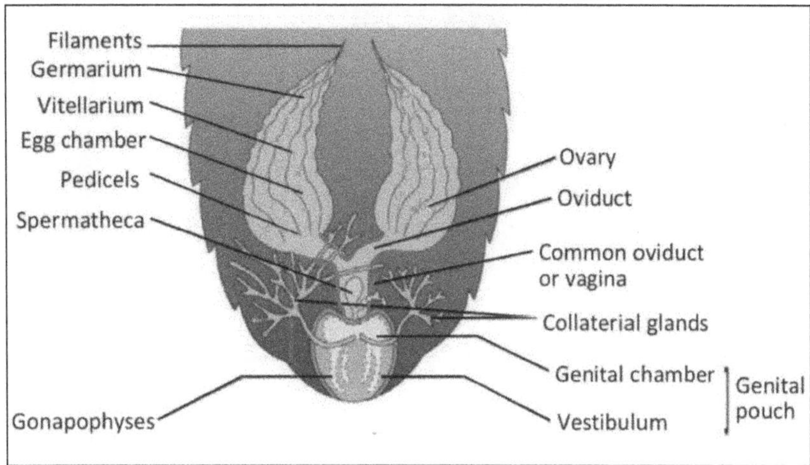

- **The female reproductive system** consists of **two large ovaries.**
- **Ovaries present laterally in the 2nd – 6th abdominal segments.**
- Each ovary is formed of a group of **eight ovarian tubules or ovarioles,** containing a chain of developing ova.
- Oviducts of each ovary unite into a single median **oviduct** (also called vagina) which opens into the genital chamber.
- **A pair of spermatheca is present in the 6th segment** which opens into the genital chamber.
- Sperms are transferred through spermatophores.

Ootheca

- **Their fertilised eggs** are encased in capsules called **oothecae.**
- **Ootheca is a dark reddish to blackish** brown capsule, about 3/8" (8 mm) long.
- Ootheca are dropped Or glued to a suitable surface, usually in a crack or crevice of high relative humidity near a food source.
- On an average, females produce **9-10 oothecae,** each containing 14-16 eggs.
- The development of **P. americana** is paurometabolous, meaning there is development through nymphal stage.

Nymph

- The **nymphs** look very much like adults.
- The nymph grows by moulting about **13 times** to convert the adult form.
- The next to last nymphal stage has wing pads but only adult cockroaches have wings.

Points to remember-

- Many species of **cockroaches** are wild and are of no economic importance.
- A few species **thrive** in and around human habitat.
- They are pests because they destroy food and **contaminate** it with their smelly excreta.
- They can **transmit** a variety of bacterial diseases by contaminating food material.

2.4 FROGS

- **Frogs can live both on land and in freshwater**.
- **Frog** belong to class Amphibia of phylum Chordata.
- The most common species of frog found in India is **_Rana tigrina_**.
- **_Rana tigrina_ also called Indian Bull frog.**
- They do not have constant body temperature i.e., their body temperature varies with the temperature of the environment so called **cold blooded or poikilotherms.**
- **Frog** can change in the colour,while they are in grasses and on dry land.
- The ability to change the colour to hide them from their enemies (camouflage).
- This protective coloration is called **mimicry.**
- The frogs are not seen **during peak summer and winter.**
- During this period they take shelter in deep burrows to protect them from extreme heat and cold.
- This is called as **summer sleep (aestivation)** and **winter sleep (hibernation).**

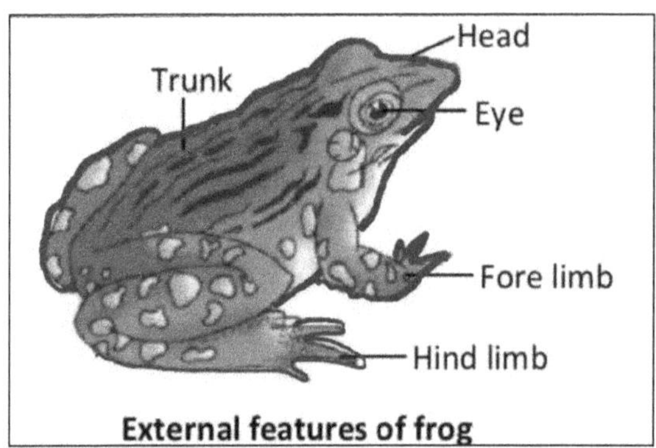

External features of frog

2.4.1 Morphology

Skin

- **The skin is smooth and slippery** due to the presence of mucus.
- **The skin is always** maintained in a moist condition.
- **The colour of dorsal side** of body is generally olive green with dark irregular spots.
- **On the ventral side** the skin is uniformly pale yellow.
- **The frog never drinks** water but absorb it through the skin.

Body division and external features

- Body of a frog is divisible **into head and trunk.**
- **A neck and tail** are absent in frog.
- Above the mouth, a pair of nostrils is present.
- Eyes are bulged and covered by a **nictitating membrane** that protects them while in water.
- On either side of eyes a **membranous tympanum (ear)** receives sound signals.

- **The forelimbs and hind limbs** help in swimming, walking, leaping and burrowing.
- **The hind limbs end in five digits** and they are larger and muscular than fore limbs that end in four digits.
- **Feet have webbed digits** that help in swimming.

Sexual dimorphism.

- Frogs exhibit sexual **dimorphism**.
- **Male** frogs can be distinguished by the presence of sound producing vocal sacs.
- **Male** also have a copulatory pad on the first digit of the fore limbs which are absent in female frogs.

2.4.2 Anatomy

- The body cavity of frogs accommodate different organ systems such as digestive, circulatory, respiratory, nervous, excretory and reproductive systems with well developed structures and functions.

Digestive system

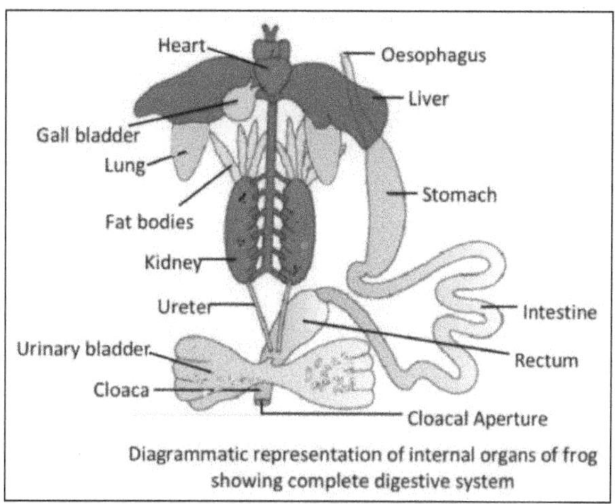

Diagrammatic representation of internal organs of frog showing complete digestive system

- **The digestive system consists** of alimentary canal and digestive glands.
- **The alimentary canal is short** because frogs are carnivores and hence the length of intestine is reduced.
- **The mouth opens into the buccal cavity** that leads to the oesophagus through pharynx.
- **Oesophagus** is a short tube that opens into the stomach which in turn continues as the intestine, rectum and finally opens outside by the cloaca.
- **Liver** secretes bile that is stored in the gall bladder.
- Pancreas, a digestive gland produces pancreatic juice containing digestive enzymes.
- Food is captured by the bilobed tongue.
- **Digestion of food takes place** by the action of HCl and gastric juices secreted from the walls of the stomach.
- **Partially digested food called chyme** is passed from stomach to the first part of the intestine, the duodenum.
- **The duodenum receives** bile from gall bladder and pancreatic juices from the pancreas through a common bile duct.

- **Bile emulsifies** fat and pancreatic juices digest carbohydrates and proteins.
- **Final digestion** takes place in the intestine.
- **Digested food** is absorbed by the numerous finger-like folds in the inner wall of intestine called villi and microvilli.
- **The undigested solid waste** moves into the rectum and passes out through cloaca.

Respiratory system

- **Frogs** respire on land and in the water by two different methods.
- **In water, skin acts** as aquatic respiratory organ (cutaneous respiration).
- **Dissolved oxygen** in the water is exchanged through the skin by diffusion.
- **On land, the buccal cavity**, skin and lungs act as the respiratory organs.
- The respiration by lungs is called pulmonary respiration.
- The lungs are a pair of elongated, **pink coloured sac-like** structures present in the upper part of the trunk region (thorax).
- Air enters through the nostrils into the buccal cavity and then to lungs.
- During **aestivation** and **hibernation** gaseous exchange takes place through skin.

Blood vascular system

- The vascular system of frog is well-developed **closed type**.
- **Lymphatic system** also found.
- The blood vascular system involves heart, blood vessels and blood.
- The lymphatic system consists of lymph, lymph channels and lymph nodes.
- **Heart is a muscular structure** situated in the upper part of the body cavity.
- **Heart is myogenic and autoexcitable.**
- It has three chambers, two atria and one ventricle and is covered by a membrane called pericardium.
- **A triangular structure** called **sinus venosus** joins the right atrium.
- Lymph receives blood through the major veins called vena cava.
- The ventricle opens into a saclike **conus arteriosus** on the ventral side of the heart.
- The blood from the heart is carried to all parts of the body by **the arteries (arterial system)**.
- The veins collect blood from **different** parts of body to the heart and form the venous system.
- Special venous connection between **liver** and **intestine** as well as the kidney and lower parts of the body are present in frogs.
- The former is called hepatic portal system and the latter is called renal portal system.
- The blood is composed of plasma and cells.
- The blood cells are **RBC (red blood cells) or erythrocytes, WBC (white blood cells) or leucocytes and platelets**.
- RBC's are nucleated and contain red **coloured** pigment namely haemoglobin.

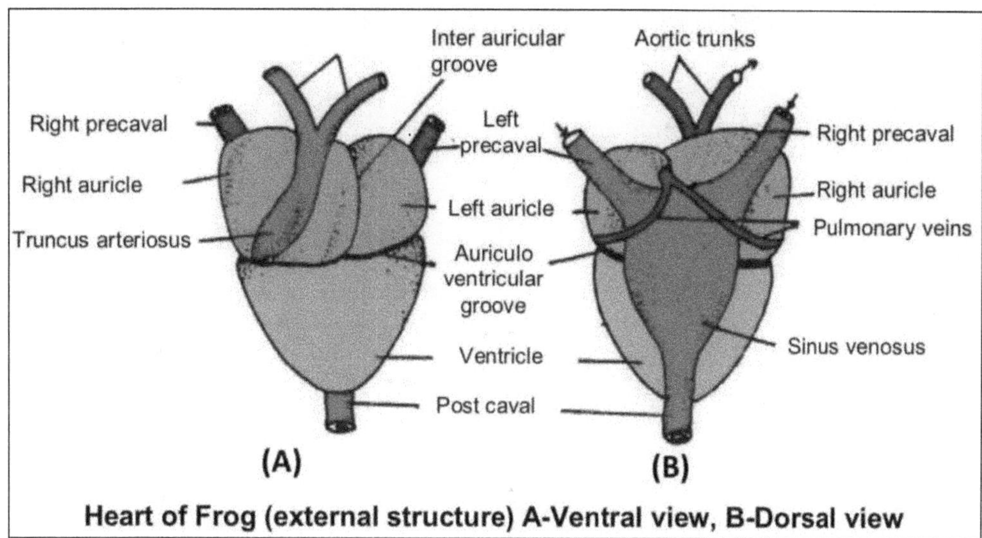

Heart of Frog (external structure) A-Ventral view, B-Dorsal view

- The lymph is different from blood.
- It lacks few **proteins** and **RBCs**.
- The blood carries nutrients, gases and water to the respective sites during the **circulation**.
- The circulation of blood is achieved by the **pumping** action of the muscular heart.

Excretory system

- Excretion by a well **developed** excretory system.
- The excretory system consists of a pair of kidneys, ureters, cloaca and urinary bladder.
- The kidneys are compact, **dark red and bean like** structures situated a little posteriorly in the body cavity on both sides of vertebral column.
- Each kidney is composed of several **structural** and functional units called uriniferous tubules or nephrons.

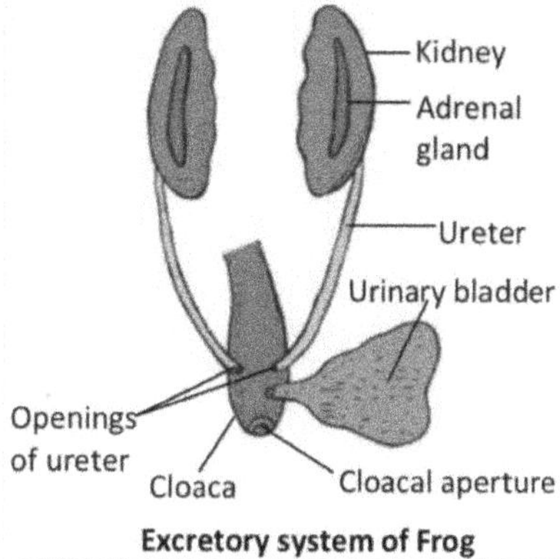

Excretory system of Frog

- Each kidney has **2000** nephrons.
- Two ureters emerge from the kidneys in the male frogs.
- The ureters act as **urinogenital** duct which opens into the cloaca.
- In females the ureters and oviduct open **seperately** in the cloaca.
- The thin-walled **urinary** bladder is present ventral to the rectum which also opens in the cloaca.
- The frog excretes urea so frog is a **ureotelic** animal.

- Excretory wastes are **carried** by blood into the kidney where it is separated and excreted.

Endocrine Sytem

- The system for **control** and coordination is highly evolved in the frog **like humans**.
- It includes both **neural** system and endocrine glands.
- The chemical **coordination** of various organs of the body is achieved by hormones which are secreted by the endocrine glands.
- The **prominent** endocrine glands found in frog are **pituitary, thyroid, parathyroid, thymus, pineal body, pancreatic islets, adrenals and gonads.**

Nervous system

- The nervous system is organised into a central nervous system (brain and spinal cord), a peripheral nervous system (cranial and spinal nerves) and an autonomic nervous system (sympathetic and parasympathetic).
- There are **ten pairs** of cranial nerves arising from the brain.
- **Ten pair** spinal nerves present.
- **Brain** is enclosed in a bony structure called brain box (cranium).
- The brain is divided into **fore-brain, mid-brain and hind-brain.**
- **Forebrain** includes olfactory lobes, paired cerebral hemispheres and unpaired diencephalon.
- The midbrain is characterised by a pair of optic lobes.
- Hind-brain consists of **cerebellum and medulla oblongata.**
- Pons absent.
- **The medulla oblongata passes out through the foramen magnum** and continues into spinal cord,which is enclosed in the vertebral column.
- Frog has different types of sense organs, namely organs of touch (sensory papillae), taste (taste buds), smell (nasal epithelium), vision (eyes) and hearing (tympanum with internal ears).
- Out of these, **eyes and internal ears are well-organised structures** and the rest are cellular aggregations around nerve endings.

Eyes and ears

- Eyes in a frog are a pair of spherical structures situated in the orbit in skull.
- These are **simple eyes (possessing only one unit).**
- External ear is absent in frogs and only tympanum can be seen externally.
- The ear is an organ of **hearing as well as balancing (equilibrium).**

Reproductive system

- Frogs have well organised male and female reproductive systems.
- Male reproductive organs consist of a pair of yellowish ovoid testes, which are found adhered to the upper part of kidneys by a double fold of peritoneum called **mesorchium.**
- **Vasa efferentia** are **10-12 in number t**hat arise from testes.

- They enter the kidneys on their side and open into Bidder's canal.

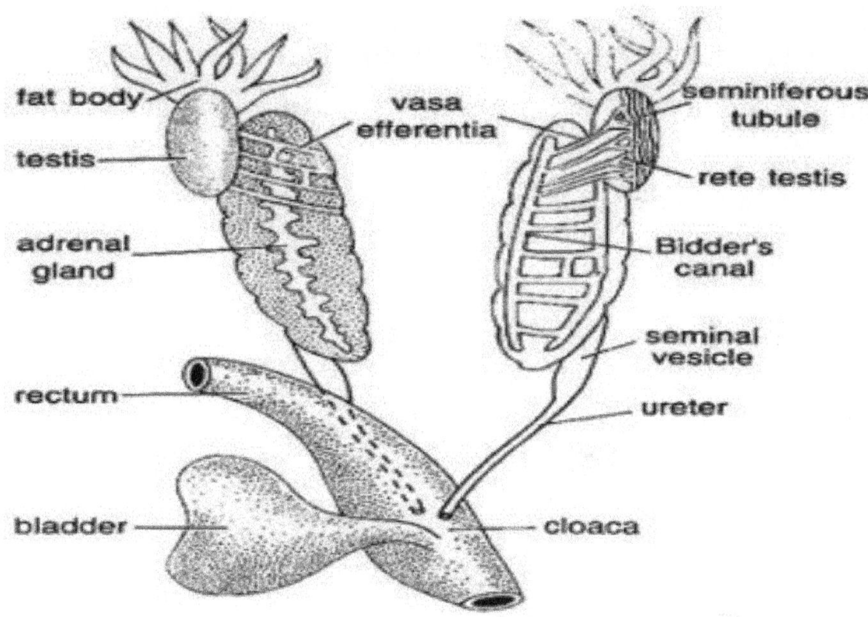

Frog. Male urinogenital organs.

- Finally it communicates with the urinogenital duct that comes out of the kidneys and opens into the cloaca.

- **The cloaca** is a small, median chamber that is used to pass faecal matter, urine and sperms to the exterior.

- The female reproductive organs include a **pair of ovaries.**

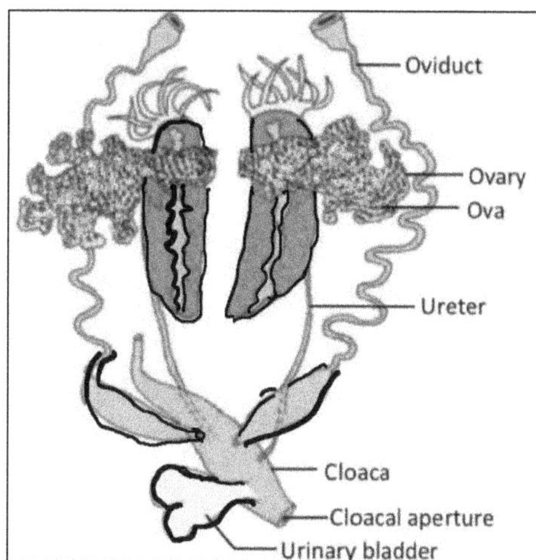

- The ovaries are situated near **kidneys** and there is no functional connection with kidneys.

- A pair of oviduct arising from the **ovaries** opens into the cloaca separately.

- A mature female can lay **2500 to 3000** ova at a time.

- Fertilisation is **external** and takes place in water.

- Development involves a **larval stage called tadpole.**

- Tadpole undergoes **metamorphosis** to form the adult.

Points to remember-

- Frogs are **beneficial** for mankind because they eat insects and protect the crop.
- Frogs maintain **ecological** balance because these serve as an important link of food chain and food web in the ecosystem.
- In some countries the **muscular** legs of frog are used as food by man.

1. Consider the following statements and find out the correct option-

A. Squamous epithelium are found in the walls of blood vessels and air sacs of lungs and are involved in a functions like forming a diffusion boundary.

B. The **cuboidal epithelium** is composed of a single layer of cube-like cells.

C. **Cuboidal epithelium** is commonly found in ducts of glands and tubular parts of nephrons in kidneys and its main functions are secretion and absorption. The epithelium of proximal convoluted tubule (PCT) of nephron in the kidney has microvilli.

D. The **columnar epithelium** is composed of a single layer of tall and slender cells.

Which of the above are correct -

1. A,B,C

2. B,C

3. D,B,A

4. A,B,C,D

2. Match the list 1 and 2-

List 1   List 2

a. **Multicellular** gland	The intestinal glands
b. **Tight junctions**	help to stop substances from leaking across a tissue.
c. **Dense connective tissues**	Fibres and fibroblasts are compactly packed

Which above of them are/is correctly matched-

1. a and b

2. b and c

3. a,b,c

4. a and c

3. Consider the following features-

a) Connective tissues are most abundant and widely distributed in the body of complex animals.

b) They are named connective tissues because of their special function of linking and supporting other tissues/organs of the body.

c) They range from soft connective tissues to specialised types, which include cartilage, bone, adipose, and blood.

d) In all connective tissues except blood, the cells secrete fibres of structural proteins called collagen or elastin.

e) The fibres provide strength, elasticity and flexibility to the tissue.

Which above features are found in Connective tissues-

1. only a and d

2. a,b,c,d,

3. only c and d

4. a,b,c,d,e

4. Read the following statement carefully with respect to Connective tissue-

a) **The areolar tissue** present beneath the skin.

b) **Loose connective tissue** contains fibroblasts (cells that produce and secrete fibres), macrophages and mast cells.

c) **Adipose tissue** is another type of loose connective tissue located mainly beneath the skin. The cells of this tissue are specialised to store fats.

d) In the dense **regular connective tissues**, the collagen fibres are present in rows between many parallel bundles of fibres.

How many of them are/is correct -

1. three

2. four

3. one

4. two

5. Consider the following statements and find out the correct option

STATEMENT 1. Blood is a fluid connective tissue containing plasma,red blood cells (RBC), white blood cells (WBC) only.

STATEMENT 2. The bone marrow in some bones is the site of production of blood cells.

1. Both are correct statements

2. Only Statement 1 correct

3. Both are wrong statements

4. Only statement 2 correct

6. Go through the following statement-

ASSERTION(A). Cardiac muscle fibers are branched muscle fibers.

REASON(R). These fibers are composed of numerous fine fibrils, called myofibrils.

1.A correct and R is correct explanation of A

2. A correct and R is also correct but R is not correct explanation of A

3. A correct but R incorrect

4. A and R both are incorrect

7. Which statement is incorrect for Cartilage-

1. The intercellular material of cartilage is hard and non pliable and resists compression.

2. Most of the cartilages in vertebrate embryos are replaced by bones in adults.

3. Cartilage is present in the tip of nose, outer ear joints, between adjacent bones of the vertebral column, limbs and hands in adults.

4. Cartilage, bones and blood are various types of specialised connective tissues.

8. Go through the following statements-

a) The bone cells (osteocytes) are present in the spaces called lacunae.

b) Limb bones, such as the long bones of the legs, serve weight-bearing functions.

c) Limb also interact with skeletal muscles attached to them to bring about movements.

d) The bone marrow in some bones is the site of production of blood cells.

How many of them are/is correct-

1. two

2. three

3. four

4. one

9. Match the list 1 and 2-

List 1	List 2
a. Tendons	j. attach one bone to another
b. Ligaments	k. the collagen fibres are present in rows between many parallel bundles of fibres
c. Dense regular connective tissues	l. attach skeletal muscles to bones
d. Areolar tissue	m. present beneath the skin

Find out the correct option –

1. a.k, b.j, c.l, d.m

2. a.k,b.l,c.j,d.m

3. a.l,b.j,c.k,d.m

4. a.l,b.j,c.m,d.k

10. Consider the following statements and find out the correct option

STATEMENT 1. Gap junctions do not facilitate the cells to communicate with each other by connecting the cytoplasm of adjoining cells.

STATEMENT 2. All cells in epithelium are held together with little intercellular material.

1. Both are wrong statements

2. Only Statement 1 correct

3. Both are correct statements

4. Only statement 2 correct

11. Read the following statements very carefully –

a) Exocrine glands secrete mucus, saliva, earwax, oil, milk, digestive enzymes and other cell products. These products are release through ducts or tubes.

b) In contrast, endocrine glands do not have ducts.

c) The products of endocrine glands called hormones are secreted directly into the fluid bathing the gland.

d) Some of the columnar or cuboidal cells get specialised for secretion and are called glandular epithelium

Which above statement are correct?

1. a and c both

2. d only

3. a,b,c,d.

4. b and d both

12. Go through the following statement-

ASSERTION(A). The **columnar epithelium** is composed of a single layer of cube like cells.

REASON(R). They are found in the lining of stomach only.

1. A correct and R is correct explanation of A

2. A correct and R is also correct but R is not correct explanation of A

3. A correct but R incorrect

4. A and R both are incorrect

13. Find out incorrect statement -

1. **Skeletal muscle** tissue is closely attached to skeletal bones.

2. The **smooth muscle** fibres taper at both ends (fusiform) and show striations.

3. Smooth muscles are 'involuntary' as their functioning cannot be directly controlled. We usually are not able to make it contract merely by thinking about it as we can do with skeletal muscles.

4. **Cardiac muscle tissue** is a contractile tissue present in the heart.

14. Read the following statements and find out correct option-

a) Neural tissue exerts the greatest control over the body's responsiveness to changing conditions. Neurons, the unit of neural system are excitable cells.

b) The neuroglial cell which constitute the rest of the neural system protect and support neurons.

c) Neuroglia make up more than one half the volume of neural tissue in our body.

d) When a neuron is suitably stimulated, an electrical disturbance is generated.

How many of them are correct-

1. four

2. one

3. two

4. three

15. Consider the following statements and find out the correct option with respect to *Periplaneta americana-*

STATEMENT 1. The female reproductive system consists of two large ovaries, lying laterally in the 2nd – 6th abdominal segments.

STATEMENT 2. Each ovary is formed of a group of eight ovarian tubules or ovarioles, containing a chain of developing ova.

1. Both are wrong statements

2. Only statement 1 correct

3. Both are correct statements

4. Only statement 2 correct

16. Match the list 1 and 2 with respect to *Periplaneta americana-*

<table><tr><td colspan="1">List 1</td><td colspan="1">List 2</td></tr><tr><td>a. Ootheca is a dark reddish to blackish brown capsule</td><td>8 cm long.</td></tr><tr><td>b. On an average, females produce</td><td>9-10 oothecae</td></tr><tr><td>c. Each Ootheca containing</td><td>14-16 eggs.</td></tr><tr><td>d. The nymph grows by moulting about</td><td>13 times to reach the adult form.</td></tr></table>

How many of them are correctly matched-

1. one

2. two

3. three

4. four

17. Consider the following statements-

a) An epithelial tissue as epithelium (pl.: epithelia) has a free surface, which faces either a body fluid or the outside environment and thus provides a covering or a lining for some part of the body.

b) There are two types of epithelial tissues namely **simple epithelium** and **compound epithelium**.

c) Simple epithelium is composed of a single layer of cells and functions as a lining for body cavities, ducts, and tubes.

d) The compound epithelium consists of two or more cell layers and protective function.

Which of the above statement are correct?

1. b and a only

2. c and a only

3. d and a only

4. a,b,c,d,

18. Match the list 1 and 2 with respect to Cockroach-

List 1   List 2

a. Proventriculus	Gizzard
b. At the junction of midgut and hindgut	malpighian tubules
c. Anal cerci	the 10th segment of abdomen
d. Gizzard	grinding the food particles

How many of them are correctly matched-

1. one   2. two

3. three   4. four

19. Consider the following statements with respect to Cockroach -

I. Heart of cockroach consists of elongated muscular tube lying along mid dorsal line of thorax and abdomen.

II. It is differentiated into funnel shaped chambers with ostia on either side.

III. Blood from sinuses enter heart through ostia and is pumped anteriorly to sinuses again.

IV. The respiratory system consists of a network of trachea, that open through 10 pairs of small holes called spiracles present on the lateral side of the body.

V. Thin branching tubes (tracheal tubes subdivided into tracheoles) carry oxygen from the air to all the parts. The opening of the spiracles is regulated by the sphincters.

VI. Exchange of gases take place at the tracheoles by diffusion.

How many of them are correct-

1. six   2. two

3. three   4. four

20. Read the following statements-

1. Excretion is performed by Malpighian tubules.

2. Each tubule is lined by glandular and ciliated cells.

3. They absorb nitrogenous waste products and convert them into uric acid which is excreted out through the hindgut so called **uricotelic**.

4. The fat body, nephrocytes and urecose glands also help in excretion.

How many of them are/is correct **statements for cockroach-**

1. two

2. three

3. four

4. one

21. Consider the following statements and find out the correct option -

STATEMENT 1. Many species of cockroaches are wild and are of no economic importance.

STATEMENT 2. They are pests because they destroy food and contaminate it with their smelly excreta.

1. Both are wrong statements

2. Only statement 1 correct

3. Both are correct statements

4. Only statement 2 correct

22. Go through the following statement and find out the correct option for *Periplaneta americana-*

ASSERTION(A). A ring of 6-8 blind tubules called hepatic or gastric caecae is present at the junction of foregut and midgut, which secrete digestive juice.

REASON(R). At the junction of midgut and hindgut 100-150 yellow coloured thin filamentous **Malphigian tubules** present.

1.A correct and R is correct explanation of A

2. A correct and R is also correct but R is not correct explanation of A

3. A. correct but R incorrect

4. A and R both are incorrect

23. Go through the following statement and find out the correct option-

a) The nervous system of cockroach consists of a series of fused, segmentally arranged ganglia joined by paired longitudinal connectives on the ventral side.

b) Three ganglia lie in the thorax, and six in the abdomen.

c) The nervous system of cockroach is spread throughout the body.

d) The head holds a bit of a nervous system while the rest is situated along the ventral (belly-side) part of its body.

e) If the head of a cockroach is cut off, it will still live for as long as one week.

Which of the above statement are correct for *Periplaneta americana-*

1. A and C only

2. C and D only

3. D and A only

4. All are correct

24. Read the statements given below with respect to *Periplaneta americana* -

A. The head is connected with thorax by a short extension of the prothorax known as the neck.

B. Each thoracic segment bears a pair of walking legs.

C. The first pair of wings arises from mesothorax and the second pair from metathorax.

D. Hindwings called tegmina are opaque dark and leathery and cover the fore wings when at rest.

Which above statement is/ are incorrect?

1. A and C only

2. D only

3. D and C only

4. A,B,C

25. Which statement are correct -

A. Cockroaches are brown or black bodied animals that are included inclass Insecta of Phylum Arthropoda.

B. Bright yellow, red and green coloured cockroaches have also been reported in tropical regions.

C. Their size ranges from ¼ inches to 3 inches (0.6-7.6 cm) and have long antenna, legs and flat extension of the upper body wall that conceals head.

D. They are nocturnal omnivores that live in damp places throughout the world.

Which of the above statement are correct?

1. A and C only

2. A only

3. D and C only

4. A,B,C,D,

26. Consider the following statements-

I. Cells, tissues, organs and organ systems split up the work in a way that ensures the survival of the body as a whole and exhibit division of labour.

II. A tissue is defined as group of cells along with intercellular substances performing one or more functions in the body.

III. Epithelia are sheet like tissues lining the body's surface and its cavities, ducts and tubes.

IV. Epithelia have one free surface facing a body fluid or the outside environment.

V. Their cells are structurally and functionally connected at junctions.

How many of them are/is correct-

1. one

2. five

3. three

4. four

27. Match the list 1 and 2-

List 1   List 2

a. Adipose tissue	reservoir of stored energy.
b. Skeletal muscle	muscle tissue attached to bones
c. Smooth muscle	component of internal organs.
d. Cardiac muscle	makes the contractile walls of the heart.

How many of them are correctly matched-

1. one

2. two

3. three

4. four

28. Read the following statements-

a) A pair of salivary gland is present near crop.

b) The blood vascular system is of open type.

c) Respiration takes place by network of tracheae.

d) Trachea opens outside with spiracles.

Which above statements are/is correct with reference to Cockroach-

1. a and c only

2. a only

3. d and c only

4. a,b,c,d

29. Consider the following statements and find out incorrect w.r.t. cockroach-

1) Nervous system is represented by segmentally arranged ganglia and ventral nerve cord.

2) Fertilisation is external.

3) Female produces 9-10 ootheca bearing developing embryos.

4) After rupturing of single ootheca about sixteen young ones, called nymphs come out.

30. Read the following facts -

   I. The body of Cockroach *(Periplaneta americana)* is covered by chitinous exoskeleton.

   II. It is divided into head, thorax and abdomen.

   III. Segments bear jointed appendages.

   IV. There are three segments of thorax, each bearing a pair of walking legs.

How many of them are/is correct with reference to Cockroach-

1. four

2. two

3. three

4. one

31. Read the following statements and find out the correct option with respect to cockroach-

STATEMENT 1. Alimentary canal is well developed with a mouth surrounded by mouth parts, a pharynx, oesophagus, crop, gizzard, midgut, hindgut and anus.

STATEMENT 2. Hepatic caecae are present at the junction of foregut and midgut.

1. Both are wrong statements

2. Both are correct statements

3. Only statement 1 correct

4. Only statement 2 correct

32. Go through the following statement and find out the correct option-

ASSERTION(A). The external genitalia of Cockroaches are represented by male gonapophysis or phallomere (chitinous asymmetrical structures, surrounding the male gonopore).

REASON(R). The sperms are stored in the seminal vesicles and are glued together in the form of bundles called spermatophores which are discharged during copulation.

1. A correct and R is correct explanation of A

2. A correct and R is also correct but R is not correct explanation of A

3. A correct but R incorrect

4. A and R both are incorrect

33. Find out the incorrect option-

1. In the head region, the brain is represented by supra-oesophageal ganglion which supplies nerves to antennae and compound eyes.

2. In cockroach, the sense organs are antennae, eyes, maxillary palps, labial palps, anal cerci, etc.

3. The compound eyes are situated at the ventral surface of the head.

4. Each eye consists of about 2000 hexagonal ommatidia (sing.: *ommatidium*).

34. Read the following events with respect to cockroach-

a. From each testis a thin vas deferens arises which opens into ejaculatory duct through seminal vesicle.

b. The ejaculatory duct opens into male gonopore situated ventral to anus.

c. A characteristic mushroom shaped gland is present in the 6th-7th abdominal segments which functions as an accessory reproductive gland.

d. Cockroaches are dioecious and both sexes have well developed reproductive organs

How many of above are correct-

1. three

2. four

3. two

4. one

35. Elucidate the following with respect to cockroaches-

a. Excretion is performed by Malpighian tubules.

b. Each tubule is lined by glandular and ciliated cells.

c. They absorb nitrogenous waste products and convert them into uric acid which is excreted out through the hindgut.

d. Blood vessels are poorly developed and open into space (haemocoel).

How many of above are correct-

1. three

2. four

3. two

4. one

36. Consider the following statements –

i. Their size ranges from ¼ inches to 3 inches (0.6-7.6 cm) and have long antenna, legs and

ii. flat extension of the upper body wall that conceals head.

iii. They are nocturnal omnivores that live in damp places throughout the world.

iv. They have become residents of human homes and thus are serious pests and vectors of several diseases.

Head is triangular in shape and lies anteriorly at right angles to the longitudinal body axis.

Which of the above statements are correct-

1. i,ii only

2. i, iii,iv only

3. i,ii,iii only

4. all are correct

37. Read the following statements-

i. A pair of thread like antennae arise from membranous sockets lying in front of eyes.

ii. Antennae have sensory receptors that help in monitoring the environment.

iii. Anterior end of the head bears appendages forming biting and lapping type of mouth parts.

iv. The mouthparts consisting of a labrum (upper lip), a pair of mandibles, a pair of maxillae and a labium (lower lip).

v. A median flexible lobe, acting as tongue (hypopharynx), lies within the cavity enclosed by the mouthparts.

Which above statements is/are incorrect for Cockroach-

1. v and ii only

2. iii And ii only

3. iii only

4. All are correct

38. Consider the following statements-

a. Thorax consists of three parts – prothorax, mesothorax and metathorax.

b. The head is connected with thorax by a short extension of the prothorax known as the neck.

c. Each thoracic segment bears two pair of walking legs.

d. The first pair of wings arises from mesothorax and the second pair from metathorax.

How many of above are/is incorrect for *Periplaneta americana*-

1. three   2. four

3. one   4. two

39. Read the following statements and find out the correct option-

STATEMENT 1. The abdomen in both males and females cockroaches consists of 10 segments.

STATEMENT 2. Males bear a pair of short, threadlike anal styles which are absent in females.

1. Both are wrong statements   2. Both are correct statements

3. Only statement 1 correct   4. Only statement 2 correct

40. Read the following statements for cockroaches-

a. The mouth opens into a short tubular pharynx, leading to a narrow tubular passage called oesophagus.

b. Oesophagus in turn opens into a sac like structure called crop used for storing of food.

c. Gizzard helps in grinding the food particles.

d. The entire foregut is lined by cuticle.

e. Gastric caecae is present at the junction of foregut and midgut, which secrete digestive juice.

Which of the above are correct statements-

1. a and b only   2. b and c only

3. c and d only   4. a,b,c,d,e

41. Go through the following statement and find out the correct option-

ASSERTION(A). The hindgut cockroach is broader than midgut and is differentiated into ileum, colon and rectum.

REASON(R). The rectum opens out through anus.

1. A correct and R is correct explanation of A

2. A correct and R is also correct but R is not correct explanation of A

3. A correct but R incorrect

4. A and R both are incorrect

42. Read the following statement and find out the suitable option with reference to cockroach-

a. The sperms are stored in the seminal vesicles and are glued together in the form of bundles called spermatophores which are discharged during copulation.

b. The female reproductive sysytem consists of two large ovaries, lying laterally in the 2nd – 6th abdominal segments.

c. Each ovary is formed of a group of eight ovarian tubules or ovarioles, containing a chain of developing ova.

d. Oviducts of each ovary unite into a single median oviduct (also called vagina) which opens into the genital chamber.

How many of above is/are correct-

1. three

2. four

3. two

4. one

43. Consider the following statements for *Periplaneta americana*-

a. Ootheca are dropped or glued to a suitable surface, usually in a crack or crevice of high relative humidity near a food source.

b. The nymphs look very much like adults.

c. The nymph grows by moulting about 2 times to reach the adult form.

d. The next to last nymphal stage has wing pads but only adult cockroaches have wings.

How many of them is/are incorrect-

1. one

2. three

3. four

4. two

44. **Read the following statements and find out the correct option with respect to** *Periplaneta americana* –

    STATEMENT 1. Heart of cockroach is differentiated into funnel shaped chambers with ostia on either side.

    STATEMENT 2. Blood from sinuses enter heart through ostia and is pumped anteriorly to sinuses again.

    1. Both are correct statements

    2. Both are wrong statements

    3. Only statement 1 correct

    4. Only statement 2 correct

45. **Which statements is incorrect -**

    1. Dense irregular connective tissue has fibroblasts and many fibres (mostly collagen) that are oriented differently.

    2. Dense irregular connective tissue is present in the bone.

    3. Cartilage, bones and blood are various types of **specialised connective tissues**.

    4. The intercellular material of **cartilage** is solid and pliable and resists compression. Cells of this tissue (chondrocytes) are enclosed in small cavities within the matrix secreted by them

46. **Read the following terms-**

    a. hard

    b. non-pliable ground substance

    c. rich in calcium salts and collagen fibres

    d. bone cells (osteocytes)

    How many of them are related with bones-

    1. one

    2. two

    3. three

    4. four

47. **Go through the following terms-**

    a. lining of stomach and intestine

    b. walls of blood vessels and air sacs of lungs

    c. ducts of glands and tubular parts of nephrons in kidneys

    d. dry surface of the skin

    Which above tissues are /is examples of simple squamous tissue-

    1. b

    2. a, b

    3. b, c

    4. c, a

48. Read the following -

a. dry surface of the skin,

b. the moist surface of buccal cavity, pharynx,

c. inner lining of ducts of salivary glands

d. inner lining of pancreatic ducts.

How many of them are example of compound epithelium-

1. one

2. two

3. three

4. four

49. Consider the following -

A. mushroom shaped gland

B. phallomere (chitinous asymmetrical structures)

C. seminal vesicles

D. spermatophores

Which above structures found in male cockroaches-

1. A and C only

2. D and A only

3. B and D only

4. All are correct

50. Read the following statements –

A. two large ovaries, lying laterally.

B. each ovary is formed of a group of eight ovarian tubules or ovarioles.

C. oviducts of each ovary unite into a single median oviduct (also called vagina) which opens into the genital chamber.

D. a pair of spermatheca is present which opens into the genital chamber.

Which of the above statements are correct for female cockroaches-

1. A and C only

2. D and A only

3. B and D only

4. A,B,C,D

51. Consider the following statements and find out the correct option-

1. Frogs can live both on land and in freshwater and belong to class Amphibia of phylum Chordata.

2. The most common species of frog found in India is *Rana tigrina.*

3. Frogs do not have constant body temperature i.e., their body temperature varies with the temperature of the environment.

4. Frogs are warm blooded animals or poikilotherms.

52. Consider the following statements and find out the correct option with respect to Frog-

STATEMENT 1. The skin is smooth and slippery due to the presence of mucus.

STATEMENT 2. The colour of dorsal side of body is generally olive green with dark irregular spots.

1. Both are correct statements

2. Only statement 1 correct

3. Both are wrong statements

4. Only statement 2 correct

53. Consider the following statements-

a. They have the ability to change the colour to hide them from their enemies (camouflage).

b. This protective coloration is called mimicry.

c. The frogs are not seen during peak summer and winter.

d. During peak summer and winter period they take shelter in deep burrows to protect them from extreme heat and cold.

e. Frogs show summer sleep (aestivation) and winter sleep (hibernation).

Which of the above are/is correct w.r.t. Frog-

1. only a and d

2. a,b,c only

3. only c and d

4. all are correct

54. Consider the following statements-

a. The frog never drinks water but absorb it through the skin.

b. Body of a frog is divisible into head and trunk.

c. A neck and tail are absent.

d. Below the mouth, a pair of nostrils is present.

Which of the above are/is incorrect w.r.t. Frog -

1. d

2. a,b

3. b,d

4. a

55. Consider the following statements and find out the correct option w.r.t. Frog -

STATEMENT 1. In Frog eyes are bulged and covered by a nictitating membrane that protects them while in water.

STATEMENT 2. On either side of eyes a membranous tympanum (ear) receives sound signals.

1. Both are correct statements

2. Only statement 1 correct

3. Both are wrong statements

4. Only statement 2 correct

56. Go through the following statements-

ASSERTION(A). The hind limbs end in five digits and they are larger and muscular than fore limbs that end in four digits.

REASON(R). Only hind limbs help in swimming, walking, leaping and burrowing.

1. A correct and R is correct explanation of A

2. A correct and R is also correct but R is not correct explanation of A

3. A correct but R incorrect

4. A and R both are incorrect

57. Which statement is incorrect –

1. Frogs exhibit sexual dimorphism.

2. Male frogs can be distinguished by the presence of sound producing vocal sacs and also a copulatory pad on the first digit of the fore limbs which are absent in female frogs.

3. The alimentary canal is short because adult frogs are herbivores and hence the length of intestine is reduced.

4. The mouth in frog opens into the buccal cavity that leads to the oesophagus through pharynx.

58. Go through the following statements w.r.t Frog-

a. Frogs respire on land and in the water by two different methods.

b. In water, skin acts as aquatic respiratory organ (cutaneous respiration).

c. Dissolved oxygen in the water is exchanged through the skin by diffusion.

d. On land, the buccal cavity, skin and lungs act as the respiratory organs.

e. The respiration by lungs is called pulmonary respiration.

f. The lungs are a pair of elongated, pink coloured sac-like structures present in the upper part of the trunk region (thorax).

How many of them are correct -

1. two

2. three

3. four

4. six

59. Consider the following statements w.r.t. Frog-

a. Male reproductive organs of Frog consist of a pair of yellowish ovoid testes, which are found adhered to the upper part of kidneys by a double fold of peritoneum called mesorchium.

b. Vasa efferentia are 10-12 in number that arise from testes.

c. They enter the kidneys on their side and open into Bidder's canal.

d. Finally it communicates with the urinogenital duct that comes out of the kidneys and opens into the cloaca.

Which of the above statement are correct?

1. b and c only

2. c and d only

3. d and a only

4. a,b,c,d

60. Consider the following statements and find out the correct option w.r.t Frog -

STATEMENT 1. Each kidney is composed of several structural and functional units called uriniferous tubules or nephrons.

STATEMENT 2. Two ureters emerge from the kidneys in the male frogs.

1. Both are wrong statements

2. Only statement 1 correct

3. Both are correct statements

4. Only statement 2 correct

BIOMOLECULE

- There is a wide **diversity** in living organisms in our biosphere.
- If we **perform** such an analysis on a plant tissue, animal tissue or a **microbial** paste, we obtain a list of elements like carbon, hydrogen, oxygen and several others and their respective content per unit mass of a **living** tissue.
- If the same analysis is performed on a piece of earth's crust as an example of non-living matter, we obtain a similar list of elements.
- In **absolute** terms, no such differences could be made out.
- All the **elements** present in a sample of **earth's crust** are also present in a sample of living tissue.
- A closer **examination** reveals that the relative abundance of carbon and hydrogen with respect to other elements is higher in any living organism than the **earth's crust**

3.1 HOW TO ANALYSE CHEMICAL COMPOSITION?

- Many types of organic compounds are found in living organisms.
- To analse them we **perform a chemical analysis**.

- We can take any living tissue (a vegetable or a piece of liver, etc.) and grind it in trichloroacetic acid (Cl_3CCOOH) by using a mortar and a pestle.

- We get a thick slurry.

- If we were to filter this through a **cheesecloth or cotton** we would obtain two fractions.

- One is called the filtrate or more technically, **the acid-soluble pool**, and the second, the **retentate or the acid-insoluble fraction**.

- Scientists have found **thousands of organic compounds** in **the acid-soluble pool**.

- All the carbon compounds that we get from living tissues can be called 'biomolecules'.

- A slightly different but destructive experiment has to be done to analyze biomolecules in an organism.

- **After drying tissue,** weighs a small amount of a living tissue (say a leaf or liver and this is called wet weight) all the water evaporates and the remaining material gives **dry weight.**

- If the tissue is fully burnt, all the **carbon compounds are oxidised to gaseous form (CO_2, water vapour)** and they are removed and 'ash' remains.

- This ash contains inorganic elements (like calcium, magnesium etc).

A List of Representative Inorganic Constituents of Living Tissues

Component	Formula
Sodium	Na^+
Potassium	K^+
Calcium	Ca^{++}
Magnesium	Mg^{++}
Water	H_2O
Compounds	$NaCl$, $CaCO_3$, PO_4^{3-}, SO_4^{2-}

- Inorganic compounds like sulphate, phosphate, etc., are also **found in the acid-soluble fraction.**

- The elemental analysis gives elemental composition of living tissues in the form of hydrogen, oxygen, chlorine, carbon etc.

- The analysis for compounds gives an idea of **Constituents of Living Tissues** the kind of organic and inorganic constituents present in living tissues.

- From a chemistry point of view, one can identify functional groups like aldehydes, ketones, aromatic compounds, etc. But from a biological point of view, we shall classify them into amino acids, nucleotide bases, fatty acids etc.

A Comparison of Elements Present in Non-living and Living Matter*

Element	% Weight of Earth's crust	Human body
Hydrogen (H)	0.14	0.5
Carbon (C)	0.03	18.5
Oxygen (O)	46.6	65.0
Nitrogen (N)	very little	3.3
Sulphur (S)	0.03	0.3
Sodium (Na)	2.8	0.2
Calcium (Ca)	3.6	1.5
Magnesium (Mg)	2.1	0.1
Silicon (Si)	27.7	negligible

* Adapted from CNR Rao, *Understanding Chemistry,* Universities Press, Hyderabad.

Amino acids

- Amino acids are organic compounds containing an amino group and an acidic group as substituents on the same carbon i.e., **the α-carbon**. Hence, they are called α-amino acids. They are substituted methanes.

- There are four substituent groups occupying the **four valency positions.**

- These are hydrogen, carboxyl group, amino group and a variable group designated as R group.

- Based on the nature of **R group** there are many amino acids.

- However, those which occur in proteins are only of twenty types.

- The R group in these proteinaceous amino acids could be a **hydrogen** (the amino acid is called glycine), **a methyl group** (alanine), **hydroxy methyl** (serine), etc

- The chemical and physical properties of amino acids are essentially of the amino, carboxyl and the R functional groups.

- Based on number of amino and carboxyl groups, **amino acids are acidic** (e.g. Aspartic acid, Glutamic acid), **basic** (Arginine, Lysine) and **neutral** (Alanine,Glycine,Valine) amino acids.

- Similarly, there are **aromatic amino acids** (Tyrosine, Phenylalanine, Tryptophan).

- A particular property of amino acids is the ionizable nature of $-NH_2$ and $-COOH$ groups.

- In solutions of different pHs, the structure of amino acids changes.

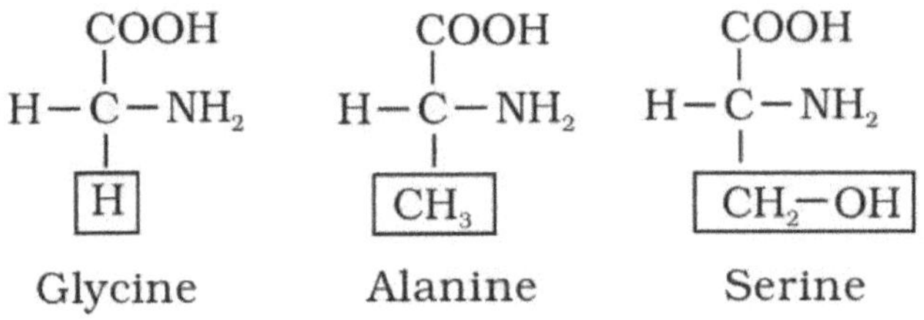

$$
\begin{array}{ccc}
\text{COOH} & \text{COOH} & \text{COOH} \\
| & | & | \\
\text{H}-\text{C}-\text{NH}_2 & \text{H}-\text{C}-\text{NH}_2 & \text{H}-\text{C}-\text{NH}_2 \\
| & | & | \\
\boxed{\text{H}} & \boxed{\text{CH}_3} & \boxed{\text{CH}_2-\text{OH}} \\
\text{Glycine} & \text{Alanine} & \text{Serine}
\end{array}
$$

Amino acids

Lipids

- Lipids are generally water **insoluble.**
- They could be simple fatty acids.
- A fatty acid has a carboxyl group attached to an R group.
- The R group could be a methyl ($-CH_3$), or ethyl ($-C_2H_5$) or higher number of $-CH_2$ groups (1 carbon to 19 carbons).
- **Palmitic acid has 16 carbons** including carboxyl carbon.
- **Stearic acid and Palmitic acids** are saturated fatty acids.
- **Oleic, Linoleic, Linolenic and Arachidonic acids** are unsaturated fatty acids.
- **Arachidonic** acid has **20** carbon atoms including the carboxyl carbon.
- Fatty acids could be saturated (without double bond) or unsaturated (with one or more C=C double bonds).
- The glycerol is **trihydroxy propane.**
- Many lipids have both glycerol and fatty acids.
- In lipids the fatty acids are found esterified with glycerol.
- They can be then **monoglycerides, diglycerides and triglycerides.**
- These are also called fats and oils based on melting point.
- Oils have lower melting point (e.g., gingely oil) and hence remain as oil in winters.
- Some lipids have phosphorous and a phosphorylated organic compound in them.
- These are phospholipids.
- Phospholipids are found in cell membrane.
- **Lecithin** and Cephalin are examples of phospholipid.
- Some tissues especially the neural tissues have lipids with more complex structures.

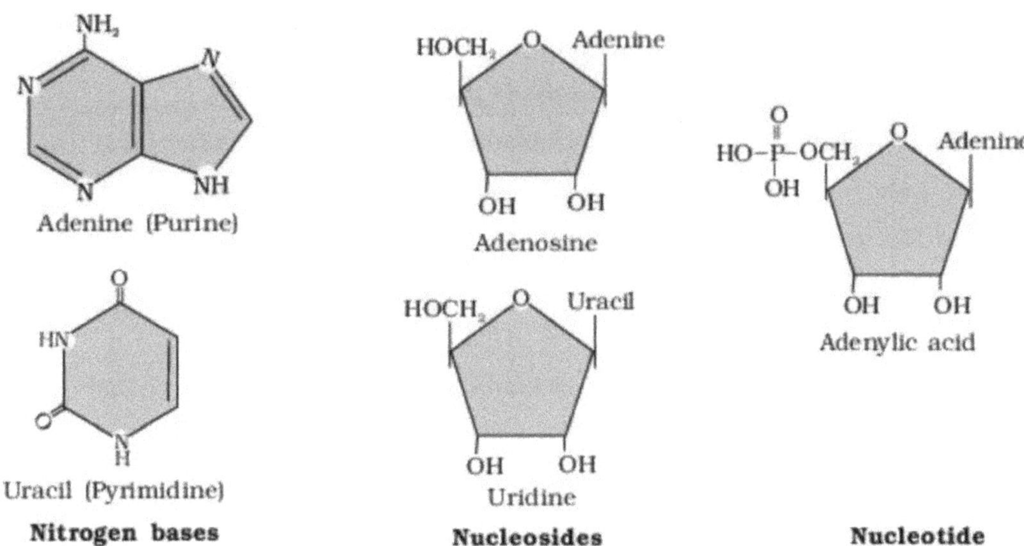

Fats and oils (lipids)

Nucleosides, Nucleosides, Nucleic acids

- In **Nucleosides, Nucleosides, Nucleic acids** heterocyclic rings present.
- Some nitrogen bases found in Living organisms are – adenine, guanine, cytosine, uracil, and thymine.
- When nitrogen bases attached to a sugar, they are called **nucleosides**.
- If a phosphate group is also found esterified to the **nucleiosides** they are called **nucleotides**.
- Adenosine, guanosine, thymidine, uridine and cytidine are **nucleosides**.
- Adenylic acid, thymidylic acid, guanylic acid, uridylic acid and cytidylic acid are nucleotides.
- Nucleic acids like DNA and RNA consist of **nucleotides** only.
- DNA and RNA function as **genetic** material.

Nitrogen bases   **Nucleosides**   **Nucleotide**

3.2 PRIMARY AND SECONDARY METABOLITES

- A thousands of organic compounds including amino acids, sugars, etc formed in living body known as '**metabolites**'.
- In animal tissues, primary metabolites have identifiable functions and play known roles in normal **physiologial processes**.

- **Alkaloides, flavonoides, rubber, essential oils, antibiotics, coloured pigments, scents, gums, spices** etc. are example of **secondary metabolites.**

- We do not know functions of all the '**secondary metabolites**' in host organisms.

- Many of **secondary metabolites** are useful to 'human welfare' (e.g., rubber, drugs, spices, scents and pigments).

- Some secondary **metabolites** have ecological importance.

Some Secondary Metabolites

Pigments	Carotenoids, Anthocyanins, etc.
Alkaloids	Morphine, Codeine, etc.
Terpenoides	Monoterpenes, Diterpenes etc.
Essential oils	Lemon grass oil, etc.
Toxins	Abrin, Ricin
Lectins	Concanavalin A
Drugs	Vinblastin, curcumin, etc.
Polymeric substances	Rubber, gums, cellulose

3.3 BIOMACROMOLECULES

- Biomicromolecules are found in the **acid soluble pool.**

- Biomicromolecules have molecular weights ranging from **18 to around 800 daltons (Da)** approximately.

- The acid insoluble fraction contain biomacromolecules, has only four types of organic compounds i.e., **proteins, nucleic acids, polysaccharides and lipids.**

- These classes of compounds with the **exception of lipids**, have molecular weights in the range of ten thousand daltons and above.

- The biomolecules, i.e., chemical compounds found in living organisms are of **two types.**

- One, those which have molecular weights less than one thousand dalton and are usually referred to as **micromolecules** or simply **biomolecules** while those which are found in the **acid insoluble** fraction are called macromolecules or **biomacromolecules.**

- **Lipids** are not a **polymeric** substances.

- The molecular weights of **lipids do not exceed 800 Da,** come under acid insoluble fraction, i.e., macromolecular fraction because **Lipids** present into structures like **cell membrane** and other membranes.

- When we **grind** a tissue, we are **disrupting** the cell structure.

- **Cell membrane** and other membranes are broken into pieces, and form vesicles which are not water soluble.

- These **vesicles** contain lipid so lipid do not comes along with **filterate** and comes along with the acid insoluble pool and hence found in the **macromolecular** fraction.

- So we can say **Lipids are not strictly macromolecules.**

- The acid soluble pool represents **roughly** the **cytoplasmic** composition.

-

Average Composition of Cells

Component	% of the total cellular mass
Water	70-90
Proteins	10-15
Carbohydrates	3
Lipids	2
Nucleic acids	5-7
Ions	1

- The macromolecules from cytoplasm and organelles become the acid insoluble fraction.

- Together they represent the entire chemical composition of living tissues or organisms.

3.4 PROTEINS

- Proteins are polypeptides.

- Proteins contain linear chains of amino acids linked by **peptide bonds.**

- **Peptide bonds are dehydrobonds.**

- Each protein is a polymer of amino acids.

- There are 20 types of amino acids (e.g., alanine, cysteine, proline, tryptophan, lysine, etc.), a protein is a **heteropolymer** and not a **homopolymer**.

- A homopolymer has only one type of monomer repeating 'n' number of times.

- Certain amino acids are essential for our health and they have to be supplied through our diet.

- These dietary proteins are the source of essential amino acids.

- The amino acids can be **essential or non-essential.**

- The **non-essential amino acids** are those which our body can make, while we get **essential amino acids** through our diet/food.

- Proteins carry out many functions in living organisms, some transport nutrients across cell membrane, some fight infectious organisms, some are hormones, some are enzymes.

TABLE 9.5 Some Proteins and their Functions

Protein	Functions
Collagen	Intercellular ground substance
Trypsin	Enzyme
Insulin	Hormone
Antibody	Fights infectious agents
Receptor	Sensory reception (smell, taste, hormone, etc.)
GLUT-4	Enables glucose transport into cells

- **Collagen** is the most abundant protein in animal world.
- **Ribulose bisphosphate Carboxylase Oxygenase (RUBISCO)** is the most abundant protein in the whole of the biosphere.

3.5 Polysaccharides

- **The acid insoluble fraction** also has polysaccharides (carbohydrates) as another class of macromolecules
- Polysaccharides are **long chains of sugars.**
- Polysaccharides are **threads (literally a cotton thread)** containing different monosaccharides as building blocks.
- In a polysaccharide chain (say glycogen), the right end is called the reducing end and the left end is called the **non-reducing end.**
- It has branches as shown in the form of a cartoon

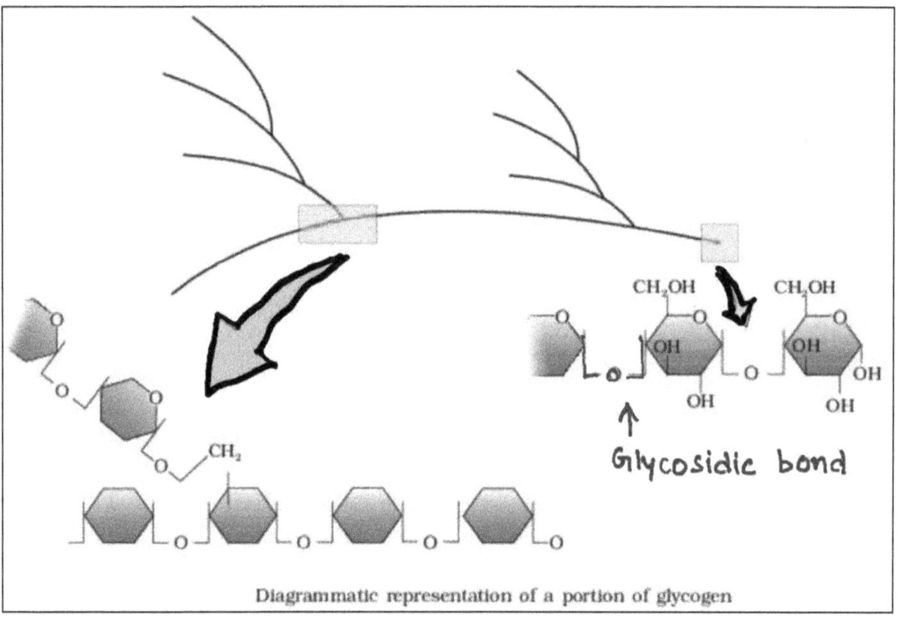

Diagrammatic representation of a portion of glycogen

Cellulose

- Cellulose is a **polymeric polysaccharide** consisting of only one type of monosaccharide i.e., glucose.
- Cellulose is a **homopolymer** of glucose.
- Cellulose does not **contain complex helices** and hence cannot hold I2.
- **Plant cell walls** are made of cellulose.
- Paper made from plant pulp is cellulose.
- **Cotton fibre** contain cellulose.

Starch

- Starch is a variant of this but present as a **store house of energy in plant tissues.**
- Animals have another variant called glycogen.
- Starch forms helical secondary structures.so starch can hold I_2 molecules in the helical portion.
- The starch-I_2 is **blue** in colour.

Inulin

- Inulin is a polymer of **fructose.**
- Inulin used to detect **GFR.**

Points to remember

- There are more complex **polysaccharides** in nature also found.
- They have as building blocks, **amino-sugars** and chemically modified sugars (e.g., glucosamine, N-acetyl galactosamine, etc.).
- Exoskeletons of **arthropods,** for example, have a complex polysaccharide called **chitin.**
- **Chitin** is a Nitrogen containing **Homopolysaccharide.**
- Heparin, Pectin, Hyaluronic acid etc. are complex polysaccharides and they are heteropolymers.

3.6 NUCLEIC ACIDS

- They are present in the acid **insoluble** fraction.
- These are **polynucleotides.**
- Like **polysaccharides** and **polypeptides** these comprise the true macromolecular fraction of any living tissue or cell.
- In nucleic acids, the building block is a **nucleotide.**
- A nucleotide has **three chemically distinct** components.
- One is a **heterocyclic compound,** the second is a monosaccharide and the third a phosphoric acid or phosphate.
- The heterocyclic compounds in nucleic acids are the nitrogenous bases named adenine, guanine, uracil, cytosine, and thymine.

- Adenine and Guanine are **substituted purines** while the uracil, cytosine, and thymine are **substituted pyrimidines.**

- The skeletal heterocyclic ring is called as purine and pyrimidine respectively.

- The sugar found in **polynucleotides** is either ribose (a monosaccharide pentose) or 2' deoxyribose.

- A nucleic acid containing **deoxyribose** is called deoxyribonucleic acid **(DNA)** while that which contains ribose is called ribonucleic acid **(RNA).**

3.7 STRUCTURE OF PROTEINS

- **Structure of molecules** can be studied in different contexts.

- In inorganic chemistry, the structure invariably refers to the molecular formulae (e.g., NaCl, $MgCl_2$, etc.).

- Organic **chemists** always write a two dimensional view of the molecules while representing the structure of the molecules (e.g., benzene, naphthalene, etc.).

- **Physicists** explain **the three dimensional views** of molecular structures while biologists describe the protein structure at four levels.

- Proteins are **heteropolymers** containing strings of amino acids.

- Proteins shows four type of structures-

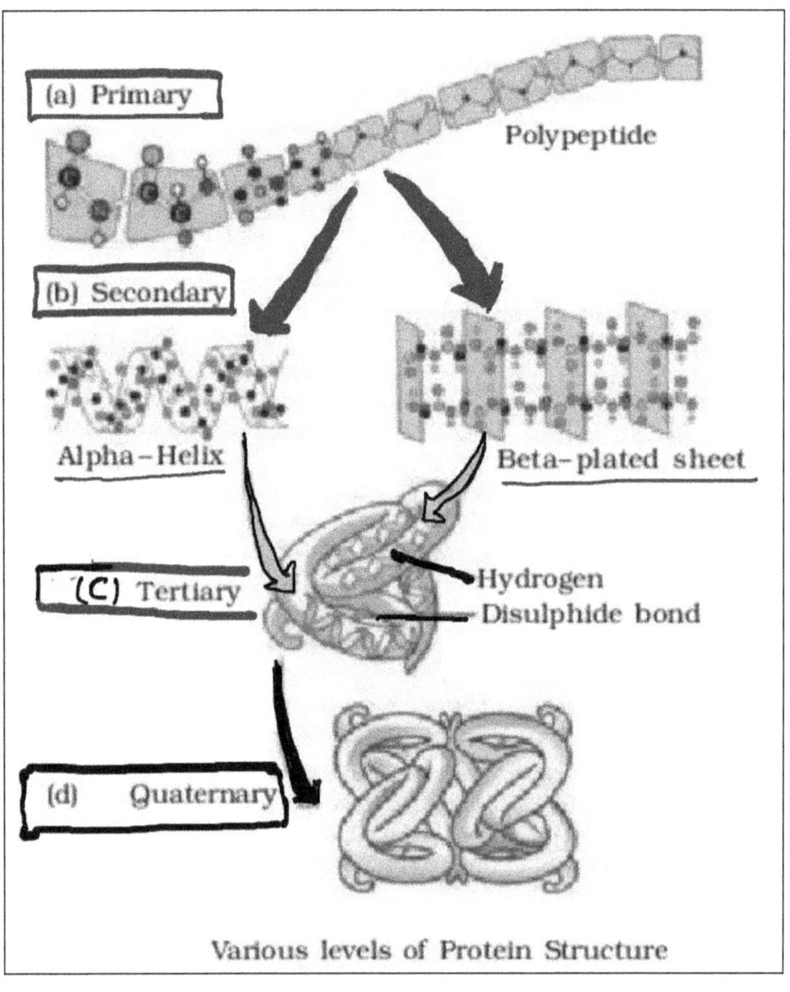

Various levels of Protein Structure

Primary structure

- The sequence of amino acids i.e., the positional information in a protein – which is the first amino acid, which is second, and so on – is called the **primary structure** of a protein.

- The **primary structure** of a protein can be seen in keratin.

- A protein is imagined as a line, the left end represented by the first amino acid and the right end represented by the last amino acid.

- The first amino acid is also called as **N-terminal amino acid.**

- The last amino acid is called the **C-terminal amino acid.**

- A protein thread does not exist throughout as an extended rigid rod.

Secondary structure

- The thread of protein is folded in the form of a helix (similar to a revolving staircase).

- Only some portions of the protein thread are arranged in the form of a helix.

- In proteins, only **right handed** helices are found.

- Other regions of the protein thread are folded into other forms in what is called the **secondary structure.** Exampl - **Alpha helix, Beta pleated sheet**

Tertiary structure

- In addition, the long protein chain is also folded upon itself like a hollow wollen ball, giving rise to the **tertiary structure.**

- This gives us a 3-dimensional view of a protein.

- Tertiary structure is absolutely necessary for the many biological activities of proteins.

  Exampl - **Myoglobin**

Quaternary structure

- Some proteins are an assembly of **more than one polypeptide** or subunits.

- The manner in which these **individual** folded polypeptides or subunits are arranged with respect to each other (e.g. **linear** string of spheres, spheres arranged one upon each other in the form of a cube or plate etc.) is the **architecture** of a protein otherwise called the **quaternary structure** of a protein.

- Eaxmple-**Human haemoglobin consists of 4 subunits**.

- **Human haemoglobin** has two subunits of α type and two subunits of β type together constitute the human haemoglobin (Hb).

3.8 NATURE OF BOND LINKING MONOMERS IN A POLYMER

Peptide bond

- In a polypeptide or a protein, amino acids are linked by a **peptide bond** which is formed when the carboxyl (-COOH) group of one amino acid reacts with the amino ($-NH_2$) group of the next amino acid with the elimination of a water moiety (the process is called dehydration).

Glycosidic bond

- In a polysaccharide the individual monosaccharides are linked by a **glycosidic bond.**
- This bond is also formed by **dehydration.**
- This bond is formed between two carbon atoms of two adjacent **monosaccharides.**

Phosphodiester bond

- In a nucleic acid a phosphate moiety links the **3'-carbon** of one sugar of one nucleotide to the **5'-carbon** of the sugar of the succeeding nucleotide.
- The bond between the **phosphate** and hydroxyl group of sugar is an ester bond.
- As there is one such ester bond on either side, it is called **phosphodiester bond.**

Watson-Crick model of DNA

- Nucleic acids exhibit a wide variety of **secondary** structures.
- One of the secondary structures exhibited by DNA is the famous **Watson-Crick model.**
- **Watson-Crick** model explains B - DNA.
- This model says that DNA exists as a **double helix.**
- The two strands of polynucleotides are **antiparallel** i.e., run in the opposite direction.
- The backbone is formed by the **sugar-phosphate-sugar chain.**
- The nitrogen bases are projected more or less **perpendicular** to this backbone but face inside.
- A and G of one strand **compulsorily** base pairs with T and C, respectively, on the other strand.
- There are **two hydrogen bonds** between A and T.
- There are **three hydrogen bonds** between G and C.
- Each strand appears like a **helical staircase.**
- Each step of **ascent** is represented by a pair of bases.
- At each step of ascent, the strand turns **36°.**
- One full turn of the **helical** strand would involve ten steps or ten base pairs.
- The pitch was **34Å.**
- The rise per base pair was **3.4Å.**
- The above mentioned salient features found in **B-DNA.**
- There are more than a **dozen** forms of DNA named after **English** alphabets with unique structural features.

3.9 DYNAMIC STATE OF BODY CONSTITUENTS – CONCEPT OF METABOLISM

- A simple **bacterial** cell, a **protozoan**, a plant or an animal, contain thousands of organic compounds.
- These compounds or biomolecules are present in certain concentrations (expressed as **mols/cell or mols/litre** etc.).

- One of the greatest discoveries ever made was the observation that all these biomolecules have a **turn over**.

- Biomolecules are constantly being changed into some other **biomolecules** and also made from some other biomolecules.

- The **breaking** and making is through chemical reactions constantly occuring in living organisms

- Together all these chemical reactions are called **metabolism**.

- Each of the **metabolic** reactions results in the transformation of biomolecules.

- **A few examples for such metabolic transformations are:**

- removal of CO2 from amino acids making an amino acid into an amine,

- removal of amino group in a nucleotide base;

- hydrolysis of a glycosidic bond in a disaccharide, etc.

- Majority of these **metabolic** reactions do not occur in isolation but are always linked to some other reactions.

- In other words, **metabolites** are converted into each other in a series of linked reactions called metabolic pathways.

- The metabolic pathways are similar to the **automobile traffic** in a city.

- The metabolic pathways are either **linear or circular**.

- The metabolic pathways crisscross each other, i.e., there are traffic junctions.

- Flow of **metabolites** through metabolic pathway has a definite rate and direction like automobile traffic.

- This metabolite flow is called the **dynamic** state of body constituents.

- What is most important is that this **interlinked** metabolic traffic is very smooth and without a single reported mishap for healthy conditions.

- Another feature of these metabolic reactions is that every chemical reaction is a **catalysed reaction**.

- There is no **uncatalysed** metabolic conversion in living systems.

- Even CO2 dissolving in water, a physical **process**, is a catalysed reaction in living systems.

$$CO_2 + H_2O \xrightleftharpoons{\text{Carbonic anhydrase}} H_2CO_3$$

carbon dioxide   water   carbonic acid

- The catalysts which hasten the rate of a given metabolic conversation are also proteins.

- These proteins with catalytic power are named **enzymes**.

3.10 METABOLIC BASIS FOR LIVING

- When during metabolic pathways a more complex structure from a simpler structure (**for example, acetic acid becomes cholesterol**) called as **anabolic** pathways.

- The formation of simpler structure from a complex structure (for example, **glucose becomes lactic acid in our skeletal muscle**) called **catabolic** pathways.

- **Anabolic** pathways consume energy.
- Formation of a protein from amino acids requires energy.
- **The catabolic pathways** lead to the release of energy. For example, **when glucose is degraded to lactic acid in our Voluntary muscle** and energy is liberated.
- This metabolic pathway **from glucose to lactic acid** which occurs in **10 metabolic steps** is called glycolysis.
- Living organisms have learnt to trap this energy liberated during degradation and store it in the form of chemical bonds.
- The energy is utilised for biosynthetic, osmotic and mechanical work that we perform.
- The most important form of energy currency in living systems is the bond energy in a chemical called **adenosine triphosphate (ATP)**.

3.11 THE LIVING STATE

- The biomolecules, are present at specific concentration in living body.
- The blood **concentration of glucose** in a normal healthy individual is **4.2-6.1 mM.**
- The hormones present in **nanograms/ mL.**
- The most important fact of biological systems is that all living organisms exist in a steady-state characterised by **concentrations** of each of these biomolecules.
- These biomolecules are in a **metabolic** flux.
- Any chemical or physical process moves **spontaneously** to equilibrium.
- **The steady state is a non-equilibirium state.**
- One should remember from physics that systems at equilibrium cannot perform work.
- As living organisms work continuously, they cannot afford to reach equilibrium.
- **The living state is a non-equilibrium steady-state to be able to perform work**; living process is a constant effort to prevent falling into equilibrium.
- Metabolism provides a mechanism for the production of energy.
- **The living state and metabolism** are synonymous.
- **Without metabolism there cannot be a living state.**

3.12 ENZYMES

- Almost **all enzymes** are proteins.
- There are some nucleic acids that behave like enzymes.
- These are called **ribozymes**.
- An enzyme like any protein has a primary structure, i.e., amino acid sequence of the protein.
- An enzyme like any protein has the secondary and the tertiary structure.

- A tertiary structure shows the backbone of the protein chain folds upon itself, the chain **criss-crosses** itself and hence, many crevices or pockets are made.

- One such pocket is the **'active site'.**

- An active site of an enzyme is a **crevice or pocket** into which the substrate fits.

- Thus enzymes, through their active site, catalyse reactions at a high rate.

- Enzyme catalysts differ from inorganic catalysts in many ways, but one major difference needs mention.

- Inorganic catalysts work **efficiently at high temperatures and high pressures**, while enzymes get damaged at high **temperatures** (say above 40°C).

- However, enzymes isolated from organisms who normally live under extremely high temperatures (e.g., hot vents and sulphur springs), are stable and retain their catalytic power even at high temperatures (upto 80°-90°C).

- **Thermal stability** is thus an important quality of such enzymes isolated from thermophilic organisms.

3.12.1 Chemical Reactions

- The physical process is a change in state of matter: when ice melts into water, or when water becomes a vapour.

- These are **physical processes.**

- Similarly, hydrolysis of starch into glucose is an organic chemical processes.

- Rate of a **physical** or **chemical** process refers to the amount of **product formed per unit time.**

- Rate can also be called velocity if the direction is specified.

- Rates of **physical** and **chemical** processes are influenced by temperature among other factors.

- **A general rule of thumb** is that rate doubles or decreases by half for every 10°C change in either direction.

- Catalysed reactions proceed at rates vastly higher than that of uncatalysed ones.

- Carbon dioxide and water combine and form carbonic acid. In the absence of any enzyme this reaction is very slow, with about **200 molecules of H_2CO_3 being formed in an hour.**

- By using the enzyme present within the cytoplasm called carbonic anhydrase, the reaction speeds dramatically with about **600,000 molecules being formed every second.**

$$CO_2 + H_2O \xrightleftharpoons{\text{Carbonic anhydrase}} H_2CO_3$$
$$\text{carbon dioxide} \qquad \text{water} \qquad\qquad\qquad \text{carbonic acid}$$

- The enzyme has **accelerated** the reaction rate by **about 10 million times.**

- The power of enzymes is incredible.

- There are thousands of types of enzymes each **catalysing** a unique chemical or metabolic reaction.

- A **multistep** chemical reaction, when each of the steps is catalysed by the same enzyme complex or different enzymes, is called a **metabolic** pathway.

- The glucose becomes pyruvic acid through ten different enzyme **catalysed** metabolic reactions.

$$Glucose \rightarrow 2\ Pyruvic\ acid$$
$$C_6H_{12}O_6 + O_2 \rightarrow 2C_3H_4O_3 + 2H_2O$$

3.12.2 How do Enzymes bring about such High Rates of Chemical Conversions?

- To **understand** this we should study enzymes a little more.
- We have already understood the idea of an 'active site'.
- The chemical or metabolic conversion refers to a reaction.
- The chemical which is converted into a product is called a 'substrate'.
- Hence enzymes, i.e. proteins with three dimensional structures including an 'active site', convert a **substrate (S)** into **a product (P)**.

Mechanism

$$E+S \rightarrow ES\ complex \rightarrow EP\ complex \rightarrow E+P$$

- The substrate 'S' has to bind the enzyme at **its 'active site'** within a given cleft or pocket.
- The substrate has to diffuse towards the 'active site'.
- Now obligatory formation of an 'ES' complex.
- E stands for enzyme.
- **'ES' complex formation is a transient phenomenon.**
- During the state where **substrate** is bound to the enzyme active site, a new structure of the substrate called transition state structure is formed known as **EP complex.**
- Very soon, after the **expected** bond breaking/making is completed, the product is released from the active site.
- In other words, the structure of **substrate** gets transformed into the structure of product(s).

Points to remember

- The energy level difference between S and P.
- **If 'P' is at a lower level than 'S', the reaction is an exothermic reaction.**
- One need not supply energy (by heating) in order to form the product.
- However, whether it is an exothermic or spontaneous reaction or an endothermic or energy requiring reaction, the **'S' has to go through a much higher energy state or transition state.**
- The difference in **average** energy content of 'S' from that of this transition state is called 'activation energy'.
- Enzymes **eventually** bring down this energy barrier making the **transition of 'S' to 'P' more easy.**

3.12.3 Nature of Enzyme Action

- Each **enzyme** (E) has a **substrate** (S) binding site in its molecule so that a highly reactive enzyme-substrate complex (ES) is produced.
-

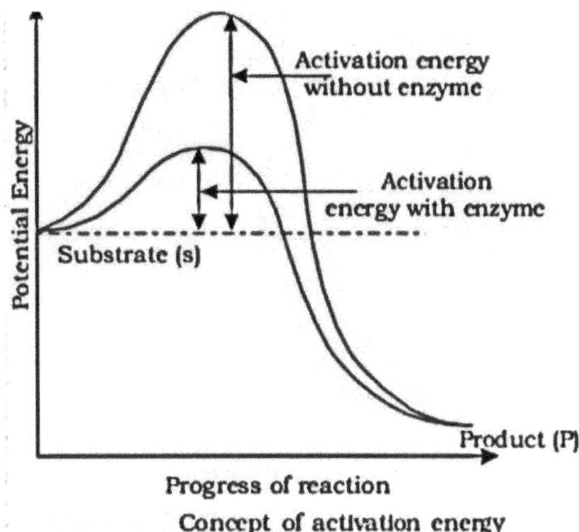

Concept of activation energy

- This complex is short-lived and **dissociates** into its product(s) P and the unchanged enzyme with an intermediate formation of the **enzyme-product** complex (EP).

- The formation of the ES complex is essential for catalysis.

- The **catalytic cycle of an enzyme action** can be described in the following steps:

  1. First, the **substrate** binds to the active site of the enzyme, fitting into the active site.

  2. The binding of the **substrate** induces the enzyme to alter its shape, fitting more tightly around the substrate.

  3. The active site of the enzyme, now in close proximity of the substrate breaks the chemical bonds of the substrate and the new **enzyme - product** complex is formed.

  4. The **enzyme** releases the **products** of the reaction and the free enzyme is ready to bind to another molecule of the **substrate** and run through the catalytic cycle once again.

3.12.4 Factors Affecting Enzyme Activity

- The activity of an enzyme can be affected by a change in the conditions which can alter the tertiary structure of the protein.

- These include **temperature, pH, change in substrate concentration** or binding of specific chemicals that regulate its activity.

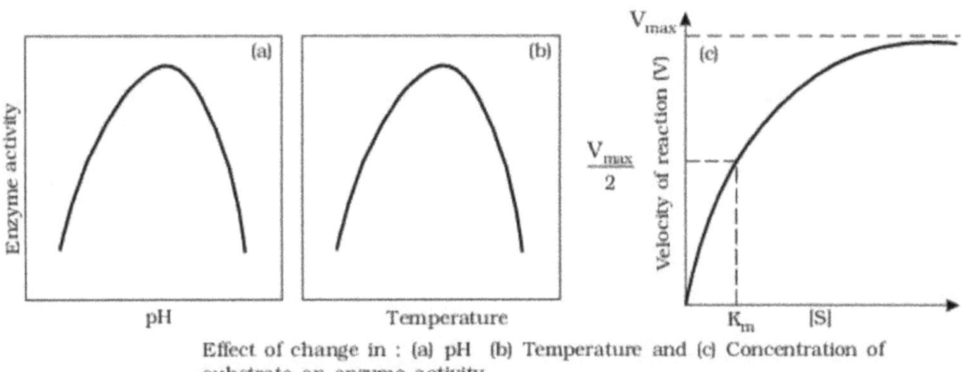

Effect of change in : (a) pH (b) Temperature and (c) Concentration of substrate on enzyme activity

Temperature and pH

- Enzymes generally function in a narrow range of **temperature** and **pH**.
- Each enzyme shows its **highest** activity at a particular **temperature** and pH called the optimum temperature and optimum **pH**.
- **Activity** declines both below and above the optimum value.
- Low temperature preserves the enzyme in a **temporarily** inactive state whereas high **temperature** destroys enzymatic activity because proteins are denatured by heat.

Concentration of Substrate

- With the increase in substrate **concentration**, the velocity of the enzymatic reaction rises at first.
- The reaction ultimately reaches a **maximum velocity** (V_{max}) which is not exceeded by any further rise in concentration of the substrate.
- This is because the **enzyme molecules** are fewer than the substrate molecules and after saturation of these molecules, there are no free enzyme molecules to bind with the additional substrate molecules.

Enzyme Inhibition

The activity of an enzyme is also **sensitive** to the presence of specific chemicals that bind to the enzyme.

- When the **binding** of the chemical shuts off enzyme activity, the process is called **inhibition** and the chemical is called an **inhibitor**.
- When the inhibitor closely resembles the substrate in its molecular structure and inhibits the activity of the enzyme, it is known as **competitive inhibitor**.
- Due to its close **structural** similarity with the substrate, the inhibitor competes with the substrate for the **substrate binding** site of the enzyme.
- Consequently, the substrate cannot bind and as a result, the enzyme action declines, e.g., **inhibition of succinic dehydrogenase by malonate which closely resembles the substrate succinate in structure.**
- Such competitive inhibitors are often used in the control of bacterial pathogens.

3.12.5 Classification and Nomenclature of Enzymes

- **Thousands** of enzymes have been discovered, isolated and studied.
- Most of these enzymes have been **classified** into different groups based on the type of reactions they catalyse.
- Enzymes are divided into **6** classes each with **4-13** subclasses and named accordingly by a four-digit number system. First digit represent class of Enzyme.

  a. **Oxidoreductases/dehydrogenases:** Enzymes which catalyse oxidoreduction between two substrates S and S'.

  b. **Transferases:** Enzymes catalysing a transfer of a group, G (other than hydrogen) between a pair of substrate S and S'.

  c. **Hydrolases:** Enzymes catalysing hydrolysis of ester, ether, peptide, glycosidic, C-C, C-halide or P-N bonds.

d. Lyases: Enzymes that catalyse removal of groups from substrates by mechanisms other than hydrolysis leaving double bonds.

e. Isomerases: Includes all enzymes catalysing inter-conversion of optical, geometric or positional isomers.

f. Ligases: Enzymes catalysing the linking together of 2 compounds, e.g., enzymes which catalyse joining of C-O, C-S, C-N, P-O etc. bonds.

3.12.6 Co-factors

- Enzymes are composed of one or several **polypeptide** chains.
- However, there are a number of cases in which **non-protein** constituents called cofactors are bound to the the enzyme to make the enzyme catalytically active.

Holoenzyme = apoenzyme + cofactor

- The protein portion of the enzymes is called the apoenzyme.
- Three kinds of cofactors are - **prosthetic groups, co-enzymes and metal ions.**

a. Prosthetic groups

- **Prosthetic groups** are organic compounds and are distinguished from other cofactors in that they are tightly bound to the apoenzyme.
- example, **in peroxidase and catalase**, which catalyze the breakdown of hydrogen peroxide to water and oxygen, **haem** is the prosthetic group and it is a part of the active site of the enzyme.

b. Co-enzymes

- **Co-enzymes** are also organic compounds but their association with the apoenzyme is only transient, usually occurring during the course of catalysis.
- **Co-enzymes** serve as co-factors in a number of different enzyme catalyzed reactions.
- The essential chemical components of many coenzymes are vitamins, e.g., coenzyme nicotinamide adenine dinucleotide **(NAD) and NADP** contain the vitamin niacin.

c. Metal ions

- A number of enzymes require **metal ions** for their activity which form coordination bonds with side chains at the active site and at the same time form one or more cordination bonds with the substrate, e.g., **zinc is a cofactor for the proteolytic enzyme carboxypeptidase.**
- Catalytic activity is lost when the co-factor is removed from the enzyme which testifies that they play a **crucial role** in the catalytic activity of the enzyme.

1. Consider the following amino acids and find out the odd one-

   1. tyrosine

   2. glycine

   3. phenylalanine

   4. cellulose

2. Match the list 1 and 2-

List 1   List 2

a. Inulin	polymer of fructose
b. Cellulose	is a homopolymer
c. Paper made from plant pulp	is cellulose
d. Collagen	is the most abundant protein in animal world

How many of them are/is correct-

   1. four

   2. three

   3. two

   4. one

3. Consider the following -

   a. adenosine,

   b. guanosine,

   c. thymidine,

   d. uridine,

   e. adenylic acid,

   f. thymidylic acid

How many of them are example of Nucleosides -

   1. only a and d

   2. only e and c

   3. only c and d

   4. a,b,c,d

4. Read the following statements carefully -

   a. Palmitic acid has 16 carbons including carboxyl carbon.

   b. Arachidonic acid has 20 carbon atoms including the carboxyl carbon.

   c. Fatty acids could be saturated (without double bond) or unsaturated (with one or more C=C double bonds).

   d. The glycerol which is trihydroxy propane.

How many of them are/is correct-

1. three	2. four
3. two	4. one

5.Consider the following statements and find out the correct option

STATEMENT 1. Lipids are generally water insoluble.

STATEMENT 2.The tyrosine and phenylalanine are aromatic amino acids.

1. Both are wrong statements	2. Only statement 1 correct
3. Both are correct statements	4. Only statement 2 correct

6. Go through the following statements-

ASSERTION(A). Cellulose is a homopolysaccharide.

REASON(R). A homopolymer has only one type of monomer repeating 'n' number of times.

1. A correct and R is correct explanation of A

2. A correct and R is also correct but R is not correct explanation of A

3. A correct but R incorrect

4. A and R both are incorrect

7. Which statement is incorrect with respect to protein-

1. Proteins are polypeptides.

2. Proteins are linear chains of amino acids linked by peptide bonds.

3. Each protein is a polymer of amino acids.

4. A protein is a homopolymer.

8. Go through the following statements-

A. Lipids are not strictly macromolecules.

B. The acid soluble pool represents roughly the cytoplasmic composition.

C. The macromolecules from cytoplasm and organelles become the acid insoluble fraction.

D. All those compounds found in the acid soluble pool have molecular weights ranging from 18 to around 800 daltons (Da) approximately.

Find out the correct statements and choose the suitable option-

1. A,C, D	2. B,C,D
3. A,B,C,D	4. C,D,

9. Match the list 1 and 2-

List1 List2

a. Chitin	NAG polymer
b. Glycine	Simplest amino acid
c. Tryptophan	Complex amino acid
d. Starch	Animal protein

How many of them are correctly matched-

1. one

2. two

3. three

4. four

10. **Consider the following statements and find out the correct option-**

    STATEMENT 1. Polysaccharides are long chains of sugars.

    STATEMENT 2. Sucrose is non reducing sugar.

    1. Both are wrong statements

    2. Only statement 1 correct

    3. Both are correct statements

    4. Only statement 2 correct

11. **Read the following statements very carefully and find out the correct-**

    a. Phospholipids have phosphorous and a phosphorylated organic compound in them.

    b. Cephalin is an example of phospholipids.

    c. Phospholipids are found in cell membrane.

    d. Lecithin is an example of phospholipid.

    Which above of the statements are correct with respect to phospholipid-

    1. a and c only

    2. c and b only

    3. a,b,c only

    4. all are correct

12. **Go through the following statements-**

    ASSERTION(A). The ash obtained by fully burnt tissue contains inorganic elements (like calcium, magnesium etc).

    REASON(R). Inorganic compounds like sulphate, phosphate, etc., are found in the acid-soluble fraction.

    1. A correct and R is correct explanation of A

    2. A correct and R is also correct but R is not correct explanation of A

    3. A correct but R incorrect

    4. A and R both are incorrect

13. **The R group in these proteinaceous amino acids could be a hydrogen (the amino acid is called X), a methyl group (the amino acid is called Y), hydroxy methyl (the amino acid is called Y).In the given paragraph X,Y,Z respectively represents-**

    1. serine, alanine, serine

    3. alanine, alanine, serine

    2. glycine, alanine, serine

    4. tryptophan, alanine, serine

14. **Read the following statements and find out correct option-**

    a. Cellulose is a polymer of glucose.

    b. Starch is a polymer of glucose present as a store house of energy in plant tissues.

    c. Inulin is a polymer of fructose.

    d. The starch-I2 complex is blue in colour.

    e. Cellulose does not contain complex helices and hence cannot hold I2.

    f. Plant cell walls are made of starch.

How many of them are correct-

1. four

2. five

3. six

4. three

15. Consider the following statements and find out the correct option

STATEMENT 1. - Amino acids are substituted methanes.

STATEMENT 2. In a polypeptide chain first amino acid is also called as C-terminal amino acid and the last amino acid is called the N-terminal amino acid.

1. Both are wrong statements

2. Only Statement 1 correct

3. Both are correct statements

4. Only statement 2 correct

16. Consider the following events during enzyme action-

a. First, the substrate binds to the active site of the enzyme, fitting into the active site.

b. The binding of the substrate induces the enzyme to alter its shape,fitting more tightly around the substrate.

c. The active site of the enzyme, now in close proximity of the substrate breaks the chemical bonds of the substrate and the new enzyme - product complex is formed.

d. The enzyme releases the products of the reaction and the free enzyme is ready to bind to another molecule of the substrate and run through the catalytic cycle once again.

How many of them are/is correct-

1. one

2. two

3. three

4. four

17. Consider the following amino acids -

a. tyrosine,

b. phenylalanine,

c. tryptophan,

d. lysine

Which of the above amino acids are/is normally basic in nature?

1. a and c only

2. c and d only

3. d only

4. a,b,c,d,

18. Match the list 1 and 2-

List 1   List 2

a. adenosine	nucleoside
b. guanosine	nucleoside
c. thymidylic acid	nucleotide
d. cytidine	nucleotide

How many of them are/is correctly matched-

1 one

2 three

3 two

4 four

19. Consider the following statements and find out the incorrect one-

1. For nucleic acids, the building block is a nucleotide.

2. A nucleotide has three chemically distinct components.

3. A nucleotide contain - one is a heterocyclic compound, the second is a monosaccharide and the third a phosphoric acid or phosphate.

4. Adenine and Guanine are substituted pyrimidines.

20. In proteins, only right handed helices are observed. Other regions of the protein thread are folded into other forms like alpha helix is called the -

1. primary structure

2. secondary structure

3. tertiary structure

4. quaternary structure

21. Consider the following statements and find out the correct option

STATEMENT 1. All the carbon compounds that we get from living tissues can be called 'biomolecules'.

STATEMENT 2. Oils have lower melting point (e.g., gingely oil) and hence remain as liquid in winters.

1. Both are wrong statements

2. Only statement 1 correct

3.Both are correct statements

4.Only statement 2 correct

22. Go through the following statements and find out the correct option-

ASSERTION(A). The heterocyclic compounds in nucleic acids are the nitrogenous bases named adenine, guanine, uracil, cytosine, and thymine.

REASON(R). The sugar found in polynucleotides is either ribose (a monosaccharide pentose) or 2' deoxyribose.

1. A correct and R is correct explanation of A

2. A correct and R is also correct but R is not correct explanation of A

3. A correct but R incorrect

4. A and R both are incorrect

23. Go through the following statements and find out the correct option-

A. A protein is imagined as a line, the left end represented by the first amino acid and the right end represented by the last amino acid.

B. The first aminoacid is also called as N-terminal amino acid.

C. The last amino acid is called the C-terminal amino acid.

D. A protein thread does not exist throughout as an extended rigid rod.

Which above statement are correct?

1. A and C only

2. C and D only

3. D and B only

4. A,B,C,D

24. Read the statements given below-

A. Organic chemists always write a two dimensional view of the molecules while representing the structure of the molecules (e.g., benzene, naphthalene, etc.).

B. Physicists conjure up the three dimensional views of molecular structures while biologists describe the protein structure at four levels.

C. The sequence of amino acids i.e., the positional information in a protein – which is the first amino acid, which is second, and so on – is called the **primary structure** of a protein.

D. A protein is imagined as a line, the left end represented by the first amino acid and the right end represented by the last amino acid.

Which of the above statement are correct?

1. A and C only

2. B and D only

3. D and A only

4. A,B,C,D,

25. Find out the incorrect statement-

1. In a polypeptide or a protein, amino acids are linked by a peptide bond which is formed when the carboxyl (-COOH) group of one amino acid reacts with the amino (-NH2) group of the next amino acid with the elimination of a water moiety (the process is called dehydration).

2. In a polysaccharide the individual monosaccharides are linked by a glycosidic bond.

3. Glycosidic bond is formed by dehydration method.

4. The glycosidic bond is formed between two carbon atoms of two adjacent amino acids.

26. Consider the following -

Alanine, Glucose, Fructose, Inulin, Glycine

How many of them are amino acids-

1. one

2. two

3. three

4. four

27. Match the list 1 and 2 with respect to average composition of cells-

List 1

List 2

a. **Water**	j. 1%
b. **Ions**	k. 2%
c. **Nucleic acid**	l. 70-90%
d. **Lipid**	m. 5-7%

Find out the correct option –

1. a.k, b.j, c.l, d.m

2. a.k,b.l,c.j,d.m

3. a.l,b.m,c.k,d.j

4. a.l,b.j,c.m,d.k

28. Read the following paragraph and find out the X and Y respectively-

X is absolutely necessary for the many biological activities of proteins. Some proteins are an assembly of more than one polypeptide or subunits. The manner in which these individual folded polypeptides or subunits are arranged with respect to each other (e.g. linear string of spheres, spheres arranged one upon each other in the form of a cube or plate etc.) is the architecture of a protein otherwise called the **Y** of a protein.

1. Primary structure, **quaternary structure**

2. Tertiary structure, **quaternary structure**

3. Tertiary structure, **primary structure**

4. Secondary structure, **quaternary structure**

29. Consider the following and find out the incorrect-

    1. Toxin - Abrin   2. Lectin - Concanavalin A

    3. Alkaloids - Rubber   4. Drug - Curcumin

30. Read the following –

    Ricin, Codeine, Gums, Cellulose, Glycine

    How many of them are secondary metabolites-

    1. five   2. two

    3. three   4. four

31. Read the following statements and find out the correct option

    STATEMENT 1. Nucleic acids exhibit a wide variety of secondary structures. For example, one of the secondary structures exhibited by DNA is the famous Watson-Crick model.

    STATEMENT 2. This model says that DNA exists as a double helix. The two strands of polynucleotides are antiparallel i.e., run in the opposite direction.

    1. Both are wrong statements   2. Both are correct statements

    3. Only statement 1 correct   4. Only statement 2 correct

32. Go through the following statements and find out the correct option-

    ASSERTION(A). In DNA the nitrogen bases are projected more or less perpendicular to this backbone but face inside.

    REASON(R). A and G of one strand compulsorily base pairs with T and C, respectively, on the other strand.

    1. A correct and R is correct explanation of A

    2. A correct and R is also correct but R is not correct explanation of A

    3. A correct but R incorrect

    4. A and R both are incorrect

33. Which statement is incorrect for Watson and Crick Model of DNA-

    1. Each strand appears like a helical staircase.

    2. Each step of ascent is represented by a pair of bases.

    3. At each step of ascent, the strand turns $136°$.

    4. One full turn of the helical strand would involve ten steps or ten base pairs.

34. Read the following statements-

    i. Almost all enzymes are proteins.

    ii. One can depict an enzyme by a line diagram.

    iii. An enzyme like any protein has a primary structure, i.e., amino acid sequence of the protein.

    iv. An enzyme like any protein has the secondary and the tertiary structure.

    v. An active site of an enzyme is a crevice or pocket into which the substrate fits.

    vi. Thus enzymes, through their active site, catalyse reactions at a high rate.

How many of above are correct-

1. three
2. four
3. five
4. six

35. Which of the following is incorrect –

1. An active site of an enzyme is a crevice or pocket into which the substrate fits.

2. Thus enzymes, through their active site, catalyse reactions at a high rate.

3. Enzyme catalysts differ from inorganic catalysts in many parameters.

4. Inorganic catalysts work efficiently only at high temperatures and high pressures, while enzymes get damaged at low temperatures (say above 40°C).

36. Which of the following is incorrect statement-

1. As living organisms work continuously, they cannot afford to reach equilibrium.

2. The living state is a equilibrium steady-state and this state not able to perform work.

3. Metabolism provides a mechanism for the production of energy.

4. The living state and metabolism are synonymous.

37. Read the following statements w.r.t. enzyme kinetics-

(i) Rate can also be called velocity if the direction is specified.

(ii) Rates of physical and chemical processes are influenced by temperature among other factors.

(iii) A general rule of thumb is that rate doubles or decreases by half for every 10°C change in either direction.

(iv) Catalysed reactions proceed at rates vastly higher than that of uncatalysed ones.

(v) When enzyme catalysed reactions are observed, the rate would be vastly higher than the same but uncatalysed reaction.

Which of the above statements are correct-

1. v and ii only
2. iii and ii only
3. iv and iii only
4. all are correct

38. Which is not a true statement-

1. Enzymes generally function in a narrow range of temperature and pH.

2. Each enzyme shows its highest activity at a particular temperature and pH called the optimum temperature and optimum pH.

3. Activity declines both below and above the optimum value.

4. High temperature preserves the enzyme in a temporarily inactive state whereas low temperature destroys enzymatic activity because proteins are denatured by heat.

39. Find out the correct statements-

A. The activity of an enzyme can be affected by a change in the conditions which can alter the tertiary structure of the protein.

B. With the increase in substrate concentration, the velocity of the enzymatic reaction rises at first.

C. The reaction ultimately reaches a maximum velocity (Vmax) which is not exceeded by any further rise in concentration of the substrate.

D. After reaching maximum velocity (Vmax) which rate of reaction can not be increases because the enzyme molecules are fewer than the substrate molecules and after saturation of these molecules, there are no free enzyme molecules to bind with the additional substrate molecules.

1. A and C only

2. D and A only

3. B and D only

4. All are correct

40. Read the following statements-

a. The activity of an enzyme is also sensitive to the presence of specific chemicals that bind to the enzyme.

b. When the binding of the chemical shuts off enzyme activity, the process is called **inhibition** and the chemical is called an **inhibitor**.

c. When the inhibitor closely resembles the substrate in its molecular structure and inhibits the activity of the enzyme, it is known as **competitive inhibitor**.

d. Due to its close structural similarity with the substrate, the inhibitor competes with the substrate for the substrate binding site of the enzyme.

Which of the above are correct?

1. a and b only

2. a, b, c only

3. c and d only

4. a,b,c,d

41. Enzymes are divided into-

1. 6 classes each with 4-13 subclasses and named accordingly by a three-digit number.

2. 6 classes each with 4-13 subclasses and named accordingly by a two-digit number.

3. 6 classes each with 4-13 subclasses and named accordingly by a one-digit number.

4. 6 classes each with 4-13 subclasses and named accordingly by a four-digit number.

42. Find out the incorrect-

1. Hydrolases: Enzymes catalysing hydrolysis of ester, ether, peptide, glycosidic, C-C, C-halide or P-N bonds.

2. Lyases: Enzymes that catalyse removal of groups from substrates by mechanism by using hydrolysis leaving double bonds.

3. Isomerases: Includes all enzymes catalysing inter-conversion of optical, geometric or positional isomers.

4. Ligases: Enzymes catalysing the linking together of 2 compounds, e.g., enzymes which catalyse joining of C-O, C-S, C-N, P-O etc. bonds.

43. Consider the given statement-

Enzymes catalysing a transfer of a group, G (other than hydrogen) between a pair of substrate S and S'.

The above statement can represents-

1. Oxidoreductases

2. Transferases

3. Hydrolases

4. Ligases

44. Consider the following statements -

A. Prosthetic groups are organic compounds and are distinguished from other cofactors in that they are tightly bound to the apoenzyme.

B. For example, in peroxidase and catalase, which catalyze the breakdown of hydrogen peroxide to water and oxygen, haem is the prosthetic group and it is a part of the active site of the enzyme.

C. Co-enzymes are organic compounds but their association with the apoenzyme is only transient, usually occurring during the course of catalysis.

D. Co-enzymes serve as co-factors in a number of different enzyme catalyzed reactions.

Which of the following are correct?

1. A and C only

2. D and C only

3. B and D only

4. All are correct

45. Consider the following statements -

A. Enzymes are composed of one or several polypeptide chains.

B. There are a number of cases in which non-protein constituents called cofactors are bound to the enzyme to make the enzyme catalytically active.

C. The protein portion of the enzymes is called the apoenzyme.

D. Three kinds of cofactors may be identified: prosthetic groups, co-enzymes and metal ions.

Which of the following are correct?

1. A and C only

2. D and A only

3. B and D only

4. All are correct

46. Read the following statements and find out the correct option

STATEMENT 1. A number of enzymes require metal ions for their activity which form coordination bonds with side chains at the active site and at the same time form one or more coordination bonds with the substrate.

STATEMENT 2. Zinc is a cofactor for the proteolytic enzyme carboxypeptidase.

1. Both are correct statements

2. Both are wrong statements.

3. Only statement 1 correct

4. Only statement 2 correct

47. Go through the following statements and find out the correct option-

ASSERTION(A). Catalytic activity is lost when the co-factor is removed from the enzyme which testifies that they play a crucial role in the catalytic activity of the enzyme.

REASON(R). The essential chemical components of many coenzymes are vitamins, e.g., coenzyme nicotinamide adenine dinucleotide (NAD) and NADP contain the vitamin niacin.

1. A correct and R is correct explanation of A

2. A correct and R is also correct but R is not correct explanation of A

3. A correct but R incorrect

4. A and R both are incorrect

48. Find out the incorrect statement –

1. Amino acids, monosaccharide and disaccharide sugars, fatty acids, glycerol, nucleotides, nucleosides and nitrogen bases are some of the organic compounds seen in living organisms.

2. There are total 10 types of amino acids and 5 types of nucleotides.

3. Fats and oils are glycerides in which fatty acids are esterified to glycerol.

4. Phospholipids contain, a phosphorylated nitrogenous compound.

49. Consider the following statements-

A. Collagen is the most abundant protein in animal world and Ribulose bisphosphate Carboxylase-Oxygenase (RUBISCO) is the most abundant protein in the whole of the biosphere.

B. Enzymes are proteins which catalyse biochemical reactions in the cells.

C. Ribozymes are nucleic acids with catalytic power.

D. Proteinaceous enzymes exhibit substrate specificity, require optimum temperature and pH for maximal activity.

1. A and C only

2. D and A only

3. B and D only

4. All are correct

50. Consider the following statements find out the correct option-

A. These metabolic pathways are similar to the automobile traffic in a city.

B. These pathways are either linear or circular.

C. These pathways crisscross each other, i.e., there are traffic junctions.

D. Flow of metabolites through metabolic pathway has a definite rate and direction like automobile traffic.

E. This metabolite flow is called the dynamic state of body constituents.

Which of the above statements are correct with respect to Metabolic pathways-

1. A,B, C only

2. D and E only

3. B and D only

4. All are correct

BREATHING AND EXCHANGE OF GASES

- **The oxygen (O_2)** is utilised by the organisms to indirectly break down simple molecules like glucose, amino acids, fatty acids, etc., to derive energy to perform various activities.

- **Carbon dioxide (CO_2)** which is harmful is also released during the above catabolic reactions.

- It is, therefore, evident that **O_2 has to be continuously provided** to the cells and CO_2 produced by the cells have to be released out.

- **This process of exchange of O_2 from** the atmosphere with CO_2 produced by the cells is called breathing, commonly known as respiration.

4.1 RESPIRATORY ORGANS

- **Mechanisms of breathing** vary among different groups of animals.

- **Mechanisms of breathing** depending mainly on their habitats and levels of organisation.

- Lower invertebrates like **porifera, coelenterates, flatworms, etc., exchange O_2 with CO_2 by simple diffusion** over their entire body surface.

- **Earthworms/Annelids** use their moist cuticle and insects have a network of tubes (tracheal tubes) to transport atmospheric air within the body.

- Special **vascularised** structures called gills (**branchial** respiration) are used by most of the aquatic arthropods and molluscs.

- The **vascularised** bags called lungs (**pulmonary respiration**) are used by the terrestrial forms for the exchange of gases.

- Book lungs present in **Scorpian.**

- Book gills present in *Limulus*.
- Among vertebrates, fishes use gills whereas **amphibians, reptiles, birds** and **mammals** respire through lungs.
- Amphibians like frogs can respire through their moist skin (cutaneous respiration) also.

4.1.1 Human Respiratory System

> External nostrils → nasal passage → nasal chamber (cavity) → pharynx → glottis → larynx → trachea → primary bronchi → secondary bronchi → tertiary bronchi → bronchioles → terminal bronchioles → respiratory bronchiole → alveolar duct.

- It includes pair of **external nostrils** opening out above the upper lips.
- It leads to a nasal chamber through the **nasal passage.**
- The nasal chamber opens into **nasopharynx**, which is a portion of pharynx, the common passage for food and air.
- Nasopharynx opens through glottis of the larynx region into the **trachea.**
- **Larynx** is a cartilaginous box.
- **Larynx** helps in sound production and hence called the **sound box.**
- On **larynx** vocal cord present.
- **Vocal cord** of males longer thicker due to testosterone.
- On **larynx** various cartilage present.
- During swallowing glottis can be covered by a thin elastic cartilaginous flap called epiglottis to prevent the entry of food into the **larynx.**
- **Trachea** is a straight tube extending up to the mid-thoracic cavity.
- **Trachea** also known as wind pipe.
- **Trachea 10-12** cm in length.
- **Trachea** divides at the level of 5th thoracic vertebra into a right and left primary **bronchi.**
- Each bronchi undergoes repeated divisions to form the secondary and tertiary bronchi and bronchioles ending up in very thin terminal **bronchioles.**
- The tracheae, primary, secondary and tertiary bronchi, and initial bronchioles are supported by **incomplete cartilaginous rings.**
- Cartilaginous rings made by **Hyaline Cartilage.**
- Each terminal bronchiole gives rise to a number of very thin, irregular walled and vascularised bag-like structures called **alveoli.**
- The branching network of **bronchi, bronchioles and alveoli** comprise the lungs.
- Origin of lungs **endodermal.**
- Weight of both lungs about **1.25 Kg.**

- Human have two lungs which are covered by a **double layered pleura**, with pleural fluid between them.

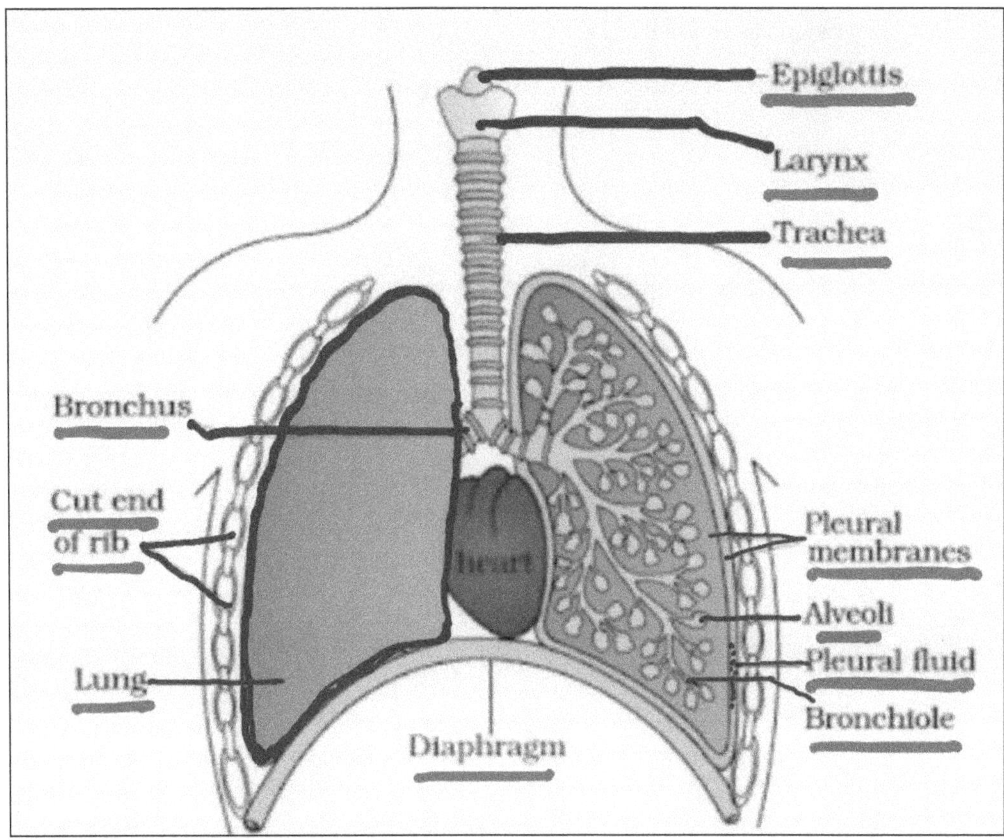

- The **pleural fluid reduces friction on the lung surface**.
- The **outer pleural membrane** is in close contact with the thoracic lining whereas the inner pleural membrane is in contact with the lung surface.
- The part starting with the **external nostrils up to the terminal bronchioles** constitute the conducting part whereas the alveoli and their ducts form the respiratory or exchange part of the respiratory system.
- **The conducting part transports** the atmospheric air to the alveoli, clears it from foreign particles, humidifies and also brings the air to body temperature.
- **Exchange part is the site** of actual diffusion of O2 and CO2 between blood and atmospheric air.
- The lungs are situated in the thoracic chamber which is **anatomically an air-tight chamber.**
- The thoracic chamber is formed dorsally by the vertebral column, ventrally by the sternum, laterally by the ribs and on the lower side by the **dome-shaped diaphragm.**
- **Diaphragm** made by phrenic muscles.
- The **anatomical setup of lungs** in thorax is such that any change in the volume of the thoracic cavity will be reflected in the lung (pulmonary) cavity.
- Such an arrangement is essential for breathing, as **we cannot directly alter the pulmonary volume.**

Respiration involves the following steps:

(a) Breathing or pulmonary ventilation by which atmospheric air is drawn in and CO2 rich alveolar air is released out.

(**b**) Diffusion of gases (O_2 and CO_2) across alveolar membrane.

(**c**) Transport of gases by the blood.

(**d**) Diffusion of O_2 and CO_2 between blood and tissues.

(**e**) Utilisation of O_2 by the cells for catabolic reactions and resultant release of CO_2

4.2 MECHANISM OF BREATHING

- Breathing involves two stages:

  a. **inspiration** during which atmospheric air is drawn in.

  b. **expiration** by which the alveolar air is released out.

- The movement of air into and out of the lungs is carried out by creating a pressure gradient between the lungs and the atmosphere.

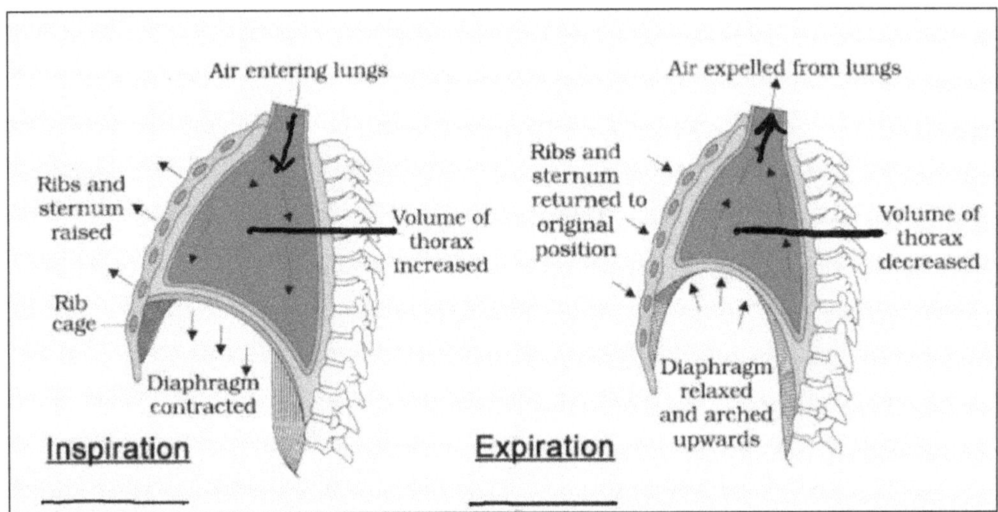

Inspiration occur

- **Inspiration** occur if the pressure within the lungs (intra-pulmonary pressure) is less than the atmospheric pressure, i.e., there is a negative pressure in the lungs with respect to atmospheric pressure.

Expiration occur

- Similarly, **expiration** takes place when the intra-pulmonary pressure is higher than the atmospheric pressure.

- The **diaphragm** and a specialised set of muscles – external and internal intercostals between the ribs, help in generation of such gradients.

Change in antero-posterior axis

- Inspiration is initiated by the contraction of diaphragm which increases the volume of thoracic chamber in the **antero-posterior axis.**

Change in dorso-ventral axis.

- The contraction of external inter-costal muscles lifts up the ribs and the sternum causing an increase in the volume of the thoracic chamber in the **dorso-ventral axis.**

- The **overall increase** in the thoracic volume causes a similar increase in pulmonary volume.

Increase in pulmonary volume

- An **increase in pulmonary volume decreases** the intra-pulmonary pressure to less than the atmospheric pressure which forces the air from outside to move into the lungs,i.e., **inspiration**.

Increase in pulmonary volume

- Relaxation of the diaphragm and the inter-costal muscles returns the diaphragm and sternum to their normal positions and reduce the thoracic volume and thereby the pulmonary volume.
- This leads to an increase in intra-pulmonary pressure to slightly above the atmospheric pressure causing the expulsion of air from the lungs, i.e., **expiration**.

Points to remember-

- Humas have the **ability** to increase the strength of inspiration and expiration with the help of additional muscles in the abdomen.
- On an average, a healthy human breathes **12-16 times**/minute.
- In fever breathing rate increases.
- The volume of air involved in breathing movements can be estimated by using a **spirometer.**
- **Spirometer** helps in clinical assessment of pulmonary functions.

4.2.1 Respiratory Volumes and Capacities

Respiratory Volumes

Tidal Volume (TV)

- Volume of air inspired or expired during a normal respiration.
- TV is approx. **500** mL.
- A healthy person can inspire or expire approximately 6000 to 8000 mL of air per minute.

Inspiratory Reserve Volume (IRV)

- Additional volume of air, a person can inspire by a forcible inspiration.
- IRV averages **2500** mL to **3000** mL.

Expiratory Reserve Volume (ERV)

- Additional volume of air, a person can expire by a forcible expiration.
- ERV averages **1000** mL to **1100** mL.

Residual Volume (RV)

- Volume of air remaining in the lungs even after a forcible expiration.
- RV averages **1100** mL to **1200** mL.

Respiratory Capacities

- By adding up a few respiratory volumes described above, one can derive various pulmonary capacities, which can be used in **clinical diagnosis.**

Inspiratory Capacity (IC):

- Total volume of air a person can **inspire** after a normal **expiration.**
- IC includes tidal volume and **inspiratory reserve volume** (TV+IRV).

Expiratory Capacity (EC):

- Total volume of air a person can expire after a normal inspiration.
- EC includes tidal volume and **expiratory reserve volume** (TV+ERV).

Functional Residual Capacity (FRC):

- Volume of air that will remain in the lungs after a normal expiration.
- FRC includes **TV+ERV.**

Vital Capacity (VC):

- The maximum volume of air a person can breathe in after a forced expiration or the maximum volume of air a person can breathe out after a forced inspiration.
- VC includes ERV, TV and IRV or the maximum volume of air a person can breathe out after a forced inspiration.

Total Lung Capacity(TLC):

- Total volume of air accommodated in the lungs at the end of a forced inspiration.
- TLC includes **RV, ERV, TV** and **IRV** or vital capacity + residual volume.

4.3 EXCHANGE OF GASES

- **Alveoli are the primary sites** of exchange of gases.
- Exchange of gases also occur between **blood and tissues.**
- O_2 and CO_2 are exchanged in these sites by **simple diffusion mainly based** on pressure/concentration gradient.
- **Solubility of the gases as well as the thickness** of the membranes involved in diffusion are also some important factors that can affect the rate of diffusion.
- **Diffusion rate directly depends upon solubility of gases and pressure difference of gases.**
- Pressure contributed by an **individual** gas in a mixture of gases is called partial pressure and is represented as pO_2 for oxygen and pCO_2 for carbon dioxide.
- Partial pressures of these two **gases** in the atmospheric air and the two sites of diffusion are given in following table-

Respiratory gas	Atmospheric air	Alveoli	Blood (deoxygenated)	Blood (oxygenated)	Tissues
O_2	159 mm Hg	104 mm Hg	40 mm Hg	95 mm Hg	40 mm Hg
CO_2	0.3 mm Hg	40 mm Hg	45 mm Hg	40 mm Hg	45 mm Hg

- The above data given in the table clearly indicates **a concentration gradient** for oxygen from alveoli to blood and blood to tissues.

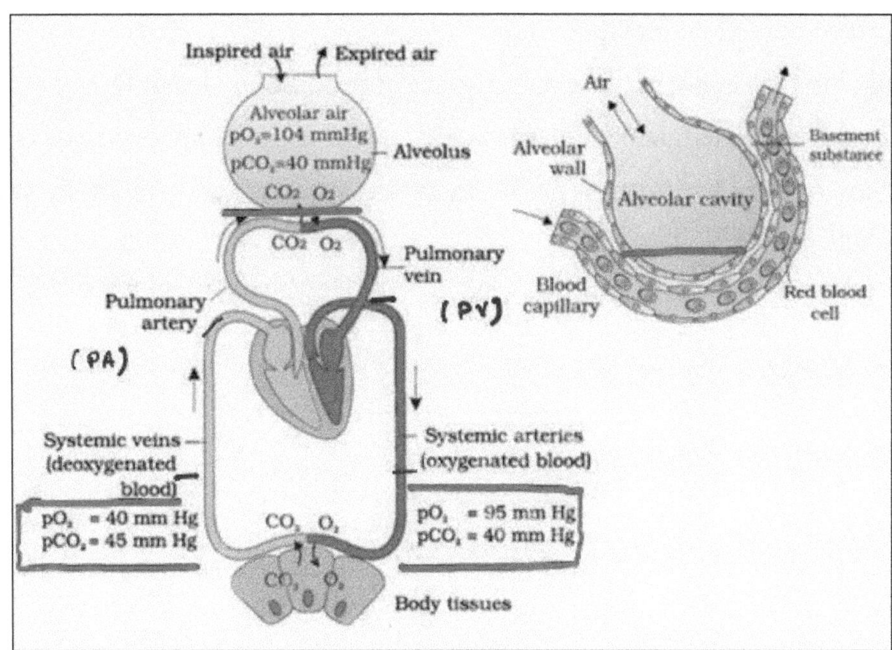

- Similarly, a **gradient** is present for CO_2 in the **opposite** direction, i.e., from tissues to blood and blood to alveoli.

- As the solubility of CO_2 is **20-25 times higher** than that of O_2, the amount of CO_2 that can diffuse through the diffusion membrane per unit difference in partial pressure is much higher compared to that of O_2.

- The **diffusion** capacity of O_2 is double than N_2.

- The diffusion **membrane** is made up of three major layers - the thin **squamous** epithelium of alveoli, the **endothelium** of alveolar capillaries and the **basement** substance in between them.

- **However, its total thickness is much less than a millimetre.**

- Therefore, all the factors in our body are **favourable** for diffusion of O_2 from alveoli to tissues and that of CO_2 from tissues to alveoli.

4.4 TRANSPORT OF GASES

- Blood is the medium of transport for O_2 and CO_2

- **97** percent of O_2 is transported by RBCs in the blood.

- **3** percent of O_2 is carried in a dissolved state through the plasma.

- **20-25 percent of CO_2 is transported by RBCs**

- **70** percent of it is carried as bicarbonate.

- **7** percent of CO_2 is carried in a dissolved state through plasma.

4.4.1 Transport of Oxygen

- **Haemoglobin(Hb)** is a red coloured iron containing pigment present in the RBCs.

- O_2 can bind with haemoglobin in a reversible manner to form **oxyhaemoglobin**.

- **100 ml**. of blood contain 12-16 gram Hb.

- **1 gram Hb** can combine 1.34 ml O_2.

- Each haemoglobin molecule can carry a maximum of **four molecules of O_2**.

- Binding of oxygen with haemoglobin is **primarily related to partial pressure of O_2**.

- **Partial pressure of CO_2, hydrogen ion concentration and temperature** are the other factors which can interfere with this binding.

- **A sigmoid curve** is obtained when percentage saturation of haemoglobin with O_2 is plotted against the pO_2.

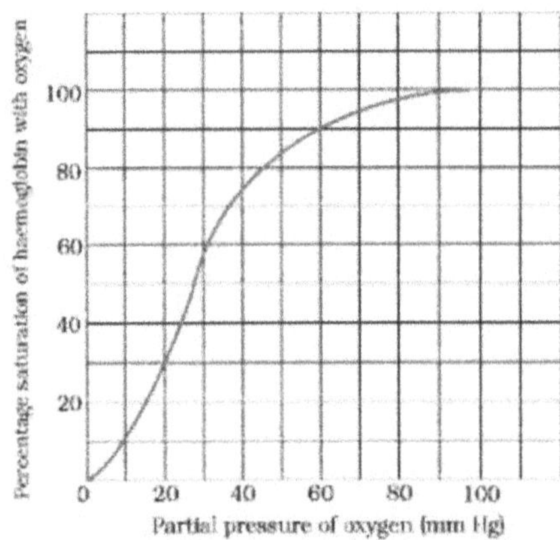

- This curve is called the Oxygen dissociation curve and is highly useful in studying the effect of factors like **pCO_2, H+** concentration, etc., on binding of O_2 with haemoglobin.

Conditions to left shift

- In the alveoli, where there is high pO_2, low pCO_2, lesser H+ concentration and lower temperature, the factors are all favourable for the formation of oxyhaemoglobin,

Conditions to right shift

- Whereas in the tissues, where **low pO_2**, high **pCO_2**, high **H·** concentration and higher temperature exist, the conditions are favourable for dissociation of oxygen from the oxyhaemoglobin.

Points to remember-

- This clearly indicates that O_2 gets bound to haemoglobin in the lung surface and gets dissociated at the tissues.

- **Every 100 ml of oxygenated blood** can deliver around 5 ml of O_2 to the tissues under normal physiological conditions.

4.4.2 Transport of Carbon dioxide

- About **20-25 per cent** CO_2 is carried by haemoglobin as **carbamino-haemoglobin**.

- This binding is related to the **partial pressure of CO_2**.

- The **pO_2 is a major factor** which could affect this binding.

- When pCO_2 is high and pO_2 is low as in the tissues, more binding of carbon dioxide occurs whereas, when the pCO_2 is low and pO_2 is high as in the alveoli, dissociation of CO_2 from carbamino-haemoglobin takes place, i.e., CO_2 which is bound to **haemoglobin** from the tissues is delivered at the alveoli.

- RBCs contain a very high concentration of the enzyme, **carbonic anhydrase** and minute quantities of the same is present in the plasma too.

$$CO_2 + H_2O \underset{\text{Carbonic anhydrase}}{\rightleftharpoons} H_2CO_3 \underset{\text{Carbonic anhydrase}}{\rightleftharpoons} HCO_3^- + H^+$$

- **Carbonic anhydrase enzyme** facilitates the following reaction in both directions.

- **At the tissue site** where partial pressure of CO_2 is high due to catabolism, CO_2 diffuses into blood (RBCs and plasma) and forms HCO_3^- and H^+

- **At the alveolar site** where pCO_2 is low, the reaction proceeds in the opposite direction leading to the formation of CO_2 and H_2O.

- Thus, CO_2 trapped as bicarbonate at the tissue level and transported to the alveoli is released out as CO_2.

- **Every 100 ml** of deoxygenated blood delivers approximately **4 ml of CO_2 to the alveoli.**

4.5 REGULATION OF RESPIRATION

- Human beings have a **significant ability** to maintain and moderate the respiratory rhythm to suit the demands of the body tissues.

- This is done by the **neural system**.

- **A specialised centre present in the medulla oblongata** region of the brain called respiratory rhythm centre is primarily responsible for this regulation.

- Respiratory rhythm centre are **DRG(Dorsal respiratory group) and VRG(Ventral respiratory group)**

- **DRG(Dorsal respiratory group)** present on dorsal side of medulla oblongata and control inspiration.

- **VRG(Ventral respiratory group)** present on dorsal side of medulla oblongata and control inspiration as well as expiration.

- A centre present in the pons varoli region of the brain called **pneumotaxic** centre can moderate the functions of the respiratory rhythm centre.

- Neural signal from this **pneumotaxic** centre can reduce the duration of inspiration and thereby alter the respiratory rate.

- **A chemosensitive area** is situated adjacent to the respiratory rhythm centre which is highly sensitive to CO_2 and hydrogen ions.

- **Increase in CO_2 and hydrogen ions** can activate this centre, which in turn can signal the rhythm centre to make necessary adjustments in the respiratory process by which these substances can be eliminated.

- Receptors associated with **aortic arch and carotid artery** also can recognise changes in CO_2 and H^+ concentration and send necessary signals to the rhythm centre for remedial actions.

- The role of oxygen in the regulation of respiratory rhythm is quite insignificant.

4.6 DISORDERS OF RESPIRATORY SYSTEM

I. Asthma

- Difficulty in **breathing** occur
- Causing **wheezing** sound
- **Inflammation** of bronchi and bronchioles seen
- **Hypersensitivity** seen

II. Emphysema

- is a **chronic** disorder
- **alveolar** walls are damaged
- **respiratory** surface is decreased
- **pCO$_2$ Level** decreases
- One of the major causes of this is **cigarette smoking**.

III. Occupational Respiratory Disorders:

- In certain **industries**, especially those involving grinding or stone-breaking, so much dust is produced that the defense **mechanism** of the body cannot fully cope with the situation.
- Long exposure can give rise to **inflammation** leading to fibrosis (proliferation of fibrous tissues) and thus **causing serious** lung damage.
- Due to silica dust **silicosis** occur.
- Workers in such **industries** should wear protective masks.

1. Consider the following statements and find out the correct option

A. Humans have a pair of external nostrils opening out above the upper lips.

B. It leads to a nasal chamber through the nasal passage.

C. The nasal chamber opens into **nasopharynx**, which is a portion of pharynx, the common passage for food and air.

D. Nasopharynx opens through glottis of the larynx region into the **trachea**.

E. Larynx is a cartilaginous box which helps in sound production and hence called the **sound box**.

Which of the above are correct for Respiration-

1. A,E,C

2. B,C

3. D,E,A

4. A,B,C,D,E

2. Match the list 1 and 2

List 1   List 2

a. **Tidal Volume (TV)**	j. 2500 mL to 3000 mL
b. **Inspiratory Reserve Volume (IRV)**	k. 1000 mL to 1100 mL
c. **Expiratory Reserve Volume (ERV)**	l. 500 mL
d. **Residual Volume (RV)**	m. 1100 mL to 1200 mL

Find out the correct option -

1. a.k, b.j, c.l, d.m

2. a.k,b.l,c.j,d.m

3. a.l,b.j,c.k,d.m

4. a.l,b.j,c.m,d.k

3. Consider the following statements-

a) During swallowing glottis can be covered by a thin elastic cartilaginous flap called epiglottis to prevent the entry of food into the larynx.

b) Trachea is a straight tube extending up to the mid-thoracic cavity, which divides at the level of 5th thoracic vertebra into a right and left primary **bronchi.**

c) Each bronchi undergoes repeated divisions to form the secondary and tertiary bronchi and bronchioles ending up in very thin terminal **bronchioles.**

d) The **tracheae, primary, secondary and tertiary** bronchi, and initial bronchioles are supported by incomplete cartilaginous rings.

How many of them are/is correct for Human-

1. one

2. two

3. three

4. four

4. **Read the following statement carefully with respect to Humans-**

I. Each terminal bronchiole gives rise to a number of very thin, irregular walled and vascularised bag-like structures called **alveoli**.

II. The branching network of bronchi, bronchioles and alveoli comprise the lungs.

III. Human have two lungs which are covered by a double layered pleura, with pleural fluid between them.

IV. Pleural fluid reduces friction on the lung surface.

V. The outer pleural membrane is in close contact with the thoracic lining whereas the inner pleural membrane is in contact with the lung surface.

How many of them are usually correct -

1. three

2. four

3. five

4. two

5. **Consider the following statements and find out the correct option-**

STATEMENT 1. The part starting with the external nostrils up to the terminal bronchioles constitute the conducting part whereas the alveoli and their ducts form the respiratory or exchange part of the respiratory system.

STATEMENT 2. The conducting part transports the atmospheric air to the alveoli, clears it from foreign particles, humidifies and also brings the air to body temperature.

1. Both are correct statements

2. Only statement 1 correct

3. Both are wrong statements

4. Only statement 2 correct

6. **Go through the following statements-**

ASSERTION(A). The lungs are situated in the thoracic chamber which is anatomically an air-tight chamber.

REASON(R). The thoracic chamber is formed ventrally by the vertebral column, dorsally by the sternum, laterally by the ribs and on the lower side by the dome-shaped diaphragm.

1. A correct and R is correct explanation of A

2. A correct and R is also correct but R is not correct explanation of A

3. A correct but R incorrect

4. A and R both are incorrect

7. Respiration do not involves-

1. Breathing or pulmonary ventilation by which atmospheric air is drawn in and CO_2 rich alveolar air is released out.

2. Diffusion of gases (O_2 and CO_2) across alveolar membrane.

3. Diffusion of O_2 and CO_2 between blood and tissues.

4. Utilisation of O_2 by the cells takes place by anabolic reactions only and resultant release of CO_2

8. Go through the following statements-

1. Breathing involves two stages: **inspiration** during which atmospheric air is drawn in and **expiration** by which the alveolar air is released out.

2. The movement of air into and out of the lungs is carried out by creating a pressure gradient between the lungs and the atmosphere.

3. Inspiration can occur if the pressure within the lungs (intra-pulmonary pressure) is less than the atmospheric pressure, i.e., there is a negative pressure in the lungs with respect to atmospheric pressure.

4. Expiration takes place when the intra-pulmonary pressure is higher than the atmospheric pressure.

How many of them are correct-

1. two

2. three

3. four

4. one

9. Match the list 1 and 2-

List1   List2

a. **Inspiratory Capacity (IC)**	j. TV+ERV
b. **Expiratory Capacity (EC)**	k. Volume of air that will remain in the lungs after a normal expiration
c. **Functional Residual Capacity (FRC)**	l. TV+IRV
d. **Vital Capacity (VC)**	m. The maximum volume of air a person can breathe in after a forced expiration

Find out the correct option –

1. a.k, b.j, c.l, d.m

2. a.k,b.l,c.j,d.m

3. a.l,b.j,c.k,d.m

4. a.l,b.j,c.m,d.k

10. Consider the following statements and find out the correct option-

STATEMENT 1.The anatomical setup of lungs in thorax is such that any change in the volume of the thoracic cavity will be reflected in the lung (pulmonary) cavity.

STATEMENT 2. Such an arrangement is essential for breathing, as we can directly alter the pulmonary volume without any effort.

1. Both are wrong statements

2. Only Statement 1 correct

3. Both are correct statements

4. Only statement 2 correct

11. Read the following statements very carefully and find out the incorrect-

a) Trachea are the primary sites of exchange of gases.

b) Exchange of gases also occur between blood and tissues.

c) O_2 and CO_2 are exchanged in these sites by simple diffusion mainly based on pressure/concentration gradient.

d) Solubility of the gases as well as the thickness of the membranes involved in diffusion are also some important factors that can affect the rate of diffusion.

Which above statement are/is incorrect?

1. a and c both

2. a,b,c,d

3. a only

4. b and d both

12. Go through the following statements-

ASSERTION(A). Pressure contributed by an individual gas in a mixture of gases is called partial pressure and is represented as pO_2 for oxygen and pCO_2 for carbon dioxide.

REASON(R). As the solubility of CO_2 is 20-25 times higher than that of O_2, the amount of CO_2 that can diffuse through the diffusion membrane per unit difference in partial pressure is much higher compared to that of O_2.

1. A correct and R is correct explanation of A

2. A correct and R is also correct but R is not correct explanation of A

3. A correct but R incorrect

4. A and R both are incorrect

13. Find out incorrect statement with respect to Humans-

1. The diffusion membrane is made up of three major layers namely, the thin squamous epithelium of alveoli, the endothelium of alveolar capillaries and the basement substance in between them.

2. The diffusion membranes total thickness is much more than a centimetre.

3. All the factors in our body are favourable for diffusion of O_2 from alveoli to tissues and that of CO_2 from tissues to alveoli.

4. Blood is the medium of transport for O_2 and CO_2

14. Read the following statements and find out correct option-

a) About 97 per cent of O_2 is transported by RBCs in the blood.

b) The remaining 3 per cent of O_2 is carried in a dissolved state through the plasma.

c) Nearly 20-25 per cent of CO_2 is transported by RBCs whereas 70 per cent of it is carried a bicarbonate.

d) About 7 per cent of CO_2 is carried in a dissolved state through plasma.

How many of them are/is correct-

1. four

2. one

3. two

4. three

15. Consider the following statements and find out the correct option-

STATEMENT 1. Haemoglobin is a red coloured iron containing pigment present in the RBCs. O_2 can bind with haemoglobin in a reversible manner to form **oxyhaemoglobin**.

STATEMENT 2. Each haemoglobin molecule can carry a maximum of six molecules of O_2.

1. Both are wrong statements

2. Only statement 1 correct

3. Both are correct statements

4. Only statement 2 correct

16. Match the list 1 and 2 -

List 1   List 2

a. **Asthma**	cigarette smoking
b. **Emphysema**	grinding or stone-breaking
c. **Occupational Respiratory Disorders**	Wheezing

Which of the above are/is incorrectly matched-

1. a only

2. b only

3. a,b only

4. a,b,c

17. Consider the following statements -

a) Inspiration and expiration are carried out by creating pressure gradients between the atmosphere and the alveoli with the help of specialised muscles – intercostals and diaphragm.

b) Volumes of air involved in these activities can be estimated with the help of spirometer and are of clinical significance.

c) Exchange of O_2 and CO_2 at the alveoli and tissues occur by diffusion.

d) Rate of diffusion is dependent on the partial pressure gradients of O_2 (pO_2) and CO_2 (pCO_2), their solubility as well as the thickness of the diffusion surface.

Which of the above statement are correct?

1. a and d only

2. c and bonly

3. d and c only

4. a,b,c,d

18. Consider the following statements-

a) Binding of oxygen with haemoglobin is primarily related to partial pressure of O_2.

b) Partial pressure of CO_2, hydrogen ion concentration and temperature are the other factors which can interfere with this binding.

c) A sigmoid curve is obtained when percentage saturation of haemoglobin with O_2 is plotted against the pO_2.

d) The above curve is also called as the Oxygen dissociation curve and is highly useful in studying the effect of factors like pCO_2, H^+ concentration, etc., on binding of O_2 with haemoglobin.

Which of the above statement are correct?

1. a and d only

2. c and a only

3. a, b,c only

4. a,b,c,d

19. Consider the following statements and find out the incorrect one-

1. The factors in our body facilitate diffusion of O_2 from the alveoli to the deoxygenated blood as well as from the oxygenated blood to the tissues.

2. The factors are favourable for the diffusion of CO_2 in the opposite direction, i.e., from tissues to alveoli.

3. Oxygen is transported mainly as carboxyhaemoglobin.

4. In the alveoli where pO_2 is higher, O_2 gets bound to haemoglobin which is easily dissociated at the tissues where pO_2 is low and pCO_2 and H^+ concentration are high.

20. Read the following statements-

1. Cells utilise oxygen for metabolism and produce energy along with substances like carbon dioxide which is harmful.

2. Animals have evolved different mechanisms for the transport of oxygen to the cells and for the removal of carbon dioxide from there.

3. Humans have a well developed respiratory system comprising two lungs and associated air passages to perform this function.

4. The first step in respiration is breathing by which atmospheric air is taken in (inspiration) and the alveolar air is released out (expiration).

How many of them are correct **statements-**

1. two   2. three

3. four   4. one

21. Consider the following statements and find out the correct option for humans-

STATEMENT 1. Human beings have a significant ability to maintain and moderate the respiratory rhythm to suit the demands of the body tissues.

STATEMENT 2. A specialised centre present in the medulla region of the brain called respiratory rhythm centre is primarily responsible for this regulation.

1. Both are wrong statements

2. Only statement 1 correct

3. Both are correct statements

4. Only statement 2 correct

22. Go through the following statements and find out the correct option-

ASSERTION(A). The centre present in the pons region of the brain called pneumotaxic centre can moderate the functions of the respiratory rhythm centre.

REASON(R). Neural signal from this centre can reduce the duration of inspiration and thereby alter the respiratory rate.

1. A correct and R is correct explanation of A

2. A correct and R is also correct but R is not correct explanation of A

3. A correct but R incorrect

4. A and R both are incorrect

23. Go through the following statement and find out the correct option-

A. A chemosensitive area is situated adjacent to the rhythm centre which is highly sensitive to CO_2 and hydrogen ions.

B. Increase in these substances can activate chemosensitive area, which in turn can signal the rhythm centre to make necessary adjustments in the respiratory process by which these substances can be eliminated.

C. Receptors associated with aortic arch and carotid artery also can recognise changes in CO_2 and H^+ concentration and send necessary signals to the rhythm centre for remedial actions.

D. Neural signal from pneumotaxic centre can reduce the duration of inspiration and thereby alter the respiratory rate.

Which of the above statements are correct -

1. A and C only
2. C and D only
3. D and A only
4. A,B,C,D

24. Read the statements given below-

A. Asthma is a difficulty in breathing causing wheezing

B. In Asthma inflammation of bronchi and bronchioles found.

C. Emphysema is not a chronic disorder.

D. In Emphysema alveolar walls are damaged due to which respiratory surface is decreased.

E. One of the major causes of Emphysema is cigarette smoking.

Which above statement are/is incorrect?

1. A and C only
2. C only
3. D and E only
4. A,B,C,D,E,

25. Which statement/s is/are correct for Occupational Respiratory Disorders (ORD)-

A. grinding or stone-breaking,
B. inflammation of lungs

C. proliferation of fibrous tissues
D. causing serious lung damage.

1. A and C only
2. A only
3. D and C only
4. A,B,C,D

26. Consider the following statements-

A. A chemosensitive area is situated adjacent to the rhythm centre which is highly sensitive to CO_2 and hydrogen ions.

B. Increase in these substances can activate chemosensitive area, which in turn can signal the rhythm centre to make necessary adjustments in the respiratory process by which these substances can be eliminated.

C. Receptors associated with aortic arch and carotid artery also can recognise changes in CO_2 and H^+ concentration and send necessary signals to the rhythm centre for remedial actions.

D. The role of oxygen in the regulation of respiratory rhythm is highly significant.

How many of them are correct-

1. one
2. two
3. three
4. four

27. Match the list 1 and 2-

List 1 | List 2

List 1	List 2
a. At the tissue site	where partial pressure of CO_2 is high due to catabolism, CO_2 diffuses into blood (RBCs and plasma) and forms HCO_3^- and H^+.
b. At the alveolar site	where pCO_2 is low, the reaction proceeds in the opposite direction leading to the formation of CO_2 and H_2O.
c. Every 100 ml of deoxygenated blood	delivers approximately 4 ml of CO2 to the alveoli.
d. Every 100 ml of oxygenated blood can	deliver around 5 ml of O_2 to the tissues under normal physiological conditions.

How many of them are correctly matched –

1. one
2. two
3. three
4. four

28. Which of the following factor/s is/are favourable for the formation of oxyhaemoglobin,In the alveoli -

a) high pO_2,

b) low pCO_2,

c) lesser H^+ concentration

d) lower temperature

1. a and c only
2. a only
3. d and c only
4. a,b,c,d

29. Consider the following statements and find out incorrect one-

1. Exchange of gases also occur between blood and tissues.

2. O_2 and CO_2 are exchanged in these sites by simple diffusion mainly based on pressure/concentration gradient.

3. Solubility of the gases as well as the thickness of the membranes involved in diffusion are also some important factors that can affect the rate of diffusion.

4. About 70 per cent of CO_2 is carried in a dissolved state through plasma

30. Read the following points -

a) The Oxygen dissociation curve and is highly useful in studying the effect of factors like pCO_2, H^+ concentration, etc., on binding of O_2 with haemoglobin.

b) In the alveoli, where there is high pO_2, low pCO_2, lesser H^+ concentration and lower temperature, the factors are all favourable for the formation of oxyhaemoglobin,

c) Whereas in the tissues, where low pO_2, high pCO_2, high H^+ concentration and higher temperature exist, the conditions are favourable for dissociation of oxygen from the oxyhaemoglobin.

d) This clearly indicates that O_2 gets bound to haemoglobin in the lung surface and gets dissociated at the tissues.

How many of them are correct –

1. four
2. two
3. three
4. one

31. Read the following statements and find out the correct option-

STATEMENT 1. We have the ability to increase the strength of inspiration and expiration with the help of additional muscles in the abdomen.

STATEMENT 2. The volume of air involved in breathing movements can be estimated by using a spirometer which helps in clinical assessment of pulmonary functions.

1. Both are wrong statements

2. Both are correct statements

3. Only statement 1 correct

4. Only statement 2 correct

32. Go through the following statements and find out the correct option-

ASSERTION(A). Relaxation of the diaphragm and the inter-costal muscles returns the diaphragm and sternum to their normal positions and reduce the thoracic volume and thereby the pulmonary volume.

REASON(R). This leads to an increase in intra-pulmonary pressure to slightly above the atmospheric pressure causing the expulsion of air from the lungs, i.e., expiration.

1. A correct and R is correct explanation of A

2. A correct and R is also correct but R is not correct explanation of A

3. A correct but R incorrect

4. A and R both are incorrect

33. Find out the incorrect option-

1. Relaxation of the diaphragm and the inter-costal muscles returns the diaphragm and sternum to their normal positions and reduce the thoracic volume and thereby the pulmonary volume.

2. This leads to an increase in intra-pulmonary pressure to slightly above the atmospheric pressure causing the expulsion of air from the lungs, i.e., expiration.

3. We have the ability to increase the strength of inspiration and expiration with the help of additional muscles in the abdomen.

4. On an average, a healthy human breathes 70-72 times/minute.

34. Read the following statements-

I. Inspiration can occur if the pressure within the lungs (intra-pulmonary pressure) is less than the atmospheric pressure, i.e., there is a negative pressure in the lungs with respect to atmospheric pressure.

II. Similarly, expiration takes place when the intra-pulmonary pressure is higher than the atmospheric pressure.

III. The diaphragm and a specialised set of muscles – external and internal intercostals between the ribs, help in generation of pressure gradients.

IV. Inspiration is initiated by the contraction of diaphragm which increases the volume of thoracic chamber in the antero-posterior axis.

How many of above is/are correct-

1. three

2. four

3. two

4. one

35. Which of the following is incorrect statement-

1. The contraction of external inter-costal muscles lifts up the ribs and the sternum causing an increase in the volume of the thoracic chamber in the dorso-ventral axis.

2. The overall increase in the thoracic volume not causes increase in pulmonary volume.

3. An increase in pulmonary volume decreases the intra-pulmonary pressure to less than the atmospheric pressure which forces the air from outside to move into the lungs, i.e., inspiration.

4. Relaxation of the diaphragm and the inter-costal muscles returns the diaphragm and sternum to their normal positions and reduce the thoracic volume and thereby the pulmonary volume.

36. Consider the following matchings –

i. **Tidal Volume (TV):** Volume of air inspired or expired during a normal respiration.

ii. **Inspiratory Reserve Volume (IRV):** Additional volume of air, a person can inspire by a forcible inspiration.

iii. **Expiratory Reserve Volume (ERV):** Additional volume of air, a person can expire by a forcible expiration.

iv. **Residual Volume (RV):** Volume of air remaining in the lungs even after a forcible expiration.

Which above statements are correct-

1. i,ii only

2. i, iii,iv only

3. i,ii,iii only

4. all are correct

37. Read the following macthings-

i. **Inspiratory Capacity (IC):** Total volume of air a person can inspire after a normal expiration.

ii. **Expiratory Capacity (EC):** Total volume of air a person can expire after a normal inspiration.

iii. **Functional Residual Capacity (FRC):** Volume of air that will remain in the lungs after a normal expiration.

iv. **Vital Capacity (VC):** The maximum volume of air a person can breathe in after a forced expiration.

Which above statements is/are correct-

1. i and ii only

2. iii And ii only

3. iv and iii only

4. All are correct

38. Consider the following statements-

I. Total Lung Capacity(TLC) is the total volume of air accommodated in the lungs at the end of a forced inspiration.

II. Total Lung Capacity(TLC) includes RV, ERV, TV and IRV

III. Total Lung Capacity(TLC) equals to vital capacity + residual volume.

IV. Total Lung Capacity(TLC) means the maximum volume of air a person can breathe out after a forced inspiration.

How many of above are correct-

1. three

2. one

3. two

4. four

39. Read the following statements and find out the correct option-

STATEMENT 1. O_2 and CO_2 are exchanged in alveoli and tissues by simple diffusion mainly based on pressure/concentration gradient.

STATEMENT 2. Solubility of the gases as well as the thickness of the membranes involved in diffusion are also some important factors that can affect the rate of diffusion.

1. Both are wrong statements

2. Both are correct statements

3. Only statement 1 correct

4. Only statement 2 correct

40. Read the following statements-

a) **Larynx** is a cartilaginous box.

b) Larynx helps in sound production and hence called the **sound box**.

c) On larynx vocal cord present.

d) Vocal cord of males longer thicker due to testosterone.

e) On larynx various cartilage present.

f) During swallowing glottis can be covered by a thin elastic cartilaginous flap called epiglottis to prevent the entry of food into the **larynx**.

Which of the following are correct?

1. a and b only

2. a,b,c,d only

3. a,b,c,d,e only

4. All are correct

41. Go through the following statements and find out the correct option-

ASSERTION(A). RBCs contain a very high concentration of the enzyme, carbonic anhydrase and minute quantities of the same is present in the plasma too.

REASON(R). At the alveolar site where pCO_2 is low, the reaction proceeds in the opposite direction leading to the formation of CO_2 and H_2O.

1. A correct and R is correct explanation of A

2. A correct and R is also correct but R is not correct explanation of A

3. A correct but R incorrect

4. A and R both are incorrect

42. Find out the incorrect statement-

1. **Asthma** is a difficulty in breathing causing wheezing due to inflammation of bronchi and bronchioles.

2. **Emphysema** is a chronic disorder in which alveolar walls are damaged due to which respiratory surface is increased.

3. One of the major causes of **Emphysema** is cigarette smoking.

4. **Occupational Respiratory Disorders:** In certain industries, especially those involving grinding or stone-breaking, so much dust is produced that the defense mechanism of the body cannot fully cope with the situation.

43. Consider the following statements-

a) Trachea is a straight tube extending up to the mid-thoracic cavity.

b) Trachea also known as wind pipe.

c) Trachea 10-12 cm in length.

d) Trachea divides at the level of 5th thoracic vertebra into a right and left primary **bronchi.**

How many of them are correct-

1. one

2. three

3. four

4. two

44. **Read the following statements and find out the correct option -**

STATEMENT 1. Receptors associated with aortic arch and carotid artery also can recognise changes in CO_2 and H^+ concentration and send necessary signals to the rhythm centre for remedial actions.

STATEMENT 2. The role of oxygen in the regulation of respiratory rhythm is quite insignificant.

1. Both are correct statements

2. Both are wrong statements

3. Only statement 1 correct

4.Only statement 2 correct

45. **Which statement is incorrect -**

1. The centre present in the pons region of the brain called pneumotaxic centre can moderate the functions of the respiratory rhythm centre.

2. Neural signal from pneumotaxic centre can reduce the duration of inspiration and thereby alter the respiratory rate.

3. A chemosensitive area is situated adjacent to the rhythm centre which is highly sensitive to Oxygen only.

4. Increase in CO_2 and H^+ substances can activate this chemosensitive area, which in turn can signal the rhythm centre to make necessary adjustments in the respiratory process by which these substances can be eliminated.

46. **Read the following statements and find out the correct option-**

STATEMENT 1. In certain industries, especially those involving grinding or stone-breaking, so much dust is produced that the defense mechanism of the body cannot fully cope with the situation.

STATEMENT 2. Long exposure can give rise to inflammation leading to fibrosis (proliferation of fibrous tissues) and thus causing serious lung damage.

1. Both are correct statements

2. Both are wrong statements.

3. Only statement 1 correct

4. Only statement 2 correct

47. **Go through the following statement and find out the correct option-**

ASSERTION(A). Nearly 70 per cent of carbon dioxide is transported as bicarbonate (HCO_3^-) with the help of the enzyme carbonic anhydrase.

REASON(R). 20-25 per cent of carbon dioxide is carried by haemoglobin as carbamino-haemoglobin.

1.A correct and R is correct explanation of A

2. A correct and R is also correct but R is not correct explanation of A

3. A correct but R incorrect

4. A and R both are incorrect

48. Find out the incorrect statement –

1. At the tissue site where partial pressure of CO_2 is high due to catabolism, CO_2 diffuses into blood (RBCs and plasma) and forms HCO_3^- and H^+.

2. At the alveolar site where pCO_2 is low, the reaction proceeds in the opposite direction leading to the formation of CO_2 and H_2O.

3. The CO_2 trapped as bicarbonate at the tissue level and transported to the alveoli and is released out as CO_2.

4. Every 100 ml of deoxygenated blood delivers approximately 40 ml of CO_2 to the alveoli.

49. Consider the following statements -

A. Residual Volume (RV) is the volume of air remaining in the lungs even after a forcible expiration.

B. RV averages 1100 mL to 1200 mL.

C. By adding respiratory volumes, various pulmonary capacities are obtained which can be used in clinical diagnosis.

D. Total Lung Capacity is the total volume of air accommodated in the lungs at the end of a forced inspiration.

Which of the above statements are correct-

1. A and C only

2. D and B only

3. B and C only

4. All are correct

50. Read the following statements-

A. The first step in respiration is breathing by which atmospheric air is taken in (inspiration) and the alveolar air is released out (expiration).

B. Exchange of O_2 and CO_2 between deoxygenated blood and alveoli is pressure gradient based.

C. Each terminal bronchiole gives rise to a number of very thin, irregular walled and vascularised bag-like structures called **alveoli.**

D. The branching network of bronchi, bronchioles and alveoli comprise the lungs.

Which of the above statements are correct-

1. A and C only

2. D and A only

3. B and D only

4. All are correct

BODY FLUIDS AND CIRCULATION

5.1 Blood

5.2 Lymph (Tissue Fluid)

5.3 Circulatory Pathways

5.4 Double Circulation

5.5 Regulation of Cardiac Activity

5.6 Disorders of Circulatory System

- All living cells have to be provided with **nutrients, O_2** and other essential substances.
- The waste or **harmful substances produced** in the body have to be removed continuously for healthy functioning of tissues.
- It is therefore, **essential to have efficient mechanisms** for the movement of these substances to the cells and from the cells.
- Different groups of animals have **different** methods for this transport.
- Simple organisms like sponges and coelenterates circulate water from their surroundings through their body cavities to **facilitate** the cells to exchange these substances.
- More complex organisms use special **fluids** within their bodies to transport such materials.
- Blood is the **most commonly** used body fluid by most of the higher organisms including humans for transport materials.
- Another **body fluid, lymph,** also helps in the transport of certain substances.

5.1 BLOOD

- Blood is a **special connective** tissue.
- Blood has two components **plasma** and **formed elements**(i.e.blood cells)

5.1.1 Plasma

- Plasma is a **straw** coloured.
- Plasma is a **viscous** fluid constituting nearly **55 per cent** of the blood.

- **90-92 per cent** of plasma is water and proteins contribute **6-8 per cent** of it.
- **Fibrinogen, globulins and albumins** are the major proteins.
- Plasma protein **fibrinogens** are needed for clotting or coagulation of blood.
- Plasma protein **globulins** primarly are involved in defense mechanisms of the body.
- The **albumins** help in osmotic balance.
- Plasma also contains small amounts of minerals like Na^+, Ca^{++}, Mg^{++}, HCO_3^-, Cl^-, etc.
- **Glucose, amino acids, lipids**, etc., are also present in the plasma as they are always in transit in the body.
- Factors for coagulation or clotting of blood are also present in the plasma in an inactive form.
- Plasma without the clotting factors is called **serum**.

5.1.2 Formed Elements

- **Erythrocytes, leucocytes and platelets** are collectively called formed elements and they constitute nearly 45 per cent of the blood.
- **Erythrocytes** or red blood cells (RBC) are the most abundant of all the cells in blood.
- A healthy adult man has, on an average, **5 millions to 5.5 millions of RBCs** mm^{-3} of blood.
- RBCs are formed in the **red bone marrow** in the adults.
- For RBC formation **Erythropoietin** hormone require.
- **Erythropoietin** hormone releases from Kidney.
- A healthy individual has **12-16 gms** of haemoglobin in every 100 ml of blood.
- These molecules play a significant role in transport of respiratory gases.
- RBCs have an average life span of **120 days**.
- After **120 days** RBCs are destroyed in the spleen (graveyard of RBCs).

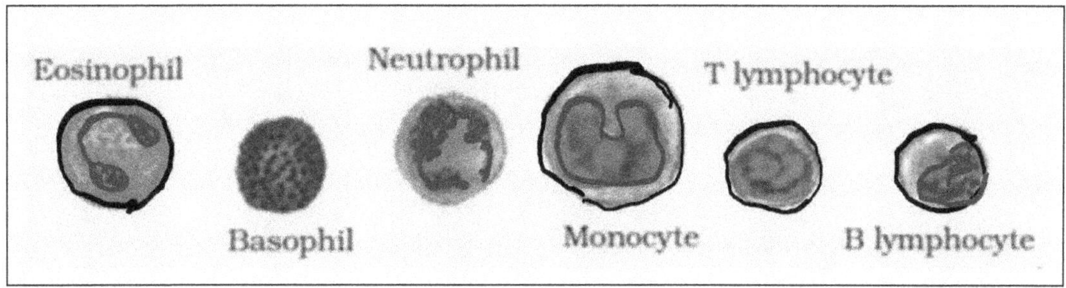

- **Leucocytes** are also known as white blood cells (WBC).
- **Leucocytes** are colourless due to the lack of haemoglobin.
- **Leucocytes** are nucleated.
- **Leucocytes** and are relatively lesser in number which averages 6000-8000 mm^{-3} of blood.
- If TLC that means total leucocyte count increases it is called **leucocytosis.**
- If TLC that means total leucocyte count decreases it is called **leucocytopenia.**

- **Leucocytes** are generally short lived.
- The two main categories of WBCs – granulocytes and agranulocytes.
- **Neutrophils, eosinophils and basophils** are different types of granulocytes, while **lymphocytes and monocytes** are the agranulocytes.
- **Neutrophils** are the most abundant cells (60-65 per cent) of the total WBCs.
- **Basophils** are the least (0.5-1 per cent) among them.
- **Neutrophils and monocytes** (6-8 per cent) are phagocytic cells which destroy foreign organisms entering the body.
- **Monocyte** known as Macro police man of blood.
- **Basophils** secrete histamine, serotonin, heparin, etc., and are involved in inflammatory reactions.
- **Eosinophils** (2-3 per cent) resist infections and are also associated with allergic reactions.
- **Lymphocytes** (20-25 per cent) are of two major types – 'B' and 'T' forms.
- Both B and T lymphocytes are responsible for immune responses of the body.
- Platelets also called **thrombocytes**, are cell fragments produced from megakaryocytes (special cells in the bone marrow).
- Blood normally contains **1,500,00-3,500,00 platelets mm^{-3}**.
- **Critical** platelet count **40,000 per mm^3**
- **Platelets** can release a variety of substances which are involved in the coagulation or clotting of blood.
- A reduction of **Platelets** below critical count can lead to clotting disorders which will lead to excessive loss of blood from the body.

5.1.3 Blood Groups

- The blood of human beings differ in **certain** aspects but it appears to be similar.
- Various types of grouping of blood has been done.
- Two such groupings – the **ABO** and Rh factors are widely used all over the world.

5.1.3.1 ABO grouping

- **ABO** grouping is based on the presence or absence of two surface antigens (chemicals that can induce immune response) on the RBCs namely A and B.
- **ABO** blood group discovered by **Landsteiner**.
- Similarly, the plasma of different **individuals** contain two natural antibodies (proteins produced in response to antigens).
- The **distribution** of antigens and antibodies in the four groups of blood, **A, B, AB** and **O** are given in Table-

Bood group	Antigen on RBCs (Donnan Membrane)	Antibodies in plasma	Donor,s group
A	A	Anti –B	A,O

B	B	Anti-A	B,O
AB	A,B	Nil	A,AB,B,O
O	Nil	Anti –A,B	O

- During **blood transfusion**, any blood cannot be used.
- The blood of a donor has to be **carefully** matched with the blood of a recipient before any blood transfusion to avoid severe problems of clumping (**destruction of RBC**)
- 'O' group individuals are called '**universal donors**'.
- Persons with '**AB' group can accept blood** from persons with AB as well as the other groups of blood.
- Therefore, such persons are called '**universal recipients**'.

5.1.3.2 Rh grouping

- Another antigen, the Rh antigen similar to one present in Rhesus **monkeys** (hence Rh), is also observed on the surface of RBCs of majority (nearly **80 per cent**) of humans.
- Rh factor discovered by **Landsteiner** and **Weiner.**
- Such individuals are called **Rh positive** (Rh+ve) and those in whom this antigen is absent are called **Rh negative** (Rh-ve).
- An **Rh-ve** person, if exposed to **Rh+ve** blood, will form specific antibodies against the Rh antigens.
- Therefore, Rh group should also be matched before transfusions.
- A special case of Rh **incompatibility** (mismatching) has been observed between the Rh-ve blood of a pregnant mother with **Rh+ve** blood of the foetus. Rh antigens of the foetus do not get exposed to the Rh-ve blood of the mother in the first pregnancy as the two bloods are well separated by the **placenta**.
- However, during the delivery of the first child, there is a possibility of exposure of the maternal blood to small amounts of the **Rh+ve** blood from the foetus.
- In such cases, the mother starts preparing antibodies against Rh in her blood.
- In case of her **subsequent** pregnancies, the Rh antibodies from the mother **(Rh-ve)** can leak into the blood of the foetus **(Rh+ve)** and destroy the foetal RBCs.
- This could be fatal to the foetus or could cause severe **anaemia** and **jaundice** to the baby.
- This condition is called ***erythroblastosis foetalis***.
- This can be avoided by **administering anti-Rh antibodies** to the mother immediately after the delivery of the first child.

5.1.4 Coagulation of Blood

- **The wound** does not continue to bleed for a long time; usually the blood stops flowing after sometime.
- Blood exhibits **coagulation** or clotting in response to an **injury or trauma.**
- This is a **mechanism** to prevent excessive loss of blood from the body.
- Best mechanism of clotting given by ***Macfarlane et.al.***
- **A dark reddish brown scum** formed at the site of a cut or an injury over a period of time.

- It is a **clot or coagulam** formed mainly of a network of threads called fibrins in which dead and damaged formed elements of blood are trapped.

- **Fibrins** are formed by the conversion of inactive fibrinogens in the plasma by the enzyme thrombin.

- **Thrombins**, in turn are formed from another inactive substance present in the plasma called prothrombin.

- An enzyme complex, **thrombokinase**, is required for the above reaction. This complex is formed by a series of linked enzymic reactions (cascade process) involving a number of factors present in the plasma in an inactive state.

- An injury or a trauma stimulates the platelets in the blood to release certain factors which activate the mechanism of coagulation.

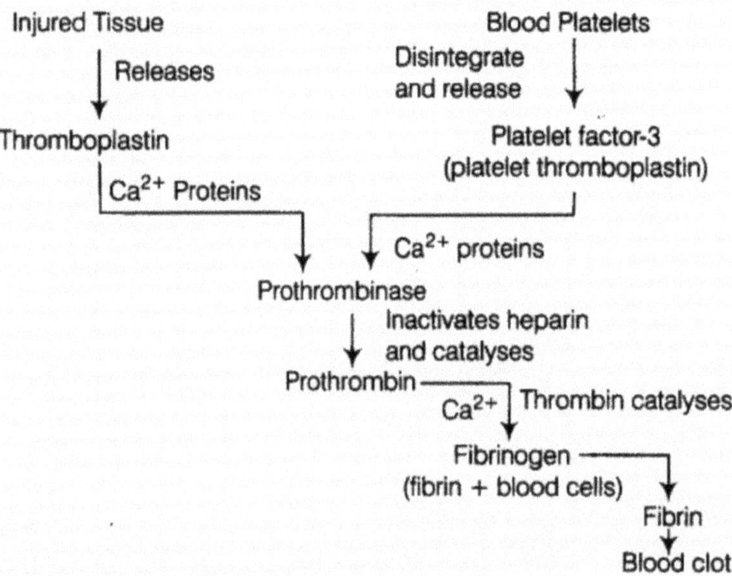

- Certain factors released by the tissues at the site of injury also can initiate **coagulation.**

- **Calcium ions** play a very important role in clotting.

5.2 LYMPH (TISSUE FLUID)

- As the blood passes through the **capillaries** in tissues, some water along with many small water soluble substances move out into the spaces **between** the cells of tissues leaving the larger proteins and most of the formed elements in the blood vessels.

- This fluid released out is called the **interstitial fluid or tissue fluid.**

- It has the same mineral distribution as that in **plasma.**

- Exchange of **nutrients**, gases, etc., between the blood and the cells always occur through this fluid.

- An **elaborate** network of vessels called the lymphatic system collects this fluid and drains it back to the major veins.

- **The fluid present** in the lymphatic system is called the lymph.

- **Lymph** is a colourless fluid containing specialised lymphocytes which are responsible for the immune responses of the body.

- **Lymph** is also an important carrier for nutrients, hormones, etc.

- **Fats are absorbed** through lymph in the lacteals present in the intestinal villi.

5.3 Circulatory Pathways

- The circulatory patterns are of two types – open or closed.

- **Open circulatory system** is present in arthropods, non-cephalopod molluscs, echinoderms, hemichordate and urochordata.

- In **Open circulatory system** blood pumped by the heart passes through large vessels into open spaces or body cavities called sinuses.

- Annelids and chordates have a **closed circulatory system** in which the blood pumped by the heart is always circulated through a closed network of blood vessels.

- **Closed circulatory system** more advantageous because the flow of fluid can be more precisely regulated.

- All vertebrates possess a **muscular chambered heart**.

- **Fishes** have a 2-chambered heart with an atrium and a ventricle.

- **Amphibians and the reptiles (except crocodiles)** have a 3-chambered heart with two atria and a single ventricle,

- The **crocodiles, birds and mammals** possess a 4-chambered heart with two atria and two ventricles.

- In **fishes** the heart pumps out deoxygenated blood which is oxygenated by the gills and supplied to the body parts from where deoxygenated blood is returned to the heart (**single circulation**).

- In **amphibians and reptiles**, the left atrium receives oxygenated blood from the gills/lungs/skin and the right atrium gets the deoxygenated blood from other body parts.

- However, **in incomplete double circulation** blood mixed up in the single ventricle.

- **In birds and mammals,** oxygenated and deoxygenated blood received by the left and right atria respectively passes on to the ventricles of the same sides.

- The **ventricles** pump it out without any mixing up, i.e., two separate circulatory pathways are present in these organisms, hence, these animals have double circulation.

5.3.1 Human Circulatory System

- Human **circulatory** system, also called the blood vascular system.

- It consists of a **muscular** chambered heart, a network of closed branching blood vessels and blood, the fluid which is circulated.

- Study of heart called as **cardiology.**

- **Heart,** the mesodermally derived organ.

- **Heart** is situated in the thoracic cavity, in between the two lungs, slightly tilted to the left.

- **Heart** has the size of a clenched fist.

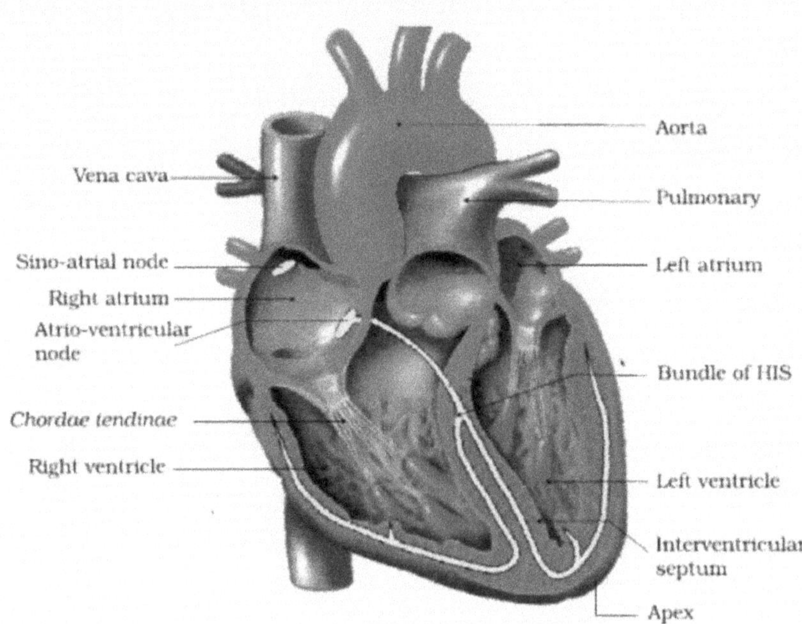

- It is protected by a double walled membranous bag, **pericardium,** enclosing the pericardial fluid.
- Our heart has **four chambers.**
- Two relatively **small upper chambers** called **atria** and two larger lower chambers called **ventricles.**
- Thickest and largest chamber is **Left ventricle.**
- A thin, muscular wall called the **interatrial septum separates** the right and the left atria, whereas a thick-walled, the inter-ventricular septum, separates the left and the right ventricles (Figure 18.2).
- The atrium and the ventricle of the same side are also separated by a **thick fibrous tissue** called the atrio-ventricular septum.
- However, each of these septa are provided with an opening through which the two chambers of the same side are connected.
- **The opening between the right atrium and the right ventricle** is guarded by a valve formed of three muscular flaps or cusps, the tricuspid valve, whereas a bicuspid or mitral valve guards the opening between the left atrium and the left ventricle.
- **The openings of the right and the left ventricles into** the pulmonary artery and the aorta respectively are provided with the semilunar valves.
- **The valves in the heart allows the flow of blood only in one direc**tion, i.e., from the atria to the ventricles and from the ventricles to the pulmonary artery or aorta.
- These valves prevent any **backward** flow.
- Superior and Inferior vena cava opens into **Right Auricle.**
- **The entire heart** is made of cardiac muscles.
- The walls of ventricles are much **thicker than** that of the atria.
- A specialised **cardiac musculature** called the nodal tissue is also distributed in the heart.

Conducting system of heart

- A patch of this tissue is present in the right upper corner of the right atrium called the **sino-atrial node** (SAN).

- Another mass of this tissue is seen in the lower left corner of the right atrium close to the atrio-ventricular septum called the **atrio-ventricular node** (AVN).

- The speed impulse couduction in SAN and AVN is 0.1-0.2 m/sec

- A bundle of nodal fibres, **atrioventricular bundle (AV bundle)** continues from the AVN which passes through the atrio-ventricular septa to emerge on the top of the interventricular septum and immediately divides into a right and left bundle.

- These branches give rise to minute fibres throughout the ventricular musculature of the respective sides and are called **purkinje fibres.**

- These fibres alongwith right and left bundles are known as **bundle of HIS.**

- **Maximum conduction speed** is found in purkinje fibres.

- **The speed in** purkinje fibres is 4 m/sec.

- The nodal musculature has the ability to generate action potentials without any external stimuli, i.e., it is **autoexcitable.**

- However, the number of action potentials that could be generated in a minute vary at different parts of the nodal system.

- The **SAN** can generate the maximum number of action potentials, i.e., **70-75 min^{-1}**, and is responsible for initiating and maintaining the rhythmic contractile activity of the heart. Therefore, it is the pacemaker.

- Our heart normally beats **70-75 times in a minute (average 72 beats min^{-1}).**

5.3.2 Cardiac Cycle

- This begins with, all the four chambers of heart are in a relaxed state, i.e., they are in joint diastole.

- Joint diastole occur in **0.4 sec.**

- As the **tricuspid** and bicuspid valves are open, blood from the pulmonary veins and vena cava flows into the left and the right ventricle respectively through the left and right atria.

- The semilunar valves are closed at this stage.

- The SAN now generates an action potential which stimulates both the atria to undergo a simultaneous contraction – the atrial systole.

- The **atrial systole** occur in **0.1 sec.**

- This increases the flow of blood into the ventricles by about **30 per cent**. The action potential is conducted to the ventricular side by the AVN and AV bundle from where **the bundle of HIS** transmits it through the entire ventricular musculature.

- This causes the ventricular muscles to contract, (ventricular systole), the atria undergoes relaxation (diastole), coinciding with **the ventricular systole.**

- Normal Systolic B.P. = 120 **mm Hg**

- Normal Diastolic B.P. = 80 **mm Hg**
- The **ventricular systole** occur in **0.3 sec.**
- **Ventricular systole increases the ventricular pressure** causing the closure of tricuspid and bicuspid valves due to attempted backflow of blood into the atria.
- As the ventricular pressure increases further, **the semilunar valves** guarding the pulmonary artery (right side) and the aorta (left side) are forced open, allowing the blood in the ventricles to flow through these vessels into the circulatory pathways.
- The ventricles now relax (ventricular diastole) and **the ventricular pressure falls causing the closure of semilunar valves** which prevents the backflow of blood into the ventricles.
- As the ventricular pressure declines further, the **tricuspid** and **bicuspid** valves are pushed open by the pressure in the atria exerted by the blood which was being emptied into them by the veins.
- The blood now once again moves freely to the **ventricles.**
- The ventricles and atria are now again comes in a relaxed (**joint diastole**) state.
- **Joint diastole = 0.8-(Auricular systole + Ventricular Systole)**
- **Joint diastole = 0.8-(0.1 + 0.3) = 0.4 sec**
- Soon the **SAN generates a new action potential** and the events described above are repeated in that sequence and the process continues.
- This sequential event in the heart which is cyclically repeated is called the **cardiac cycle** and it consists of **systole** and **diastole** of both the atria and ventricles.
- As mentioned earlier, the heart beats **72 times per minute**, i.e., that many cardiac cycles are performed per minute. From this it could be deduced that the duration of a cardiac cycle is 0.8 seconds.
- During a cardiac cycle, each ventricle pumps out **approximately 70 mL of blood** which is called the stroke volume.
- **The stroke volume** multiplied by the heart rate (no. of beats per min.) gives the cardiac output. Therefore, the cardiac output can be defined as the volume of blood pumped out by each ventricle per minute and averages **5000 mL or 5 litres** in a healthy individual.
- **Cardiac output = stroke volume multiplied heart beat per minute**
- The body has the ability to alter the stroke volume as well as the heart rate and thereby the cardiac output.
- For example, **the cardiac output of an athlete will be much higher** than that of an ordinary man.
- During each cardiac cycle two prominent sounds are produced which can be easily heard through a stethoscope.
- **The first heart sound (lub)** is associated with the closure of the tricuspid and bicuspid valves whereas **the second heart sound (dub)** is associated with the closure of the semilunar valves.
- These sounds are of clinical diagnostic significance.

5.3.3 Electrocardiograph (ECG)

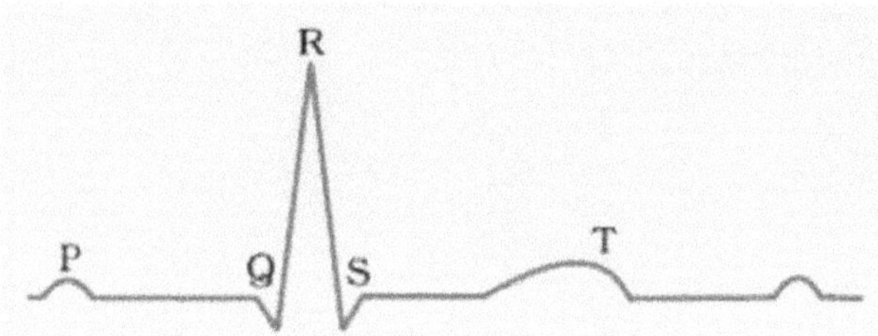

- A patient is hooked up to a monitoring machine that shows voltage traces on a screen and makes the sound **"... pip... pip... pip..... peeeeeeeeeeeeeeeeeeeeeee"** as the patient goes into cardiac arrest.

- The machine called as electro-cardiograph is used to obtain an **electrocardiogram (ECG).**

- **ECG** is a graphical representation of the electrical activity of the heart during a cardiac cycle.

- To obtain a standard **ECG** a patient is connected to the machine with three electrical leads (one to each wrist and to the left ankle) that continuously monitor the heart activity.

- **For a detailed evaluation of the heart's function, multiple leads are attached to the chest region.**

- Now we talk only about a **standard ECG.**

- In standard **ECG,** P,Q,R,S,T waves present.

- Each peak in the **ECG** is identified with a letter from P to T that corresponds to a specific electrical activity of the heart.

- The P-wave represents the electrical **excitation (or depolarisation) of the atria,** which leads to the contraction of both the atria.

- The QRS complex represents the **depolarisation of the ventricles,**which initiates the ventricular contraction.

- The contraction starts shortly **after Q** and marks the beginning of the systole.

- The **T-wave** represents the return of the ventricles from excited to normal state (**repolarisation**).

- The end of the **T-wave marks the end of systole.**

- T-P segment represents repolarization of heart.

- By counting the number of **QRS** complexes that occur in a given time period, one can determine the heart beat rate of an individual.

- Since the ECGs obtained from different individuals have roughly the same shape for a given lead configuration, any deviation from this shape indicates a possible abnormality or disease.

- **Hence, ECG has a great clinical significance.**

5.4 Double Circulation

- The blood **pumped by the right ventricle** enters the pulmonary artery, whereas the left ventricle pumps blood into the aorta.

- The deoxygenated blood **pumped into the pulmonary artery** is passed on to the lungs from where the oxygenated blood is carried by the pulmonary veins into the left atrium.

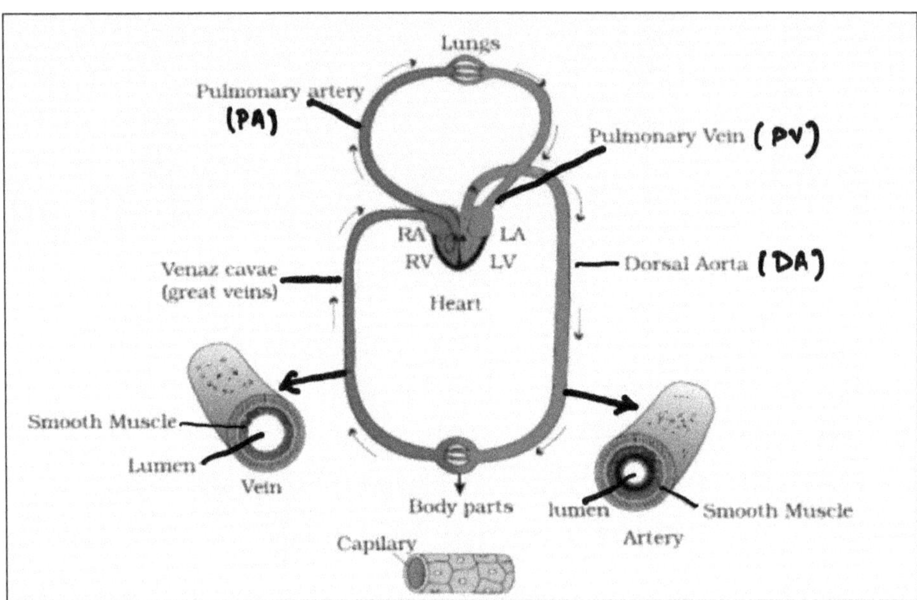

- This pathway constitutes the pulmonary circulation.

- The oxygenated blood entering the aorta is carried by a network of **arteries, arterioles and capillaries to the tissues** from where the deoxygenated blood is collected by a system of venules, veins and vena cava and emptied into the right atrium.

- This is the **systemic circulation.**

- The systemic circulation provides nutrients, O_2 and other essential substances to the tissues and takes CO_2 and other harmful substances away for elimination.

Points to remember-

- A unique vascular connection exists between the digestive tract and liver **called hepatic portal system.**

- The **hepatic portal vein carries blood from intestine to the liver** before it is delivered to the systemic circulation.

- Renal portal system absent in Humans.

- **Pulse rate = Heart beat rate**

- **Pulse** measured from superficial arteries of **wrist, neck** and **temporal** region.

- A special coronary system of blood vessels is present in our body exclusively for the circulation of blood to and from the **cardiac musculature.**

- **Vasa vassorum** are blood vessels which supply blood to blood vessels.

- If heart beat increases called as **Tachycardia.**

- If heart beat decreases called as **Bradycardia.**

5.5 REGULATION OF CARDIAC ACTIVITY

- Normal activities of the heart are regulated intrinsically, i.e., auto regulated by specialised muscles (nodal tissue), hence **the heart is called myogenic.**

- A special neural centre in the **medulla oblangata** can moderate the cardiac function through autonomic nervous system (ANS).

- Neural signals through the **sympathetic nerves (part of ANS) can increase the rate of heart beat**, the strength of ventricular contraction and thereby the cardiac output.
- On the other hand, **parasympathetic neural signals (another component of ANS) decrease the rate of heart beat**, speed of conduction of action potential and thereby the cardiac output.
- 10th cranial nerve is vagus nerve which is a component of **parasympathetic nervous system.**
- **Adrenal medullary hormones** can also increase the cardiac output.

5.6 Disorders of Circulatory System

I. High Blood Pressure (Hypertension):

- Hypertension is the term for **blood pressure that is highe**r than normal **(120/80).**
- In this measurement 120 mm Hg (millimetres of mercury pressure) is the systolic, or pumping, pressure and 80 mm Hg is the diastolic, or resting, pressure.
- **If repeated checks of blood pressure** of an individual is **140/90 (140 over 90) or higher, it shows hypertension.**
- High blood pressure leads to **heart diseases** and also affects vital organs **like brain and kidney.**

II. Coronary Artery Disease (CAD):

- Coronary Artery Disease, often referred to as **atherosclerosis**, affects the vessels that supply blood to the heart muscle.
- It is caused by **deposits of calcium, fat, cholesterol and fibrous tissues,** which makes the lumen of arteries narrower.

III. Angina:

- It is also called 'angina pectoris'.
- **Acute chest pain** appears when no enough oxygen is reaching the heart muscle.
- **Angina** can occur in men and women of any age but it is more common among the middle-aged and elderly.
- It occurs due to **conditions** that affect the blood flow.

IV. Heart Failure:

- Heart **failure** means the state of heart when it is **not** pumping blood effectively enough to meet the needs of the body.
- It is sometimes called **congestive heart failure** because congestion of the lungs is one of the main symptoms of this disease.

V. Cardiac Arrest:

- **Cardiac** arrest when the **heart stops beating.**
- **Heart failure** is not the same as **cardiac arrest.**

VI. Heart attack

- When the **heart muscle is suddenly damaged** by an inadequate blood supply.

1. Consider the following statements and find out the correct option-

A. Fibrinogens are needed for clotting or coagulation of blood.

B. Globulins primarly are involved in defense mechanisms of the body and the albumins help in osmotic balance.

C. Plasma also contains small amounts of minerals.

D. Glucose, amino acids, lipids, etc., are also present in the plasma as they are always in transit in the body.

Which of the above statement is/are correct for Human blood-

1. A,C only

2. B,C only

3. D,A only

4. A,B,C,D

2. Match the list 1 and 2-

List1	List2
a. Erythrocytes, leucocytes and platelets are	j. 5 millions to 5.5 millions mm^{-3} of blood
b. A healthy adult man has RBCs	k. 45%
c. A healthy individual has Platelets	l. 12-16 gms
d. Blood normally contains haemoglobin in every 100 ml	m. 1,500,00-3,500,00 mm^{-3}.

Find out the correct option –

1. a.k, b.j, c.l, d.m

2. a.k,b.l,c.j,d.m

3. a.l,b.j,c.k,d.m

4. a.l,b.j,c.m,d.k

3. Consider the following statements-

a) Leucocytes are generally short lived.

b) Neutrophils, eosinophils and basophils are different types of granulocytes, while lymphocytes and monocytes are the agranulocytes.

c) Neutrophils are the most abundant cells of the total WBCs and basophils are the least (0.5-1 per cent) among them.

d) Neutrophils and monocytes are phagocytic cells which destroy foreign organisms entering the body.

Which of the above statements are correct –

1. only a and d

2. a,b,c,d

3. only c and d

4. a,b,c only

4. Read the following statement carefully -

I. Basophils secrete histamine.

II. Eosinophils (2-3 per cent) resist infections and are also associated with allergic reactions.

III. Lymphocytes (20-25 per cent) are of two major types – 'B' and 'T' forms.

IV. Both B and T lymphocytes are responsible for immune responses of the body.

V. Platelets also called leucocytes, are cell fragments produced from megakaryocytes (special cells in the bone marrow).

How many of them are correct -

1. three

2. four

3. five

4. two

5. Consider the following statements and find out the correct option

STATEMENT 1. Factors for coagulation or clotting of blood are also present in the plasma.

STATEMENT 2. Plasma without the clotting factors is called serum.

1. Both are correct statements

2. Only statement 1 correct

3. Both are wrong statements

4. Only statement 2 correct

6. Go through the following statement-

ASSERTION(A). Erythrocytes or red blood cells (RBC) are the most abundant of all the cells in blood.

REASON(R). RBCs have an average life span of 120 days after which they are destroyed in the spleen (graveyard of RBCs).

1. A correct and R is correct explanation of A

2. A correct and R is also correct but R is not correct explanation of A

3. A correct but R incorrect

4. A and R both are incorrect

7. Find out the incorrect statement -

1. Leucocytes are also known as white blood cells (WBC) as they are colourless due to the lack of haemoglobin.

2. Leucocytes are nucleated and are relatively lesser in number which averages 16000-800000 mm^{-3} of blood.

3. Leucocytes are generally short lived.

4. We have two main categories of WBCs – granulocytes and agranulocytes

8. Go through the following statements-

1. Basophils found 0.5-1 per cent in blood.

2. Neutrophils are phagocytic cells which destroy foreign organisms entering the body.

3. Basophils secrete heparin and are involved in inflammatory reactions.

4. Eosinophils resist infections and are also associated with allergic reactions.

How many of them are/is correct-

1. two   2. three

3. four   4. One

9. Match the list 1 and 2-

List 1   List 2

a. Neutrophils	j. 0.5 – 1.0%
b. Basophils	k. 2-3%
c. Eosinophils	l. 60-65%
d. Monocytes	m. 6-8%

Find out the correct option –

1. a.k, b.j, c.l, d.m   2. a.k,b.l,c.j,d.m

3. a.l,b.j,c.k,d.m   4. a.l,b.j,c.m,d.k

10. Consider the following statements and find out the correct option-

STATEMENT 1. ABO grouping is based on the presence or absence of two surface antigens (chemicals that can induce immune response) on the RBCs namely A and B.

STATEMENT 2. The plasma of different individuals contain natural antibodies (proteins produced in response to antigens).

1. Both are wrong statements   2. Only Statement 1 correct

3. Both are correct statements   4. Only statement 2 correct

11. Read the following statements very carefully and find out the correct-

a) Platelets also called thrombocytes, are cell fragments produced from megakaryocytes (special cells in the bone marrow).

b) Blood normally contains 1,500,00-3,500,00 platelets mm^{-3}.

c) Platelets can release a variety of substances most of which are involved in the coagulation or clotting of blood.

d) A reduction in Platelet numbers can lead to clotting disorders which will lead to excessive loss of blood from the body.

Which of the above statement is/are correct?

1. a and c both   2. d only

3. a,b,c,d.   4. b,c,d only

12. Go through the following statement-

ASSERTION(A). 'O' blood group individuals are called 'universal donors'.

REASON(R). Persons with 'AB' group can accept blood from persons with AB as well as the other groups of blood. Therefore, persons with AB blood group are called 'universal recipients'.

1. A correct and R is correct explanation of A

2. A correct and R is also correct but R is not correct explanation of A

3. A correct but R incorrect

4. A and R both are incorrect

13. Find out incorrect statement with respect to Heart-

    1. During a cardiac cycle, each ventricle pumps out approximately **70** mL of blood which is called the stroke volume.
    2. The cardiac output can be defined as the volume of blood pumped out by each ventricle per minute and averages **50** litres in a healthy individual.
    3. The body has the ability to alter the stroke volume as well as the heart rate and thereby the cardiac output.
    4. The cardiac output of an athlete will be much higher than that of an ordinary man.

14. Read the following statements and find out correct option-

    I. The fluid present in the lymphatic system is called the lymph.
    II. Lymph is a colourless fluid containing specialised lymphocytes which are responsible for the immune responses of the body.
    III. Lymph is also an important carrier for nutrients, hormones, etc.
    IV. Fats are absorbed through lymph in the lacteals present in the intestinal villi.

    How many of them are/is correct-

    1. four   2. one

    3. two   4. three

15. **Consider the following statements and find out the correct option-**

    STATEMENT 1. Exchange of nutrients, gases, etc., between the blood and the cells can occur through plasma.

    STATEMENT 2. An elaborate network of vessels called the lymphatic system collects plasma and drains it back to the major veins.

    1. Both are wrong statements   2. Only Statement 1 correct

    3. Both are correct statements   4. Only statement 2 correct

16. **Match the list 1 and 2 -**

    List 1   List 2

a. Coronary Artery Disease	Atherosclerosis
b. Angina	acute chest pain
c. Heart Failure	not pumping blood effectively
d. High Blood Pressure	Hypertension

    How many of them are correctly matched-

    1. one   2. two

    3. three   4. four

17. **Consider the following statements-**

    a) Vertebrates circulate blood, a fluid connective tissue, in their body, to transport essential substances to the cells and to carry waste substances from there.

    b) Lymph (tissue fluid) is used for the transport of certain substances.

    c) Blood comprises of a fluid matrix, plasma and formed elements.

d) Blood of humans are grouped into A, B, AB and O systems based on the presence or absence of two surface antigens, A, B on the RBCs.

Which of the above statements are correct?

1. a,b,c only

2. a,c,d only

3. b, c, d only

4. a,b,c,d

18. Consider the following statements -

   I. The spaces between cells in the tissues contain a fluid derived from blood called tissue fluid.

  II. The lymph is almost similar to blood except for the protein content and the formed elements.

 III. All vertebrates and a few invertebrates have a closed circulatory system

 IV. Our circulatory system consists of a muscular pumping organ, heart, a network of vessels and a fluid, blood.

  V. Heart has two atria and two ventricles.

How many of them are correct for Humans-

1. one

2. five

3. three

4. four

19. Consider the following statements with respect to humans-

A. Cardiac musculature is auto-excitable.

B. Sino-atrial node (SAN) called as Pacesetter.

C. AVN called as pacemaker.

D. The systole forces the blood to move from the atria to the ventricles and to the pulmonary artery and the aorta.

How many of them are incorrect-

1. one

2. two

3. three

4. four

20. Read the following statements-

A. Human have a complete double circulation, i.e., two circulatory pathways, namely, pulmonary and systemic are present.

B. The pulmonary circulation starts by the pumping of deoxygenated blood by the right ventricle which is carried to the lungs where it is oxygenated and returned to the left atrium.

C. The systemic circulation starts with the pumping of oxygenated blood by the left ventricle to the aorta which is carried to all the body tissues and the deoxygenated blood from there is collected by the veins and returned to the right atrium.

D. The heart is autoexcitable, its functions can be moderated by neural and hormonal mechanisms.

How many of them are correct **statements w.r.t. Humans-**

1. two

2. three

3. four

4. one

21. Consider the following statements and find out the correct option for humans-

STATEMENT 1. The electrical activity of the heart can be recorded from the body surface by using electrocardiograph and the recording is called electrocardiogram (ECG) which is of clinical importance.

STATEMENT 2. Angina pectoris can occur in men and women of any age but it is more common among the middle-aged and elderly.

1. Both are wrong statements

2. Only Statement 1 correct

3. Both are correct statements

4. Only statement 2 correct

22. Go through the following statement and find out the correct option-

ASSERTION(A). If repeated checks of blood pressure of an individual is 140/90 (140 over 90) or higher, it shows hypertension.

REASON(R). High blood pressure leads to heart diseases and also affects vital organs like brain and kidney.

1. A correct and R is correct explanation of A

2. A correct and R is also correct but R is not correct explanation of A

3. A correct but R incorrect

4. A and R both are incorrect

23. Go through the following statement and find out the correct option-

A. Normal activities of the heart are regulated intrinsically, i.e., auto regulated by specialised muscles (nodal tissue), hence the heart is called myogenic.

B. A special neural centre in the medulla oblangata can moderate the cardiac function through autonomic nervous system (ANS).

C. Neural signals through the sympathetic nerves (part of ANS) can increase the rate of heart beat, the strength of ventricular contraction and thereby the cardiac output.

D. Parasympathetic neural signals (another component of ANS) decrease the rate of heart beat, speed of conduction of action potential and thereby the cardiac output.

E. Adrenal medullary hormones can also increase the cardiac output.

Which above statement are correct -

1. A,B,C,D only

2. C and D only

3. D and A only

4. All are correct

24. Read the statements given below-

A. Coronary Artery Disease, often referred to as atherosclerosis, affects the vessels that supply blood to the heart muscle.

B. Coronary Artery Disease is caused by deposits of calcium, fat, cholesterol and fibrous tissues, which makes the lumen of arteries narrower.

C. Angina is also called 'angina pectoris'.

D. In angina symptom of acute chest pain appears when no enough oxygen is reaching the heart muscle.

Which of the above statement are correct?

1. A and C only

2. A only

3. D and A only

4. A,B,C,D

25. Consider the following statements -

   A. Heart failure means the state of heart when it is not pumping blood effectively enough to meet the needs of the body.

   B. It is sometimes called congestive heart failure because congestion of the lungs is one of the main symptoms of this disease.

   C. Heart failure is not the same as cardiac arrest (when the heart stops beating) or a heart attack (when the heart muscle is suddenly damaged by an inadequate blood supply).

Which of the above statement are correct?

1. A and C only

2. A only

3. C only

4. A,B,C

26. Consider the following statements-

   I. Open circulatory system is present in arthropods and molluscs.

   II. Annelids and chordates have a closed circulatory system in which the blood pumped by the heart is circulated through a closed network of blood vessels.

   III. Closed circulatory system more advantageous as the flow of fluid can be more precisely regulated.

   IV. All vertebrates possess a muscular chambered heart.

   V. Fishes have a 2-chambered heart with an atrium and a ventricle.

How many of them are/is correct-

1. five

2. two

3. three

4. four

27. Match the list 1 and 2-

List 1   List 2

a. amphibians	3-chambered heart
b. crocodiles	3-chambered heart
c. birds	4-chambered heart
d. mammals	4-chambered heart

How many of them are correctly matched-

1. one   2. two

3. three   4. four

28. Read the following statements-

   a) In fishes the heart pumps out deoxygenated blood which is oxygenated by the gills and supplied to the body parts from where deoxygenated blood is returned to the heart (single circulation).

   b) In amphibians and reptiles, the left atrium receives oxygenated blood from the gills/lungs/skin and the right atrium gets the deoxygenated blood from other body parts.

   c) However, they get mixed up in the single ventricle which pumps out mixed blood (incomplete double circulation).

   d) In birds and mammals, oxygenated and deoxygenated blood received by the left and right atria respectively passes on to the ventricles of the same sides.

   Which of the above statements are correct-

   1. a and c only

   2. a only

   3. d and c only

   4. a,b,c,d

29. Consider the following statements and find out incorrect one-

   1. Human circulatory system, also called the blood vascular system consists of a muscular chambered heart, a network of closed branching blood vessels and blood, the fluid which is circulated.

   2. Heart, the endodermal organ, is situated in the thoracic cavity, in between the two lungs, slightly tilted to the left.

   3. Heart has the size of a clenched fist.

   4. Heart is protected by a double walled membranous bag, pericardium, enclosing the pericardial fluid.

30. Read the following facts -

   I. Our heart has four chambers, two relatively small upper chambers called atria and two larger lower chambers called ventricles.

   II. A thin, muscular wall called the interatrial septum separates the right and the left atria, whereas a thick-walled, the inter-ventricular septum, separates the left and the right ventricles.

   III. The atrium and the ventricle of the same side are also separated by a thick fibrous tissue called the atrio-ventricular septum.

   IV. Atrio-ventricular septa are provided with an opening through which the two chambers of the same side are connected.

   How many of them are correct –

   1. four

   2. two

   3. three

   4. one

31. Read the following statements and find out the correct option

   STATEMENT 1. *Erythroblastosis foetalis* could cause severe anaemia and jaundice to the baby.

   STATEMENT 2. This can be avoided by administering anti-Rh antibodies to the mother immediately after the delivery of the first child.

1. Both are wrong statements

2. Both are correct statements

3. Only statement 1 correct

4. Only statement 2 correct

32. Go through the following statement and find out the correct option-

ASSERTION(A). A special case of Rh incompatibility (mismatching) has been observed between the Rh^{-ve} blood of a pregnant mother with Rh^{+ve} blood of the foetus.

REASON(R). During the delivery of the first child, there is a possibility of exposure of the maternal blood to small amounts of the Rh^{+ve} blood from the foetus. In such cases, the mother starts preparing antibodies against Rh in her blood.

1. A correct and R is correct explanation of A

2. A correct and R is also correct but R is not correct explanation of A

3. A correct but R incorrect

4. A and R both are incorrect

33. Find out the incorrect option w.r.t. blood clotting mechanism-

1. Fibrins are formed by the conversion of inactive fibrinogens in the plasma by the enzyme thrombin. Thrombins, in turn are formed from another inactive substance present in the plasma called prothrombin.

2. An enzyme complex, thrombokinase, is required for the above reaction.

3. Thrombokinase complex is formed by a series of linked enzymic reactions (cascade process) involving a number of factors present in the plasma in an inactive state.

4. An injury or a trauma stimulates the Fat cells in the blood to release certain factors which activate the mechanism of coagulation.

34. Read the following events with respect to Human heart-

I. The opening between the right atrium and the right ventricle is guarded by a valve formed of three muscular flaps or cusps, the tricuspid valve, whereas a bicuspid or mitral valve guards the opening between the left atrium and the left ventricle.

II. The openings of the right and the left ventricles into the pulmonary artery and the aorta respectively are provided with the semilunar valves.

III. The valves in the heart allows the flow of blood only in one direction, i.e., from the atria to the ventricles and from the ventricles to the pulmonary artery or aorta.

IV. These valves do not prevent backward flow of blood.

How many of above are incorrect-

1. three

2. four

3. two

4. one

35. Which of the following is/are correct with respect to Human heart -

I. The walls of ventricles are much thicker than that of the atria.

II. A specialised cardiac musculature called the nodal tissue is also distributed in the heart.

III. A patch of this tissue is present in the right upper corner of the right atrium called the **sino-atrial node** (SAN).

IV. Another mass of this tissue is seen in the lower left corner of the right atrium close to the atrio-ventricular septum called the **atrio-ventricular node** (AVN).

V. A bundle of nodal fibres, atrioventricular bundle (AV bundle) continues from the AVN which passes through the atrio-ventricular septa to emerge on the top of the interventricular septum and immediately divides into a right and left bundle.

How many of above are correct-

1. three

2. four

3. two

4. five

36. Consider the following statements w.r.t. conducting system of Human heart-

i. The branches give rise to minute fibres throughout the ventricular musculature of the respective sides and are called purkinje fibres.

ii. These fibres alongwith right and left bundles are known as bundle of HIS.

iii. The nodal musculature has the ability to generate action potentials without any external stimuli, i.e., it is autoexcitable.

iv. The number of action potentials that could be generated in a minute vary at different parts of the nodal system.

Which above statements are correct-

1. i,ii only

2. i, iii,iv only

3. i,ii,iii only

4. all are correct

37. Read the following statements-

i. The SAN can generate the maximum number of action potentials, i.e., 70-75 min^{-1}, and is responsible for initiating and maintaining the rhythmic contractile activity of the heart. Therefore, it is the pacemaker.

ii. Our heart normally beats 70-75 times in a minute (average 72 beats min^{-1}).

iii. The entire heart is made of cardiac muscles.

iv. The walls of ventricles are much thicker than that of the atria.

Which of the above statements is/are incorrect-

1. iii and ii only

2. iii And iv only

3. i and ii only

4. All are correct

38. Consider the following statements w.r.t. ECG-

   I. A patient is hooked up to a monitoring machine that shows voltage traces on a screen and makes the sound "... pip... pip... pip..... peeeeeeeeeeeeeeeeeeeeeee" as the patient goes into cardiac arrest.

   II. ECG is a graphical representation of the electrical activity of the heart during a cardiac cycle.

   III. To obtain a standard ECG a patient is connected to the machine with three electrical leads (one to each wrist and to the left ankle) that continuously monitor the heart activity.

   IV. For a detailed evaluation of the heart's function, multiple leads are attached to the leg region only.

How many of above are/is incorrect-

1. three

2. four

3. two

4. one

39. Read the following statements and find out the correct option-

STATEMENT 1. Each peak in the ECG is identified with a letter from P to T that corresponds to a specific electrical activity of the heart.

STATEMENT 2. The P-wave represents the electrical **excitation (or depolarisation) of the atria**, which leads to the contraction of both the atria.

1. Both are wrong statements

2. Both are correct statements

3. Only statement 1 correct

4. Only statement 2 correct

40. Read the following statements-

   a) The QRS complex represents the **depolarisation of the ventricles,**which initiates the ventricular contraction.

   b) The contraction starts shortly after Q and marks the beginning of the systole.

   c) The T-wave represents the return of the ventricles from excited to normal state (**repolarisation**).

   d) The end of the T-wave marks the end of systole.

Which of the above statements are correct?

1. a and b only	2. b and c only
3. c and d only	4. a,b,c,d

41. Go through the following statement and find out the correct option w.r.t. ECG-

ASSERTION(A). ECG is a graphical representation of the electrical activity of the heart during a cardiac cycle.

REASON(R). To obtain a standard ECG a patient is connected to ECG machine with three electrical leads (one to each wrist and to the left ankle) that continuously monitor the heart activity.

1. A correct and R is correct explanation of A

2. A correct and R is also correct but R is not correct explanation of A

3. A correct but R incorrect

4. A and R both are incorrect

42. Read the following statement and find out the suitable option-

I. The contraction starts shortly after Q and marks the beginning of the systole.

II. The T-wave represents the return of the ventricles from excited to normal state (**repolarisation**).

III. The end of the T-wave marks the end of systole

IV. The ECGs obtained from different individuals have roughly the same shape for a given lead configuration, any deviation from this shape indicates a possible abnormality or disease.

How many of above are correct for Human ECG -

1. three

2. four

3. two

4. one

43. Consider the following statements-

I. The systemic circulation provides nutrients, O2 and other essential substances to the tissues and takes CO2 and other harmful substances away for elimination.

II. A unique vascular connection exists between the digestive tract and liver called hepatic portal system.

III. The hepatic portal vein carries blood from intestine to the liver before it is delivered to the systemic circulation.

IV. A special coronary system of blood vessels is present in our body exclusively for the circulation of blood to and from the cardiac musculature.

How many of them are correct-

1. one

2. three

3. four

4. two

44. Read the following statements and find out the correct option-

STATEMENT 1. Neural signals through the sympathetic nerves (part of ANS) can increase the rate of heart beat, the strength of ventricular contraction and thereby the cardiac output.

STATEMENT 2. The parasympathetic neural signals (another component of ANS) decrease the rate of heart beat, speed of conduction of action potential and thereby the cardiac output.

1. Both are correct statements

2. Both are wrong statements

3. Only statement 1 correct

4. Only statement 2 correct

45. Find out the incorrect statements-

1. Hypertension is the term for blood pressure that is higher than normal (120/80).

2. In this measurement 120 mm Hg (millimetres of mercury pressure) is the systolic, or pumping, pressure and 80 mm Hg is the diastolic, or resting, pressure.

3. If repeated checks of blood pressure of an individual is 140/90 (140 over 90) or higher, it shows hypertension.

4. High blood pressure leads to heart diseases and but not affects vital organs like brain and kidney.

46. Read the following statements and find out the correct option-

STATEMENT 1. Sino-atrial node (SAN) generates the maximum number of action protentials per minute (70-75/min) and therefore, it sets the pace of the activities of the heart.

STATEMENT 2. About 70 mL of blood is pumped out by each ventricle during a cardiac cycle and it is called the stroke or beat volume.

1. Both are correct statements

2. Both are wrong statements.

3. Only statement 1 correct

4. Only statement 2 correct

47. Go through the following statement and find out the correct option-

ASSERTION(A). All vertebrates and a few invertebrates have a closed circulatory system.

REASON(R). Our circulatory system consists of a muscular pumping organ, heart, a network of vessels and a fluid, blood.

1. A correct and R is correct explanation of A

2. A correct and R is also correct but R is not correct explanation of A

3. A correct but R incorrect

4. A and R both are incorrect

48. Read the following statements with respect to Angina-

I. It is also called 'angina pectoris'.

II. Angina pectoris shows symptom of acute chest pain appears when no enough oxygen is reaching the heart muscle.

III. Angina can occur in men and women of any age but it is more common among the middle-aged and elderly.

IV. It occurs due to conditions that affect the blood flow.

How many of them are correct-

1. one   2. two

3. three   4. four

49. Consider the following statements -

A. A specialised cardiac musculature called the nodal tissue is also distributed in the heart.

B. A patch of this tissue is present in the right lower corner of the right atrium called the **sino-atrial node** (SAN).

C. Another mass of this tissue is seen in the upper left corner of the right atrium close to the atrio-ventricular septum called the **atrio-ventricular node** (AVN).

D. A bundle of nodal fibres, atrioventricular bundle (AV bundle) continues from the AVN which passes through the atrio-ventricular septa to emerge on the top of the interventricular septum and immediately divides into a right and left bundle.

Which above statements are correct-

1. A and C only   2. A,B,C only

3. B and C only   4. All are correct

50. Read the following with respect to Blood-

A. Basophils are involved in inflammatory reactions.

B. Eosinophils associated with allergic reactions.

C. B and T lymphocytes are responsible for immune responses of the body.

D. Platelets are cell fragments produced from megakaryocytes

Which of the above statements are correct-

1. A and C only   2. D and A only

3. A,B,C,D   4. A,B,C only

EXCRETORY PRODUCTS AND THEIR ELIMINATION

- In animal kingdom a variety of **excretory** structures present.

- In most of the **invertebrates**, these structures are simple tubular forms whereas vertebrates have complex tubular organs called kidneys.

- **Protonephridia or flame cells** are the excretory structures in Platyhelminthes/Flatworms, rotifers, some annelids and the cephalochordate/*Amphioxus*.

- **Renette cells** are the excretory structures in round worm.

- **Flame cells and Renette** cells are comes under protonephridia category.

- **Protonephridia** are primarily concerned with ionic and fluid volume regulation, i.e., osmoregulation.

- **Nephridia** are the tubular excretory structures of earthworms and other annelids.

- **Nephridia** help to remove nitrogenous wastes and maintain a fluid and ionic balance.

- **Malpighian tubules** are the excretory structures of most of the insects including cockroaches.

- **Malpighian tubules** help in the removal of nitrogenous wastes and osmoregulation.

- **Antennal glands or green glands** perform the excretory function in crustaceans like prawns.

6.1 HUMAN EXCRETORY SYSTEM

- In humans, the excretory system consists of **a pair of kidneys, one pair of ureters, a urinary bladder and a urethra.**

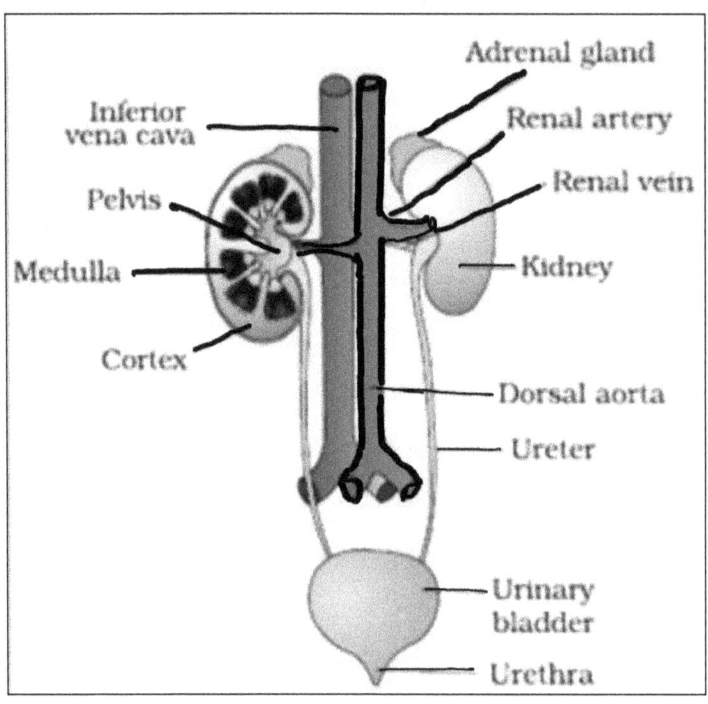

Kidneys

- **Kidneys** are reddish brown, bean shaped structures.

- **Kidneys** are mesodermal in origin.

- **Kidneys** situated between the levels of last thoracic (T_{12}) and third lumbar(L_3) vertebra close to the dorsal inner wall of the abdominal cavity.

a. Size of kidney

- Each kidney of an adult human measures-

  10-12 cm in length, 5-7 cm in width, 2-3 cm in thickness with an average weight of 120- 170 g.

b. Hilum

- Towards the centre of the inner concave surface of the kidney is a notch called hilum.

- Through hilum ureter, blood vessels and nerves passes.

- Inner to the hilum is a broad funnel shaped space called the renal pelvis with projections called calyces.

c. Tough capsule

- The outer layer of kidney is a tough capsule.

- This is made by WFCT.

d. Zones in kidney

- Inside the kidney, there are two zones, an outer *cortex* and an inner *medulla*.

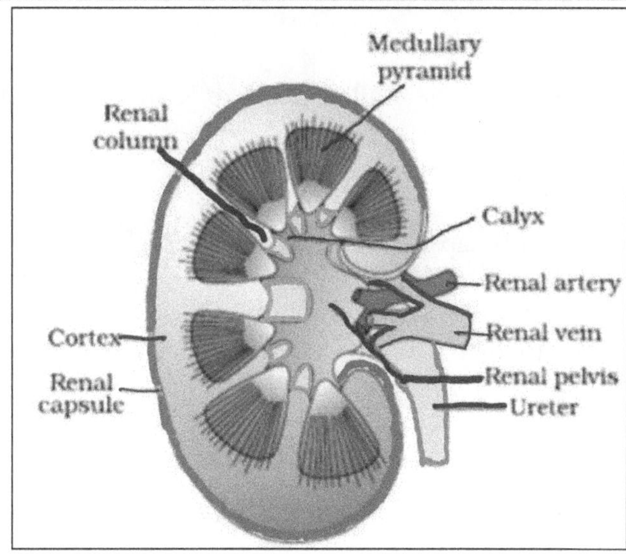

- The medulla is divided into a few conical masses (medullary pyramids) projecting into the calyces (sing.: calyx).

d. Columns of Bertini

- The cortex extends in between the duct and tubule medullary pyramids as renal columns called **Columns of Bertini**
- Columns of Bertini are **pillar like structure.**
- These are extensions **renal cortex.**
- Each kidney has nearly one million complex tubular structures called **nephrons**, which are the functional units.

Nephron

- Each nephron has two parts – the **glomerulus** and the **renal tubule.**

a. Glomerulus

- Glomerulus is a tuft of capillaries formed by the **afferent arteriole** – a fine branch of renal artery.
- Blood from the glomerulus is carried away by an **efferent arteriole.**
- **Diameter** of **efferent arteriole** is more than afferent arteriole.

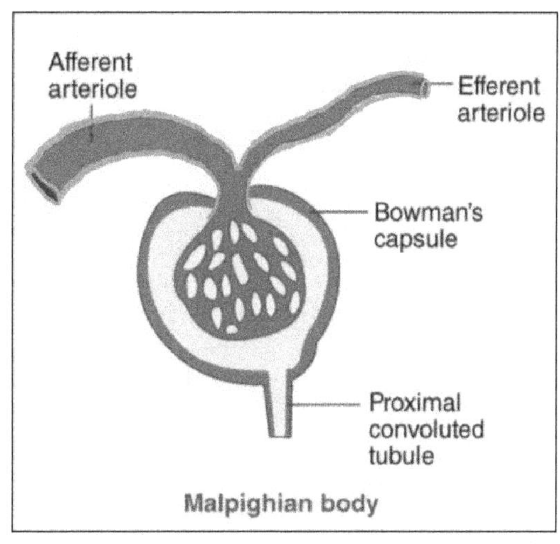

b. Renal tubule

- The renal tubule begins with a double walled cup-like structure called **Bowman's capsule**, which encloses the glomerulus.

c. Malpighian body or renal corpuscle

- Glomerulus along with Bowman's capsule, is called the *malpighian body* or *renal corpuscle.*

d. Proximal convoluted tubule(PCT)

- The tubule continues further to form a highly coiled network – **proximal convoluted tubule(PCT)**.
- PCT lined by cuboidal Epithelium.

e. Henle's loop

- A hairpin shaped **Henle's loop** is the next part of the tubule which has a descending and an ascending limb.

f. Distal convoluted tubule

- The ascending limb continues as another highly coiled tubular region called **distal convoluted tubule (DCT)**.
- DCT lined by Cuboidal epithelium.
- The DCTs of many nephrons open into a **straight tube called *collecting duct,*** many of which converge and open into the renal pelvis through medullary pyramids in the calyces.
- **The Malpighian corpuscle, PCT and DCT of the nephron are situated in the cortical region** of the kidney whereas the **loop of Henle dips into the medulla.**

Points to remember

- In majority of **nephrons**, the loop of Henle is too short and extends only very little into the medulla. Such nephrons are called **cortical** nephrons.
- In some of the **nephrons**, the loop of Henle is very long and runs deep into the medulla.
- These nephrons are called **juxta medullary nephrons.**
- The **efferent arteriole** emerging from the glomerulus forms a fine capillary network around the renal tubule called the peritubular capillaries.
- A minute vessel of this network runs parallel to the **Henle's loop** forming a 'U' shaped *vasa recta*.
- *Vasa recta* is absent or highly reduced in cortical nephrons.

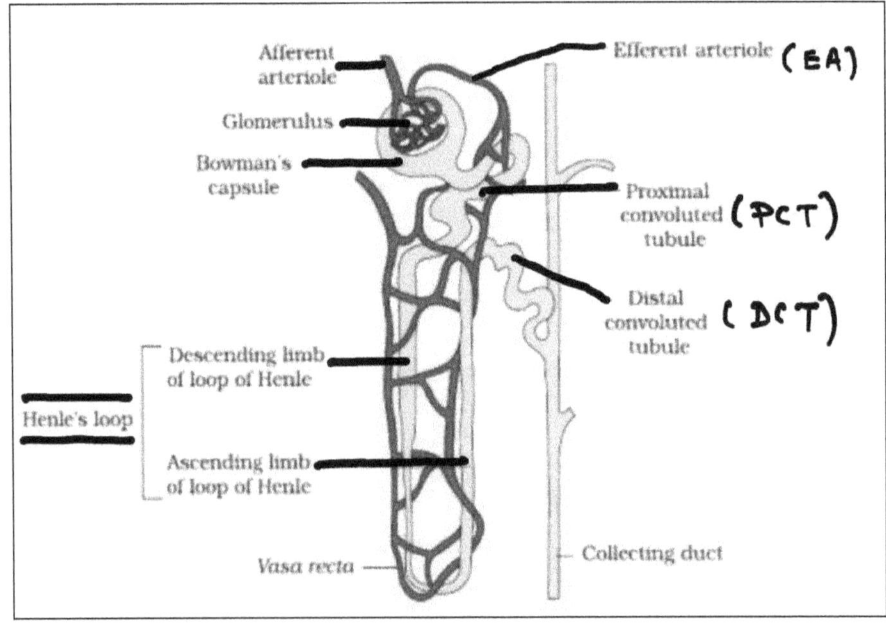

6.2 URINE FORMATION

- Urine formation involves three main processes namely, glomerular filtration, reabsorption and secretion, that takes place in different parts of the nephron.

a. Glomerular filtration/ ultra filtration

- The first step in urine formation is the filtration of blood, which is carried out by the glomerulus and is called **glomerular filtration.**

- On an average, **1100-1200** ml of blood is **filtered** by the **kidneys** per minute which constitute roughly 1/5th of the blood **pumped** out by each **ventricle** of the heart in a minute.

- The **glomerular** capillary blood pressure causes **filtration** of blood through **3** layers, i.e., the **endothelium** of glomerular blood vessels, the **epithelium** of Bowman's capsule and a **basement membrane** between these two layers.

- The epithelial cells of **Bowman's capsule** called **podocytes** are arranged in an intricate manner so as to leave some minute spaces called filtration slits or slit pores.

- Blood is filtered so finely through these membranes,that almost all the constituents of the plasma except the proteins pass onto the lumen of the **Bowman's capsule.**

- Therefore, it is considered as a process of **ultra filtration.**

b. Selective Reabsorption.

- A comparison of the volume of the filtrate formed per day (180 litres per day) with that of the urine released **(1.5 litres)**, suggest that nearly 99 per cent of the filtrate has to be reabsorbed by the renal tubules.

- This process is called **reabsorption.**

- The tubular epithelial cells in different segments of nephron perform **reabsorption** either by active or passive mechanisms.

- For example, substances like **glucose, amino acids, Na$^+$**, etc., in the filtrate are reabsorbed actively whereas the **nitrogenous** wastes are absorbed by **passive transport.**

- **Reabsorption** of **water** also occurs passively in the initial segments of the nephron.

c. Tubular secretion

- During urine formation, the tubular cells secrete substances like **H$^+$, K$^+$ and ammonia** into the filtrate.

- **Tubular secretion** is also an important step in urine formation as it helps in the maintenance of ionic and acid base **balance** of **body fluids.**

Points to remember-

- The amount of the filtrate formed by the kidneys per minute is called **glomerular filtration rate (GFR).**

- **GFR** in a healthy individual is approximately **125** ml/minute, i.e., 180 litres per day.

- The kidneys have built-in mechanisms for the regulation of **glomerular filtration rate.**

- One such efficient mechanism is carried out by juxta glomerular apparatus (**JGA**).

- **JGA** is a special sensitive region formed by cellular modifications in the distal convoluted tubule and the afferent arteriole at the location of their contact

- .A fall in **GFR** can activate the **JG** cells to release renin which can stimulate the glomerular blood flow and thereby the **GFR** back to normal.

6.3 FUNCTION OF THE TUBULES

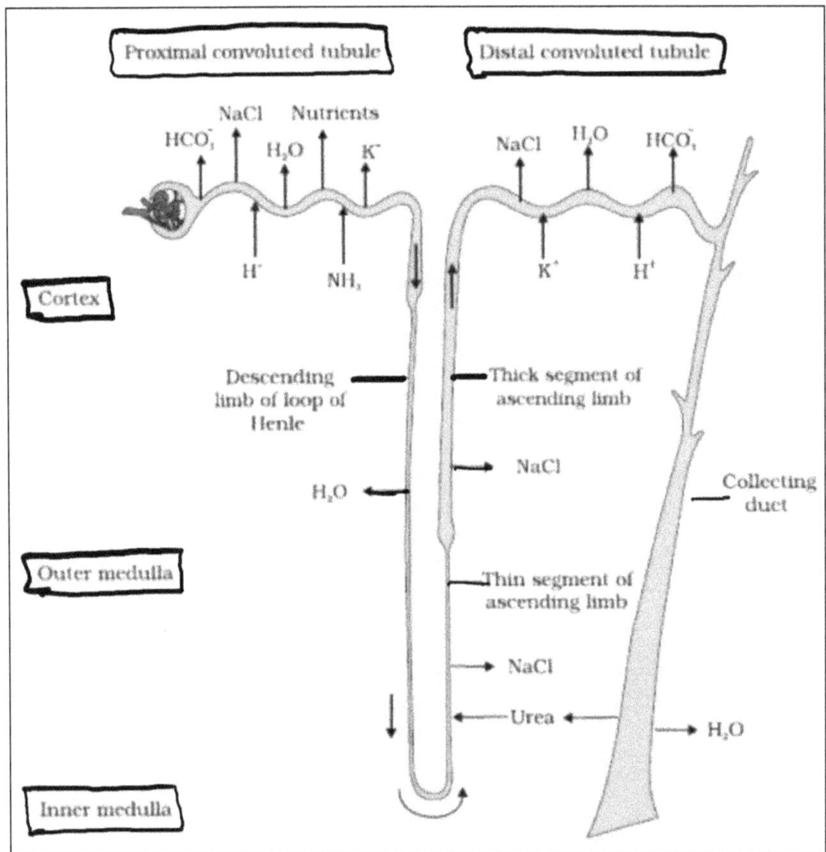

a. Proximal Convoluted Tubule (PCT):

- PCT is lined by simple **cuboidal brush** border epithelium which increases the surface area for reabsorption.
- Nearly all of the essential nutrients, and **70-80** per cent of electrolytes and water are reabsorbed by this segment.
- PCT also helps to maintain the **pH** and **ionic balance** of the body fluids by selective secretion of hydrogen ions, ammonia and potassium ions into the filtrate and by **absorption** of HCO3⁻ from it.

b. Henle's Loop:

- Reabsorption in this segment is **minimum**.
- Henle loop region plays a significant role in the maintenance of high osmolarity of medullary **interstitial fluid**.
- The **descending limb** of loop of Henle is **permeable** to water but almost **impermeable** to electrolytes.
- The **descending** limb of loop of Henle is **permeable concentrates** the filtrate as it moves down.
- The ascending limb is **impermeable** to **water** but allows transport of electrolytes actively or passively.
- Therefore, as the **concentrated** filtrate pass upward, it gets diluted due to the passage of electrolytes to the medullary fluid.

c. Distal Convoluted Tubule (DCT):

- Conditional reabsorption of **Na⁺** and **water** takes place in this segment.
- DCT is also capable of reabsorption of **HCO3 ⁻** and selective secretion of hydrogen and **potassium** ions and NH3 to **maintain** the pH and **sodium-potassium** balance in blood.

d. Collecting Duct:

- This long duct extends from the **cortex** of the **kidney** to the inner parts of the medulla.
- Large amounts of water could be **reabsorbed** from this region to produce a concentrated urine.
- This segment allows passage of **small amounts** of urea into the medullary interstitium to keep up the osmolarity.
- It also plays a role in the maintenance of pH and ionic balance of blood by the selective secretion of **H⁺** and **K⁺** ions.

6.4 MECHANISM OF CONCENTRATION OF THE FILTRATE

- Mammals have the **ability** to produce a **concentrated** urine.
- The Henle's loop and *vasa recta* play a significant role to produce a **concentrated** urine.
- The flow of filtrate in the two limbs of Henle's loop is in **opposite directions** and thus forms a counter current.
- The flow of blood through the two limbs of *vasa recta* is also in a **counter current** pattern.
- The **proximity** between the **Henle's loop** and *vasa recta*, as well as the **counter current** in them help in maintaining an increasing **osmolarity** towards the inner medullary interstitium, i.e., from **300 mOsmolL⁻¹** in the cortex to about **1200 mOsmolL⁻¹** in the inner medulla.
- This gradient is mainly caused by **NaCl** and **urea**.
- NaCl is **transported** by the **ascending** limb of Henle's loop which is exchanged with the descending limb of *vasa recta*.
- NaCl is returned to the interstitium by the **ascending** portion of *vasa recta*.
- The **small amounts** of urea enter the thin segment of the ascending limb of Henle's loop which is transported back to the **interstitium** by the collecting tubule.
- The above described **transport** of substances **facilitated** by the special arrangement of Henle's loop and *vasa recta* is called the **counter current mechanism** in the **medullary interstitium**.

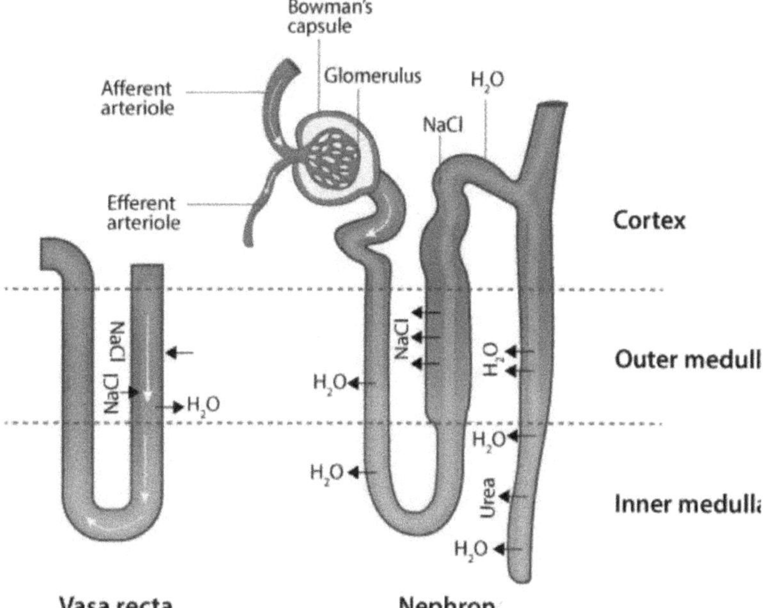

- Presence of such **interstitial** gradient helps in an easy passage of water from the collecting tubule thereby **concentrating** the filtrate (urine).
- Human kidneys can produce urine nearly **four times** concentrated than the initial filtrate formed.

6.5 REGULATION OF KIDNEY FUNCTION

The functioning of the kidneys is efficiently monitored and regulated by hormonal feedback mechanisms involving the **ADH, Renin-Angiotensin mechanism** and **ANF.**

a. ADH

- Osmoreceptors in the body are activated by changes in blood volume, body fluid volume and ionic concentration.
- An excessive loss of fluid from the body can activate these **receptors** which stimulate the **hypothalamus** to release antidiuretic hormone (**ADH**) or **vasopressin** from the neurohypophysis.
- **ADH** facilitates water reabsorption from latter parts of the tubule, thereby preventing diuresis.
- An increase in body fluid volume can switch off the osmoreceptors and suppress the ADH release to complete the feedback.
- **ADH** can also affect the kidney function by its constrictory effects on blood vessels.
- This causes an increase in blood pressure

b. Renin-Angiotensin mechanism

- An **increase** in blood pressure can increase the glomerular blood flow and thereby the GFR.
- The JGA plays a **complex regulatory** role.
- A fall in glomerular blood flow/glomerular blood pressure/GFR can activate the JG cells to release **renin** which converts **angiotensinogen** in blood to **angiotensin** I and further to angiotensin II.
- Angiotensin II, being a **powerful vasoconstrictor**, increases the glomerular blood pressure and thereby GFR.
- **Angiotensin** II also activates the adrenal cortex to release Aldosterone.
- Aldosterone causes reabsorption of Na^+ and water from the distal parts of the tubule.
- This also leads to an increase in blood pressure and GFR.
- This complex mechanism is generally known as the **Renin-Angiotensin** mechanism.

c. **Atrial Natriuretic Factor**

- An increase in blood flow to the atria of the heart can cause the release of **Atrial Natriuretic Factor** (ANF).
- **ANF** can cause vasodilation (dilation of blood vessels) and thereby decrease the blood pressure.
- **ANF** mechanism acts as a check on the renin-angiotensin mechanism.

6.6 MICTURITION

- Urine formed by the nephrons is ultimately carried to the urinary bladder where it is stored till a voluntary signal is given by the central nervous system (**CNS**).

- This **signal** is initiated by the **stretching** of the **urinary bladder** as it gets filled with urine.

- In response, the stretch receptors on the walls of the bladder send signals to the CNS.

- The **CNS passes** on **motor messages** initiate the contraction of smooth muscles of the bladder and simultaneous relaxation of the **urethral sphincter** causing the release of urine.

- **Detrusor** muscles present in the wall of **urinary bladder** which helps urine to push down.

- The process of release of urine is called **micturition** and the neural mechanisms causing it is called the micturition reflex.

Urine

- **An adult human excretes, on an average, 1 to 1.5 litres of urine per day.**

- The urine formed is a light yellow coloured watery fluid which is slightly acidic (pH-6.0) and has a characterestic odour.

- On an average, **25-30** gm of urea is excreted out per day.

- Various conditions can affect the characteristics of urine.

Analysis of urine helps in clinical diagnosis

- Analysis of **urine** helps in clinical diagnosis of many **metabolic** discorders as well as malfunctioning of the kidney.

- For example, **presence of glucose (Glycosuria) and ketone bodies (Ketonuria)** in urine are indicative of diabetes mellitus.

6.7 ROLE OF OTHER ORGANS IN EXCRETION

- Other than the kidneys, lungs, liver and skin also help in the elimination of excretory wastes.

Lungs

- Our lungs remove **large amounts** of CO_2 and also **significant** quantities of water every day.

Liver

- Liver, the largest gland in our body, secretes bile-containing substances like bilirubin, **biliverdin,cholesterol,** degraded **steroid** hormones, **vitamins** and **drugs**.

- Most of these substances ultimately pass out alongwith digestive wastes.

Skin

- The **sweat** and **sebaceous** glands in the skin can eliminate certain substances through their secretions.

- Sweat produced by the sweat glands is a watery fluid containing **NaCl, small amounts of urea, lactic acid,** etc.

- Though the primary function of **sweat** is to facilitate a cooling effect on the body surface, it also helps in the removal of some of the wastes mentioned above.

- Sebaceous glands eliminate certain substances like **sterols, hydrocarbons** and waxes through sebum.
- This secretion provides a protective **oily** covering for the skin.
- **Small amounts** of nitrogenous wastes could be eliminated through saliva too.

6.8 DISORDERS OF THE EXCRETORY SYSTEM

Uremia

- **Malfunctioning** of kidneys can lead to accumulation of urea in blood, a condition called **uremia**, which is highly harmful and may lead to kidney failure.
- In such **patients**, urea can be removed by a process called **hemodialysis**.

Hemodialysis

- Blood drained from a **convenient artery** is pumped into a dialysing unit after adding an anticoagulant like **heparin**.
- The unit contains a coiled **cellophane tube**.
- These tubes surrounded by a fluid (dialysing fluid) having the **same composition as that of plasma** except the nitrogenous wastes.
- The porous cellophane membrane of the tube allow the passage of molecules **based on concentration gradient**.
- The **nitrogenous wastes are absent** in the dialysing fluid, these substances freely move out, thereby clearing the blood.
- The cleared blood is pumped back to the body through a vein after **adding anti-heparin** to it.
- This method is a boon for thousands of uremic patients all over the world.

Kidney transplantation

- Kidney transplantation is the **ultimate** method in the correction of acute **renal failures** (kidney failure).
- A functioning kidney is used in **transplantation** from a donor, preferably a close relative, to minimise its chances of **rejection** by the immune system of the host.
- Modern clinical methods have **increased** the success rate of such a complicated technique.

Renal calculi:

- Stone or insoluble mass of **crystallised** salts (oxalates, etc.) formed within the kidney.

Glomerulonephritis:

- Inflammation of **glomeruli** of kidney.

1. Consider the following statements and find out the correct option-

A. In humans, the excretory system consists of a pair of kidneys, one pair of ureters, a urinary bladder and a urethra.

B. Kidneys are reddish brown, bean shaped structures situated between the levels of last thoracic and third lumbar vertebra close to the dorsal inner wall of the abdominal cavity.

C. Each kidney of an adult human measures 10-12 cm in length, 5-7 cm in width, 2-3 cm in thickness with an average weight of 120- 170 g.

D. Towards the centre of the inner convex surface of the kidney is a notch called hilum through which ureter, blood vessels and nerves enter.

Which of the above are correct with respect to humans-

1. A,D,C

2. B,C

3. A,B,C

4. A,B,C,D

2. Match the list 1 and 2-

List 1   List 2

a. Protonephridia	j. leech
b. Nephridia	k. insects
c. Malpighian tubules	l. flatworm
d. Antennal glands	m. crustacea

Find out the correct option –

1. a.k, b.j, c.l, d.m

2. a.k,b.l,c.j,d.m

3. a.l,b.j,c.k,d.m

4. a.l,b.j,c.m,d.k

3. Consider the following statements-

    I. JGA is a special sensitive region formed by cellular modifications in the distal convoluted tubule and the afferent arteriole at the location of their contact

    II. A fall in GFR can activate the JG cells to release renin which can stimulate the glomerular blood flow and thereby the GFR back to normal.

    III. A comparison of the volume of the filtrate formed per day (180 litres per day) with that of the urine released (1.5 litres).

    IV. Nearly 20 per cent of the filtrate has to be reabsorbed by the renal tubules.

How many of them are/is correct w.r.t. Human-

1. one

2. two

3. three

4. four

4. Read the following statement carefully with respect to Humans-

    I. The substances like glucose, amino acids, Na^+, etc., in the filtrate are reabsorbed actively whereas the nitrogenous wastes are absorbed by passive transport.

    II. Reabsorption of water also occurs passively in the initial segments of the nephron.

    III. During urine formation, the tubular cells secrete substances like H^+, K^+ and ammonia into the filtrate.

    IV. Tubular secretion is also an important step in urine formation as it helps in the maintenance of ionic and acid base balance of body fluids.

How many of them are/is correct -

1. three

2. four

3. one

4. two

5. Consider the following statements and find out the correct option-

STATEMENT 1. Each kidney of an adult human measures 10-12 cm in length.

STATEMENT 2. Towards the centre of the inner concave surface of the kidney is a notch called hilum through which ureter, blood vessels and nerves passes.

5. Both are correct statements

6. Only Statement 1 correct

7. Both are wrong statements

8. Only statement 2 correct

6. Go through the following statement and find out the correct -

ASSERTION(A). The medulla is divided into a few conical masses (medullary pyramids) projecting into the calyces (sing.: calyx).

REASON(R). The cortex extends in between the duct and tubule medullary pyramids as renal columns called **Columns of Bertini.**

1. A correct and R is correct explanation of A

2. A correct and R is also correct but R is not correct explanation of A

3. A. correct but R incorrect

4. A and R both are incorrect

7. Which one is an incorrect statement -

1. Each kidney has nearly one million complex tubular structures called **nephrons** which are the functional units.

2. Each nephron has two parts – the glomerulus and the renal tubule.

3. Glomerulus is a tuft of capillaries formed by the afferent arteriole – a fine branch of renal artery.

4. Blood from the glomerulus is carried away by an afferent arteriole.

8. Go through the following statements-

I. In some of the nephrons, the loop of Henle is very long and runs deep into the medulla.

II. These above nephrons are called juxta medullary nephrons.

III. The efferent arteriole emerging from the glomerulus forms a fine capillary network around the renal tubule called the peritubular capillaries.

IV. A minute vessel runs parallel to the Henle's loop forming a 'U' shaped *vasa recta*.

V. *Vasa recta* is absent or highly reduced in cortical nephrons.

How many of them are correct-

1. two

2. three

3. four

4. five

9. Match the list 1 and 2-

List 1	List 2
a. An adult human excretes, on an average urine per day	j. 6.0
b. The pH of urine	k. 25-30 gm
c. On an average urea is excreted out per day	l. 1 to 1.5 litres
d. Presence of glucose in urine	m. Glycosuria

Find out the correct option –

1. a.k, b.j, c.l, d.m

2. a.k,b.l,c.j,d.m

3. a.l,b.j,c.k,d.m

4. a.l,b.j,c.m,d.k

10. Consider the following statements and find out the correct option

STATEMENT 1. Urine formed by the nephrons is ultimately carried to the urinary bladder where it is stored till a voluntary signal is given by the central nervous system (CNS).

STATEMENT 2. This signal is initiated by the stretching of the urinary bladder as it gets filled with urine.

1. Both are wrong statements

2. Only statement 1 correct

3. Both are correct statements

4. Only statement 2 correct

11. Read the following statements very carefully and find out the incorrect-

a) Angiotensin II, being a powerful vasoconstrictor, increases the glomerular blood pressure and thereby GFR. Angiotensin II also activates the adrenal cortex to release Aldosterone.

b) Aldosterone causes reabsorption of Na+ and water from the distal parts of the tubule.

c) Aldosterone also leads to an decrease in blood pressure and GFR.

d) The above mechanism is generally known as the **Renin-Angiotensin** mechanism.

Which of the above statement are/is incorrect?

1. a and c both

2. a,b,c,d

3. c only

4. b and d both

12. Go through the following statement-

ASSERTION(A). An increase in blood flow to the atria of the heart can cause the release of **Atrial Natriuretic Factor** (ANF).

REASON(R). ANF can cause vasodilation (dilation of blood vessels) and thereby decrease the blood pressure

1. A correct and R is correct explanation of A

2. A correct and R is also correct but R is not correct explanation of A

3. A correct but R incorrect

4. A and R both are incorrect

13. Find out incorrect statement with respect to Humans-

1. Urine formed by the nephrons is ultimately carried to the urinary bladder where it is stored till a voluntary signal is given by the central nervous system (CNS).

2. This signal is initiated by the stretching of the urinary bladder as it gets filled with urine.

3. In response, the stretch receptors on the walls of the bladder send signals to the CNS.

4. The CNS passes on motor messages to initiate the contraction of smooth muscles of the bladder and simultaneous contraction of the urethral sphincter causing the release of urine.

14. Read the following statements and find out correct option-

I. Other than the kidneys, lungs, liver and skin also help in the elimination of excretory wastes.

II. Our lungs remove large amounts of CO_2 and also significant quantities of water every day.

III. Liver, the largest gland in our body, secretes bile-containing substances like bilirubin, biliverdin, cholesterol, degraded steroid hormones, vitamins and drugs.

IV. Most of these substances ultimately pass out alongwith digestive wastes.

How many of them are correct-

1. four

2. one

3. two

4. three

15. Consider the following statements and find out the correct option

STATEMENT 1. The sweat and sebaceous glands in the skin can eliminate certain substances through their secretions.

STATEMENT 2. Sweat produced by the sweat glands is a watery fluid containing NaCl, small amounts of urea, lactic acid, etc.

1. Both are wrong statements

2. Only Statement 1 correct

3. Both are correct statements

4. Only statement 2 correct

16. Match the list 1 and 2 -

List 1   List 2

a. **Renal calculi**	Stone or insoluble mass of crystallised salts (oxalates, etc.) formed within the kidney.
b. **Glomerulonephritis**	Inflammation of glomeruli of kidney.
c. **Acute renal failures**	Kidney transplantation is the ultimate method in the correction

Which of the above are correctly matched-

1. a and b

2. b and c

3. c and a

4. a, b, c

17. Consider the following statements w.r.t. Haemodialysis-

a) The unit contains a coiled cellophane tube surrounded by a fluid (dialysing fluid) having the same composition as that of plasma except the nitrogenous wastes.

b) As nitrogenous wastes are absent in the dialysing fluid, these excretory substances freely move out, thereby clearing the blood.

c) The cleared blood is pumped back to the body through a vein after adding anti-heparin to it.

Which of the above statement are correct?

1. a and b only

2. c and b only

3. a and c only

4. a,b,c

18. Consider the following statements-

a) Sweat produced by the sweat glands is a watery fluid containing NaCl, small amounts of urea, lactic acid, etc.

b) The sweat facilitates a cooling effect on the body surface and also helps in the removal of some of the wastes mentioned above.

c) Sebaceous glands eliminate certain substances like sterols, hydrocarbons and waxes through sebum.

d) The secretion of oil glands provides a protective oily covering for the skin.

Which of the above statement are correct?

1. a and d only

2. c and a only

3. d and b only

4. a,b,c,d

19. Consider the following statements and find out the incorrect one-

1. An excessive loss of fluid from the body can activate these receptors which stimulate the hypothalamus to release antidiuretic hormone (ADH) or vasopressin from the neurohypophysis.

2. ADH facilitates water reabsorption from latter parts of the tubule, thereby preventing diuresis.

3. An increase in body fluid volume can switch off the osmoreceptors and suppress the ADH release to complete the feedback.

4. ADH can also affect the kidney function by its dilatory effects on blood vessels.

20. Read the following statements-

I. A fall in glomerular blood flow/glomerular blood pressure/GFR can activate the JG cells to release renin which converts angiotensinogen in blood to angiotensin I and further to angiotensin II.

II. Angiotensin II, being a powerful vasoconstrictor, increases the glomerular blood pressure and thereby GFR. Angiotensin II also activates the adrenal cortex to release Aldosterone.

III. Aldosterone causes reabsorption of Na^+ and water from the distal parts of the tubule.

IV. Reabsorption of Na^+ and water from the distal parts of the tubule leads to an increase in blood pressure and GFR.

How many of them are/is correct **statements-**

1. two

2. three

3. four

4. one

21. Consider the following statements and find out the correct option for humans-

STATEMENT 1. The functioning of the kidneys is efficiently monitored and regulated by hormonal feedback mechanisms involving the hypothalamus, JGA and to a certain extent, the heart.

STATEMENT 2. Osmoreceptors in the body are activated by changes in blood volume, body fluid volume and ionic concentration.

1. Both are wrong statements

2. Only statement 1 correct

3. Both are correct statements

4. Only statement 2 correct

22. Go through the following statement and find out the correct option-

ASSERTION(A). Angiotensin II, being a powerful vasoconstrictor, increases the glomerular blood pressure and GFR.

REASON(R). Angiotensin II also activates the adrenal cortex to release Aldosterone.

1. A correct and R is correct explanation of A

2. A correct and R is also correct but R is not correct explanation of A

3. A correct but R incorrect

4. A and R both are incorrect

23. Go through the following statement and find out the correct option-

A. Mammals have the ability to produce a concentrated urine.

B. The Henle's loop and *vasa recta* play a significant role in this.

C. The flow of filtrate in the two limbs of Henle's loop is in opposite directions and thus forms a counter current.

D. The flow of blood through the two limbs of *vasa recta* is also found in a counter current pattern.

Which of the above statement are/is correct -

1. A and C only

2. A,B,C only

3. B,C only

4. A,B,C,D

24. Read the statements given below-

A. The proximity between the Henle's loop and *vasa recta*, as well as the counter current in them help in maintaining an increasing osmolarity towards the inner medullary interstitium, i.e., from 300 mOsmolL^{-1} in the cortex to about 1200 mOsmolL^{-1} in the inner medulla.

B. This gradient is mainly caused by NaCl and urea.

C. NaCl is transported by the ascending limb of Henle's loop which is exchanged with the descending limb of *vasa recta*.

D. NaCl is returned to the interstitium by the ascending portion of *vasa recta*.

E. The small amounts of urea enter the thin segment of the ascending limb of Henle's loop which is transported back to the interstitium by the collecting tubule.

F. The above described transport of substances facilitated by the special arrangement of Henle's loop and *vasa recta* is called the **counter current mechanism** in the medullary interstitium.

Which above statement are correct?

1. A,B,C,D only

2. B,C only

3. A,B,C,D,E only

4. A,B,C,D,E,F

25. Consider the following-

A. Henle's Loop: Reabsorption in this segment is maximum.

B. Henle's Loop plays a significant role in the maintenance of high osmolarity of medullary interstitial fluid.

C. The descending limb of loop of Henle is permeable to water but almost impermeable to electrolytes.

Which of the above statement are/is correct?

1. A,B only

2. A only

3. B and C only

4. A,B,C

26. Consider the following statements-

I. Distal Convoluted Tubule (DCT): Conditional reabsorption of Na^+ and water takes place in this segment.

II. DCT is also capable of reabsorption of bicarbonate ions and selective secretion of hydrogen and potassium ions and NH3 to maintain the pH and sodium-potassium balance in blood.

III. Collecting duct extends from the cortex of the kidney to the inner parts of the medulla.

IV. Large amounts of water could be reabsorbed from collecting duct to produce a concentrated urine.

How many of them are correct-

1. one

2. two

3. three

4. four

27. Match the list 1 and 2-

List 1   List 2

a. *Amphioxus*	Protonephridia
b. Earthworms	Nephridia
c. Prawns	Antennal glands
d. Insects	Malpighian tubules

How many of them are correctly matched –

1. one

2. two

3. three

4. four

28. Consider the following statements-

a) The cortex extends in between the duct and tubule medullary pyramids as renal columns called **Columns of Bertini**

b) Each kidney has nearly one million complex tubular structures called **nephrons**, which are the functional units.

c) Each nephron has two parts – the glomerulus and the renal tubule.

d) Glomerulus is a tuft of capillaries formed by the afferent arteriole – a fine branch of renal artery.

e) Blood from the glomerulus is carried away by an efferent arteriole.

f) The renal tubule begins with a double walled cup-like structure called **Bowman's capsule**, which encloses the glomerulus.

Which of the above statements are correct-

1. a and c only

2. a,b,c,d,e only

3. d and c only

4. all are correct

29. Consider the following statements and find out incorrect one-

1. Glomerulus along with PCT, is called the *malpighian body* or *renal corpuscle.*

2. The tubule continues further to form a highly coiled network – **proximal convoluted tubule**(PCT).

3. A hairpin shaped part of nephron is called **Henle's loop.**

4. The ascending limb continues as another highly coiled tubular region called **distal convoluted tubule** (DCT).

30. Read the following points -

a) The DCTs of many nephrons open into a straight tube called *collecting duct*, many of which converge and open into the renal pelvis through medullary pyramids in the calyces.

b) The Malpighian corpuscle, PCT and DCT of the nephron are situated in the cortical region of the kidney whereas the loop of Henle dips into the medulla.

c) In majority of nephrons, the loop of Henle is too short and extends only very little into the medulla.

d) Such nephrons are called cortical nephrons.

e) In some of the nephrons, the loop of Henle is very long and runs deep into the medulla.

f) The above nephrons are called juxta medullary nephrons.

How many of them are correct –

1. four 2. six

3. three 4. two

31. Read the following statements and find out the correct option

STATEMENT 1. A minute vessel of network runs parallel to the Henle's loop forming a 'U' shaped *vasa recta.*

STATEMENT 2. *Vasa recta* is absent or highly reduced in cortical nephrons.

1. Both are wrong statements 2. Both are correct statements

3. Only statement 1 correct 4. Only statement 2 correct

32. Go through the following statement and find out the correct option-

ASSERTION(A). On an average, 1100-1200 ml of blood is filtered by the kidneys per minute which constitute roughly 1/5th of the blood pumped out by each ventricle of the heart in a minute.

REASON(R). The glomerular capillary blood pressure causes filtration of blood through 3 layers, i.e., the endothelium of glomerular blood vessels, the epithelium of Bowman's capsule and a basement membrane between these two layers.

1. A correct and R is correct explanation of A

2. A correct and R is also correct but R is not correct explanation of A

3. A. correct but R incorrect

4. A and R both are incorrect

33. Find out the incorrect statement-

1. On an average, 1100-1200 ml of blood is filtered by the kidneys per minute which constitute roughly 1/5th of the blood pumped out by each ventricle of the heart in a minute.

2. The glomerular capillary blood pressure causes filtration of blood through 3 layers, i.e., the endothelium of glomerular blood vessels, the epithelium of Bowman's capsule and a basement membrane between these two layers.

3. The epithelial cells of Bowman's capsule called podocytes are arranged in an intricate manner so as to leave some minute spaces called filtration slits or slit pores.

4. Blood is filtered so finely through these membranes and the proteins pass onto the lumen of the Bowman's capsule.

34. Read the following –

I. The amount of the filtrate formed by the kidneys per minute is called **glomerular filtration rate** (GFR). GFR in a healthy individual is approximately 125 ml/minute, i.e., 180 litres per hour.

II. The kidneys have built-in mechanisms for the regulation of glomerular filtration rate.

III. JGA is a special sensitive region formed by cellular modifications in the PCT and the afferent arteriole at the location of their contact

IV. A fall in GFR can activate the JG cells to release renin which can stimulate the glomerular blood flow and thereby the GFR back to normal.

How many of above is/are incorrect-

1. three	2. four
3. two	4. one

35. Renal calculi mostly made by-

1. Ca-oxalate	2. Ca-Carbonate
3. $KmnO_4$	4. Uric acid

36. Consider the following statements –

i. The tubular epithelial cells in different segments of nephron perform **reabsorption** either by active or passive mechanisms.

ii. The substances like glucose, amino acids, Na+, etc., in the filtrate are reabsorbed actively whereas the nitrogenous wastes are absorbed by passive transport.

iii. Reabsorption of water also occurs passively in the initial segments of the nephron.

iv. During urine formation, the tubular cells secrete substances like H^+, K^+ and ammonia into the filtrate.

Which of the above statements are correct w.r.t. Nephron-

1. i,ii only	2. i, iii,iv only
3. i,ii,iii only	4. all are correct

37. Read the following statements-

   i. A fall in GFR can activate the JG cells to release renin which can stimulate the glomerular blood flow and thereby the GFR back to normal.

   ii. A comparison of the volume of the filtrate formed per day (180 litres per day) with that of the urine released (1.5 litres).

   iii. Nearly 99 per cent of the filtrate has to be reabsorbed by the renal tubule process is called **reabsorption**.

   iv. The tubular epithelial cells in different segments of nephron perform **reabsorption** either by active or passive mechanisms.

Which above statements is/are correct-

1. i and ii only	2. iii And ii only
3. iv and iii only	4. All are correct

38. Consider the following statements-

   a) Proximal Convoluted Tubule (PCT) is lined by simple cuboidal brush border epithelium

   b) This tissue increases the surface area for reabsorption.

   c) Nearly all of the essential nutrients, and 70-80 per cent of electrolytes and water are reabsorbed by this segment.

   d) PCT also helps to maintain the pH and ionic balance of the body fluids by selective secretion of hydrogen ions, ammonia and potassium ions into the filtrate and by absorption of HCO_3^- from it.

How many of above are correct-

1. three	2. four
3. two	4. one

39. Read the following statements and find out the correct option-

STATEMENT 1. DCT is also capable of reabsorption of HCO_3^- and selective secretion of hydrogen and potassium ions and NH_3 to maintain the pH and sodium-potassium balance in blood.

STATEMENT 2. PCT also helps to maintain the pH and ionic balance of the body fluids by selective secretion of hydrogen ions, ammonia and potassium ions into the filtrate and by absorption of HCO_3^- from it.

1. Both are wrong statements	2. Both are correct statements
3. Only statement 1 correct	4. Only statement 2 correct

40. Read the following statements-

   a) ADH can also affect the kidney function by its constrictory effects on blood vessels which causes an increase in blood pressure

   b) An increase in blood pressure can increase the glomerular blood flow and thereby the GFR.

   c) The JGA plays a complex regulatory role.

   d) A fall in glomerular blood flow/glomerular blood pressure/GFR can activate the JG cells to release **renin** which converts angiotensinogen in blood to angiotensin I and further to angiotensin II.

e) Angiotensin II, being a powerful vasoconstrictor, increases the glomerular blood pressure and thereby GFR.

Which of the above are correct?

1. a and b only

2. b and c only

3. a, b, c, d only

4. All are correct

41. Go through the following statement and find out the correct option-

ASSERTION. Sebaceous glands eliminate certain substances like sterols, hydrocarbons and waxes through sebum.

REASON. Sweat produced by the sweat glands is a watery fluid containing NaCl, small amounts of urea, lactic acid, etc.

1. A correct and R is correct explanation of A

2. A correct and R is also correct but R is not correct explanation of A

3. A correct but R incorrect

4. A and R both are incorrect

42. Find out the incorrect statement-

1. Malfunctioning of kidneys can lead to accumulation of urea in blood, a condition called **uremia,** which is highly harmful and may lead to kidney failure.

2. In such patients, urea can be removed by a process called **hemodialysis.**

3. Blood drained from a convenient vein is pumped into a dialysing unit after removing an anticoagulant like heparin.

4. The unit contains a coiled cellophane tube surrounded by a fluid (dialysing fluid) having the same composition as that of plasma except the nitrogenous wastes.

43. Consider the following statements-

a) Kidney transplantation is the ultimate method in the correction of acute **renal failures** (kidney failure).

b) A functioning kidney is used in transplantation from a donor, preferably a close relative, to minimise its chances of rejection by the immune system of the host.

c) Modern clinical procedures have increased the success rate of such a complicated technique.

d) Renal calculi: Stone or insoluble mass of crystallised salts (oxalates, etc.) formed within the kidney.

e) Glomerulonephritis: Inflammation of glomeruli of kidney.

How many of them are correct-

1. five

2. three

3. four

4. two

44. Read the following statements and find out the correct option –

STATEMENT 1. Protonephridia, nephridia, malpighian tubules, green glands and the kidneys are the common excretory organs in animals.

STATEMENT 2. Protonephridia, nephridia, malpighian tubules, green glands and the kidneys not only eliminate nitrogenous wastes but also help in the maintenance of ionic and acid-base balance of body fluids.

1. Both are correct statements

2. Both are wrong statements

3. Only statement 1 correct

4.Only statement 2 correct

45. Which statements is incorrect -

1. The process of release of urine is called micturition and the neural mechanisms causing it is called the micturition reflex.

2. An adult human excretes, on an average, 1 to 1.5 litres of urine per day.

3. On an average, 25-30 gm of urea is excreted out per day.

4. Various conditions of body can not affect the characteristics of urine.

46. Read the following statements and find out the correct option

STATEMENT 1. The presence of glucose (Glycosuria) and ketone bodies (Ketonuria) in urine are indicative of diabetes mellitus.

STATEMENT 2. Urine formed by the nephrons is ultimately carried to the urinary bladder where it is stored till a voluntary signal is given by the central nervous system (CNS).

1.Both are correct statements

2. Both are wrong statements.

3. Only statement 1 correct

4. Only statement 2 correct

47. Go through the following statement and find out the correct option-

ASSERTION(A). A fall in glomerular blood flow/glomerular blood pressure/GFR can activate the JG cells to release **renin** which converts angiotensinogen in blood to angiotensin I and further to angiotensin II.

REASON(R). ADH facilitates water reabsorption from latter parts of the tubule, so preventing diuresis.

1. A correct and R is correct explanation of A

2. A correct and R is also correct but R is not correct explanation of A

3. A correct but R incorrect

4. A and R both are incorrect

48. Find out the incorrect statement –

1. Mammals do not have the ability to produce a concentrated urine.

2. The Henle's loop and *vasa recta* play a significant role to produce a concentrated urine.

3. The flow of filtrate in the two limbs of Henle's loop is in opposite directions and thus forms a counter current.

4. The flow of blood through the two limbs of *vasa recta* is also in a counter current pattern.

49. Consider the following statements -

A. The proximity between the Henle's loop and *vasa recta*, as well as the counter current in them help in maintaining an increasing osmolarity towards the inner medullary interstitium, i.e., from 300 mOsmolL^{-1} in the cortex to about 1200 mOsmolL^{-1} in the inner medulla.

B. The small amounts of urea enter the thin segment of the ascending limb of Henle's loop which is transported back to the interstitium by the collecting tubule.

C. The above described transport of substances facilitated by the special arrangement of Henle's loop and *vasa recta* is called the **counter current mechanism** in the medullary interstitium.

Which of the above statements are/is correct-

1. A and C only

2. B and A only

3. B and C only

4. All are correct

50. Read the following -

A. **Collecting Duct** extends from the cortex of the kidney to the inner parts of the medulla.

B. The water could be reabsorbed from **Collecting Duct** helps to produce a concentrated urine.

C. **Collecting Duct** segment allows passage of small amounts of urea into the medullary interstitium to keep up the osmolarity.

D. **Collecting Duct** also plays a role in the maintenance of pH and ionic balance of blood by the selective secretion of H$^+$ and K$^+$ ions

Which of the above statements are/is correct-

1. A and C only

2. D and A only

3. B and D only

4. All are correct

LOCOMOTION AND MOVEMENT

7.1 Types of Movement

7.2 Muscle

7.3 Skeletal System

7.4 Joints

7.5 Disorders of Muscular and Skeletal System

- **Movement** is one of the significant features of living organisms.
- Animals and plants **shows** a wide range of movements.
- Streaming of **protoplasm** in the unicellular organisms like *Amoeba* is a simple form of movement.
- Movement of cilia, flagella and **tentacles** are shown by many organisms.
- **Human** beings can move limbs, jaws, eyelids, tongue, etc.
- The change in position on same place known as **movement**. Example plants
- The change in place is called **locomotion**. Example animals
- Walking, **running**, climbing, flying, swimming are some forms of locomotory movements.
- **Locomotory** structures need not be different from those affecting other types of movements.
- In *Paramoecium*, cilia helps in the movement of food through cytopharynx and in locomotion as well.
- *Hydra* can use its tentacles for capturing its prey and also use them for locomotion.
- We use limbs for **changes** in body postures and locomotion as well.
- The movements and **locomotion** cannot be studied separately.
- The two may be linked by stating that all **locomotions** are movements but all movements are not locomotions.
- Methods of locomotion **performed** by animals vary with their habitats and the demand of the situation.
- The locomotion is **generally** for search of food, shelter, mate, suitable breeding grounds, **favourable** climatic conditions or to escape from enemies/predators.

7.1 TYPES OF MOVEMENT

- Cells of the human body exhibit three main types of movements, namely, amoeboid, ciliary and muscular.

a. Amoeboid movement.

- Some **specialised** cells in our body like macrophages and leucocytes in blood exhibit amoeboid movement.
- This **movement** is effected by pseudopodia formed by the streaming of protoplasm (as in *Amoeba*).
- **Cytoskeletal** elements like microfilaments are also involved in amoeboid movement.

b. Ciliary movement

- **Ciliary** movement occurs in most of our internal tubular organs which are lined by ciliated epithelium.
- The **coordinated** movements of cilia in the trachea help us in removing dust particles and some of the foreign substances inhaled alongwith the atmospheric air.
- **Passage** of ova through the female reproductive tract is also facilitated by the ciliary movement.

b. Muscular movement

- **Movement** of our limbs, jaws, tongue, etc, require muscular movement.
- The **contractile** property of muscles are effectively used for locomotion and other movements by human beings and majority of multicellular organisms.
- Locomotion **requires** a perfect **coordinated** activity of muscular, skeletal and neural systems.

7.2 MUSCLE

- Muscles are mostly of **mesodermal** origin.
- About **40-50** per cent of the body weight of a human adult is contributed by muscles.
- They have special properties like **excitability, contractility, extensibility and elasticity.**
- Muscles have been classified using different **criteria**, namely location, appearance and nature of regulation of their activities.
- **Based** on their location, three types of muscles are three types: (i) **Skeletal** (ii) **Visceral** and (iii) **Cardiac.**

a. Skeletal muscles/striated muscle /skeletal muscle

- **Skeletal muscles** are closely associated with the skeletal components of the body.
- They have a **striped** appearance under the microscope and hence are called **striated muscles**.
- As their activities are under the voluntary control of the nervous system, they are known as **voluntary** muscles too.
- They are **primarily** involved in locomotory actions and changes of body postures.
- Distinct A and I **bands** present.

b. Visceral muscles/Non-striated muscle /Non-skeletal muscle/Smooth muscle

- **Visceral muscles** are located in the inner walls of hollow visceral organs of the body like the alimentary canal, reproductive tract, etc.
- A and I bands absent.
- They do not **exhibit** any striation and are smooth in appearance.
- Hence, they are called **smooth muscles (nonstriated muscle)**.
- Their **activities** are not under the voluntary control of the nervous system and are therefore known as involuntary muscles.
- They assist, for example, in the **transportation** of food through the digestive tract and gametes through the genital tract.

c. Cardiac muscles

- **Cardiac muscles** are the muscles of heart.
- **Intercalated disc present.**
- A and I bands **present** but they are not distinct.
- Many **cardiac** muscle cells assemble in a branching pattern to form a cardiac muscle.
- Based on **appearance**, cardiac muscles are striated.
- They are **involuntary** in nature as the nervous system does not control their activities directly.

d. Structure of skeletal muscles

- Each organised skeletal muscle in our body is made of a number of **muscle bundles** or **fascicles** held together by a common collagenous connective tissue layer called **fascia**.

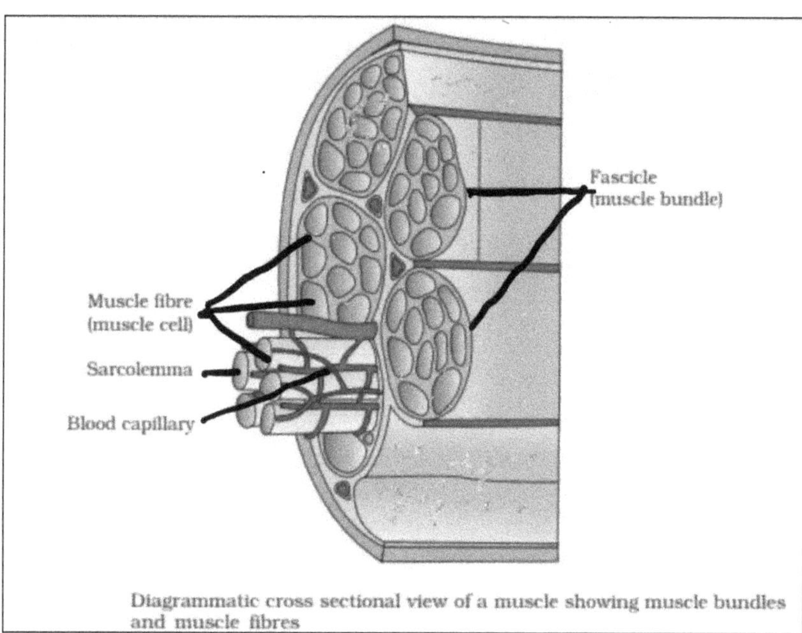

Diagrammatic cross sectional view of a muscle showing muscle bundles and muscle fibres

- Each muscle **bundle** contains a number of muscle fibres.
- Muscle fibre also called **Myocyte**.

- Each muscle fibre is lined by the plasma membrane called **sarcolemma** enclosing the sarcoplasm. **Muscle** fibre is a syncytium as the sarcoplasm contains many nuclei.
- The **endoplasmic** reticulum, i.e., **sarcoplasmic reticulum** of the muscle fibres is the store house of calcium ions.

e. Myofibrils

- A characteristic feature of the muscle fibre is the presence of a large number of **parallelly** arranged filaments in the **sarcoplasm** called myofilaments or **myofibrils**.
- Each myofibril has **alternate dark and light band**s on it.
- **A detailed study of the myofibril** has established that the striated appearance is due to the distribution pattern of two important proteins – **Actin** and **Myosin**.
- The **light bands** contain actin and is called I-band or Isotropic band,
- The **dark band** called 'A' or Anisotropic band contains myosin.
- Both proteins are arranged as **rod-like structures**, parallel to each other and also to the **longitudinal axis of the myofibrils.**
- **Actin filaments are thinner** as compared to the **myosin filaments**, hence are commonly called **thin and thick** filaments respectively.
- In the centre of each **'I' band** is an elastic fibre called **'Z' line** which bisects it.
- The thin filaments are firmly attached to the **'Z' line**.
- The thick filaments in the **'A' band** are also held together in the middle of this band by a thin fibrous membrane called **'M' line.**
- The **'A' and 'I' bands** are arranged alternately throughout the length of the myofibrils.

f. Sarcomere

- The portion of the myofibril between two successive 'Z' lines is considered as the functional unit of contraction and is called a **sarcomere**.
- **Sarcomere** is structural and functional unit of voluntary muscles.
- In a **resting state**, the edges of **thin filaments on either side of the thick filaments partially overlap** the free ends of the thick filaments leaving the central part of the thick filaments.
- The central part of thick filament, which is not overlapped by thin filaments is called **the 'H' zone.**

7.2.1 Structure of Contractile Proteins

a. Actin

- Each actin (thin) **filament** is made of two 'F' (filamentous) actins helically wound to each other. Each 'F' actin is a polymer of **monomeric 'G'** (Globular) actins.

b. Tropomyosin

- Two filaments of another protein, **tropomyosin** also run close to the 'F' actins throughout its length.

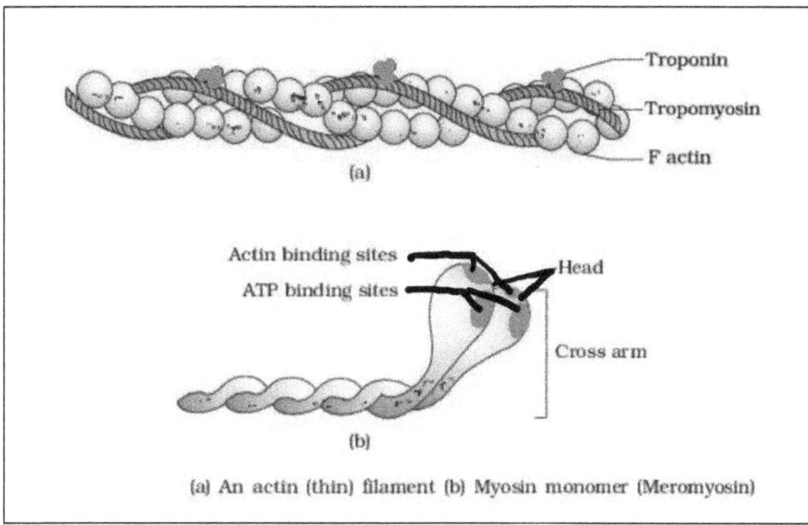

(a) An actin (thin) filament (b) Myosin monomer (Meromyosin)

c. Troponin

- A complex protein **Troponin** is distributed at regular intervals on the tropomyosin.

- In the resting state a subunit of **troponin** masks the active binding sites for myosin on the actin filaments.

d. Myosin

- Each myosin (thick) filament is also a **polymerised** protein.

- Many monomeric proteins called **Meromyosins** constitute one thick filament.

- Each **meromyosin** has two important parts, a globular head with a short arm and a tail, the former being called the heavy **meromyosin** (HMM) and the latter, the light **meromyosin** (LMM).

- The **HMM** component, i.e.; the head and short arm projects **outwards** at regular distance and angle from each other from the surface of a **polymerised** myosin filament and is known as cross arm.

- The globular head is an **active** ATPase enzyme and has binding sites for ATP and active sites for actin.

7.2.2 Mechanism of Muscle Contraction

- Mechanism of muscle contraction is best explained by the **sliding filament theory**.

- The sliding filament theory given by **Huxley, Huxley and Hanson**.

- **The sliding filament theory** states that contraction of a muscle fibre takes place by the sliding of the thin filaments over the **thick filaments.**

Muscle contraction takes place in following manner-

1. Muscle contraction is initiated by **a signal sent by** the **central nervous system (CNS)** via a motor neuron.

2. **A motor neuron** alongwith the muscle fibres connected to it constitute a motor unit.

3. The junction between a motor neuron and the sarcolemma of the muscle fibre is called the **neuromuscular junction or motor-end plate.**

4. A neural signal reaching this junction releases a **neurotransmitter (Acetyl choline)** which generates an action potential in **the sarcolemma.**

5. This **spreads** through the muscle fibre and causes the release of **calcium** ions into the sarcoplasm.

6. Increase in **Ca⁺⁺** level leads to the binding of calcium with a subunit of troponin on actin filaments and thereby remove the masking of active sites for myosin.

7. **Utilising** the energy from **ATP hydrolysis**, the myosin head now binds to the exposed active sites on actin to form a cross bridge.

8. This pulls the attached actin **filaments** towards the **centre of 'A' band**.

9. **The 'Z' line** attached to these actins are also pulled **inwards** thereby causing a shortening of the sarcomere, i.e., contraction.

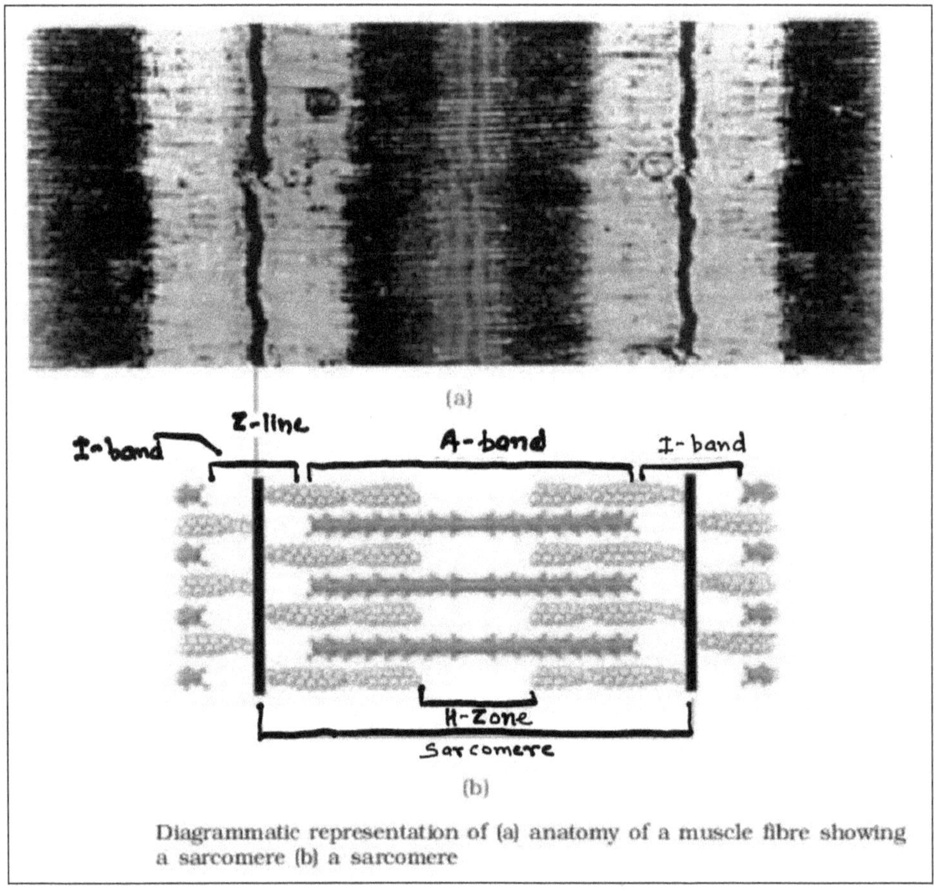

Diagrammatic representation of (a) anatomy of a muscle fibre showing a sarcomere (b) a sarcomere

1. It is clear from the above steps, that **during shortening** of the muscle, i.e., contraction, the 'I' bands get reduced, whereas the 'A' bands retain the length.

2. The myosin, releasing the **ADP** and **P1 goes** back to its relaxed state.

   A new **ATP binds** and the **cross-bridge is broken**.

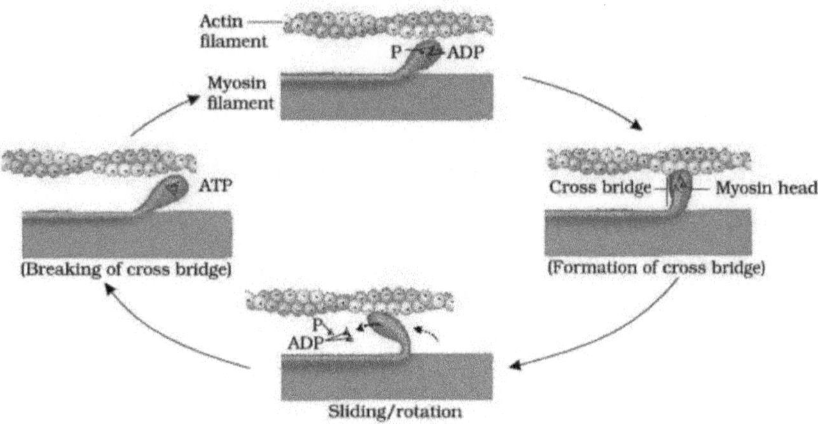

Stages in cross bridge formation, rotation of head and breaking of cross bridge

- **The ATP is again hydrolysed** by the myosin head and the cycle of cross bridge formation and breakage is repeated causing further sliding.

- The process continues till the **Ca⁺⁺ ions are pumped back** to the sarcoplasmic cisternae resulting in the masking of actin filaments. This causes the return of **'Z' lines back to their original position,** i.e., relaxation.

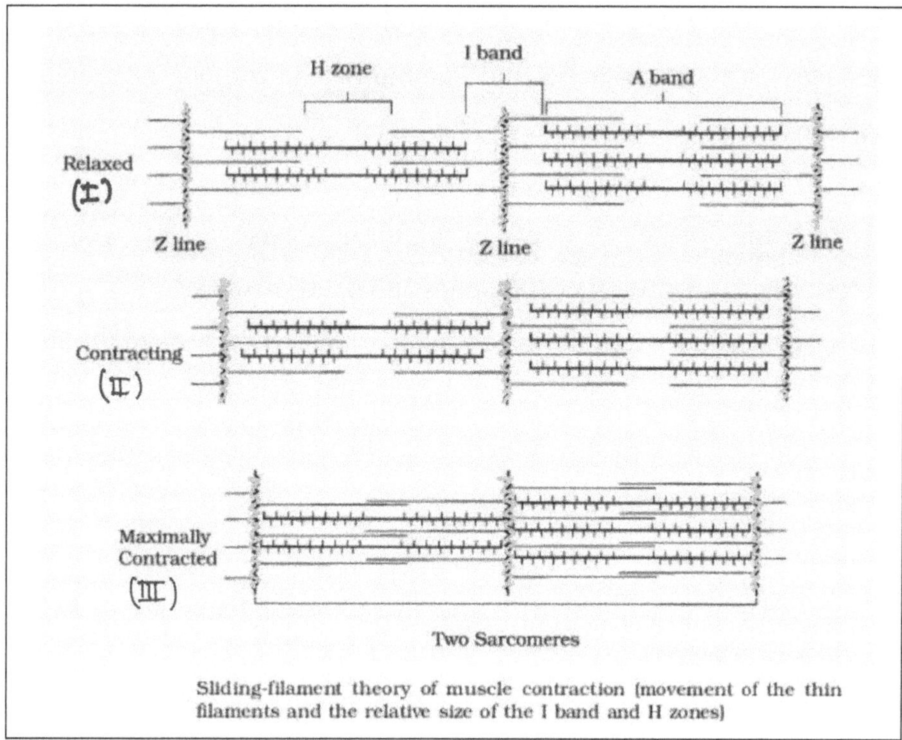

Sliding-filament theory of muscle contraction (movement of the thin filaments and the relative size of the I band and H zones)

Points to remember-

- **The reaction time** of the fibres can vary in different muscles.

- **Repeated activation** of the muscles can lead to the accumulation of lactic acid due to anaerobic breakdown of glycogen in them, causing fatigue.

Aerobic muscles

- Muscle contains a **red coloured oxygen** storing pigment called myoglobin.
- **Myoglobin** content is high in some of the muscles which gives a reddish appearance. Such muscles are called the **Red fibres**.
- These muscles also contain plenty of **mitochondria** which can utilise the **large amount of oxygen stored** in them for ATP production.
- These muscles, therefore, can also be **called aerobic muscles**.

Anaerobic muscles

- Some of the muscles possess very **less quantity of myoglobin** and so, appear pale or whitish. These are the White fibres.
- Number of **mitochondria are few** in these muscles.
- The amount of **sarcoplasmic reticulum** is **high**.
- They depend on **anaerobic process** for energy.

7.3 Skeletal System

- **Skeletal system** consists of a framework of bones and a few cartilages.
- **Skeletal system** has a significant role in movement shown by the body.
- Imagine chewing food without jaw bones and walking around without the limb bones.
- **Bone and cartilage** are specialised connective tissues.
- The bone has a very **hard matrix** due to calcium salts in it.
- The cartilage has **slightly pliable** matrix due to chondroitin salts.
- In human skeletal system is made up of **206** bones and a few cartilages.
- Human skeletal system grouped into two principal divisions – the axial and the appendicular skeleton.

Axial skeleton

- **Axial skeleton** comprises 80 bones distributed along the main axis of the body.
- The skull, vertebral column, sternum and ribs constitute axial skeleton.

a. Skull

- The **skull** is composed of two sets of bones – **cranial and facial**, that totals to **22** bones.
- Cranial bones are **8** in number.
- Cranial bones are - Frontal(1), Parietal(2),Temporal(2),Occipital(1),Sphenoid(1),Ethmoid(1).
- Cranial bones form the hard protective outer covering, cranium for the brain.
- The **facial region** is made up of **14 skeletal elements** which form the front part of the skull.
- Facial bones are-Nasal(2), Maxilla(2), Zygomatic(2), Lacrimal(2), Palatine(2), Inferior nasal bone(2), Vomer(1), Mandible(1)
- A single **U-shaped bone** called **hyoid** is present at the base of the buccal cavity and it is also included in the skull.

- Each middle ear contains three tiny bones – **Malleus, Incus and Stapes**.
- **Malleus, Incus and Stapes** collectively called **Ear Ossicles**.
- Total number of Ear ossicles in human-6
- The skull region articulates with the superior region of the vertebral column with the help of two occipital condyles.
- So human skull is dicondylic skull.

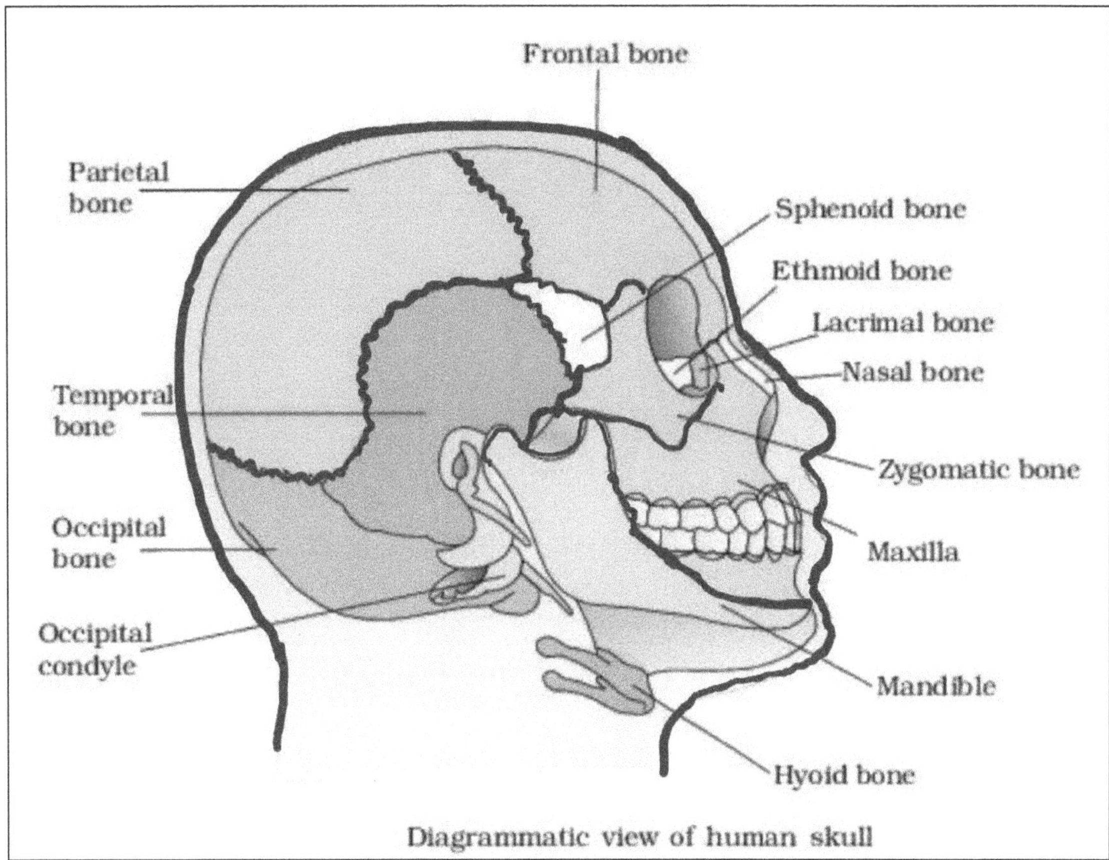

Diagrammatic view of human skull

b. Vertebral column

- Our **vertebral column** is formed by **26** serially arranged units called vertebrae.
- These are present dorsally.
- It extends from the base of the skull and constitutes the main framework of the trunk.
- Each vertebra has a **central hollow portion (neural canal)** through which the spinal cord passes.
- First vertebra is the **atlas**.
- **Atlas** with the occipital condyles.
- **Axis** is 2nd vertebra of human body.
- The **vertebral column** is differentiated into **cervical (7), thoracic (12), lumbar (5), sacral (1-fused) and coccygeal (1-fused)** regions starting from the skull.
- The number of cervical vertebrae are seven in **almost all mammals** including human beings.

- The vertebral column protects the spinal cord, supports the head and serves as the point of attachment for the ribs and musculature of the back.

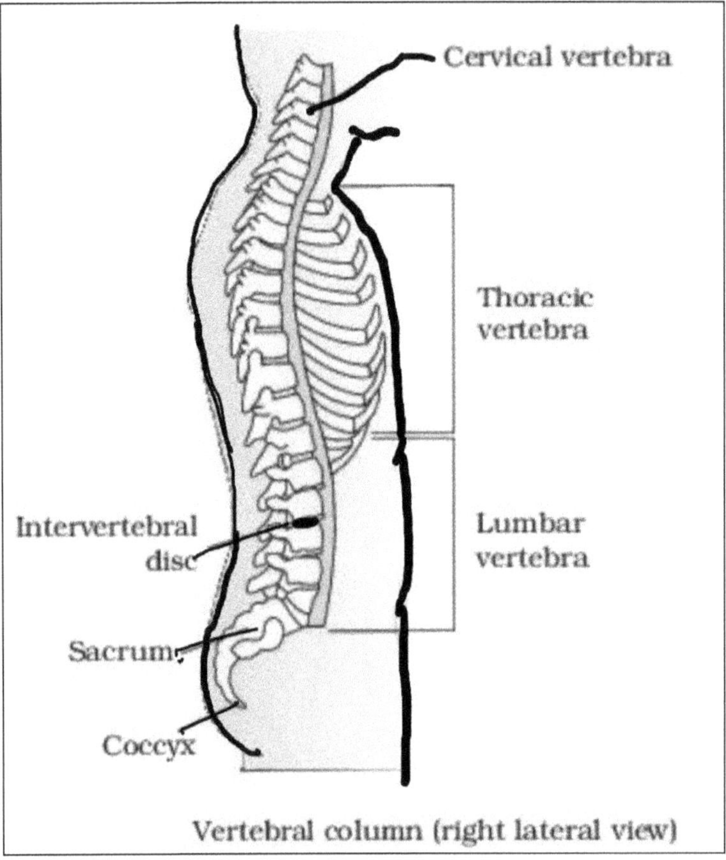

Vertebral column (right lateral view)

c. Sternum

- **Sternum** is a flat bone.
- One in number.
- **Sternum present** on the ventral midline of thorax.

d. Ribs

- There are 12 pairs of **Ribs.**
- Each rib is a thin flat bone connected dorsally to the vertebral column and ventrally to the sternum.
- It has two articulation surfaces on its dorsal end and is hence **called bicephalic.**
- **First seven pairs** of ribs are called true ribs.
- **Dorsally** true ribs are attached to the thoracic vertebrae.
- **Ventrally** true ribs connected to the sternum with the help of hyaline cartilage.
- The 8th, 9th and 10th pairs of ribs do not articulate directly with the sternum but join the seventh rib with the help of hyaline cartilage.
- The 8th, 9th and 10th pairs of ribs are called vertebrochondral (false) ribs.
- Last **2 pairs (11th and 12th)** of ribs are not connected ventrally and are therefore, called floating ribs.
- **Floating ribs** protects kidney.

- Thoracic vertebrae, ribs and sternum together form the rib cage.

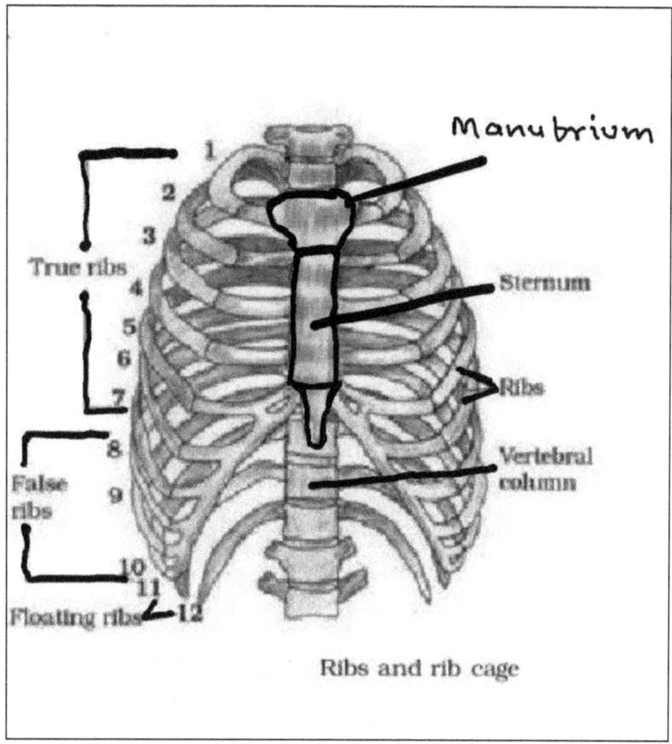

Ribs and rib cage

Appendicular skeleton.

- The bones of the **limbs** alongwith their **girdles** constitute the **appendicular skeleton.**

a. Limbs

- Each **limb** is made of **30 bones.**
- The bones of the hand (fore limb) are-
- **Humerus, radius and ulna, carpals** (wrist bones – 8 in number), **metacarpals** (palm bones – 5 in number) and **phalanges** (digits – 14 in number).
- Humerus has **deltoid ridge**.
- The bones of the leg (hind limb) are-

    Femur (thigh bone – the longest bone), tibia and fibula, tarsals (ankle bones – 7 in number), patella (knee cap), metatarsals (5 in number) and phalanges (digits – 14 in number) are the bones of the legs (hind limb).

b. Patella

- A cup shaped bone.
- Patella cover the knee ventrally.
- Also called knee cap.

c. Girdles

- **Pectoral (shoulder girdle)** and **Pelvic girdle(Hip girdle)** bones helps to join the upper and the lower limbs respectively with the axial skeleton.

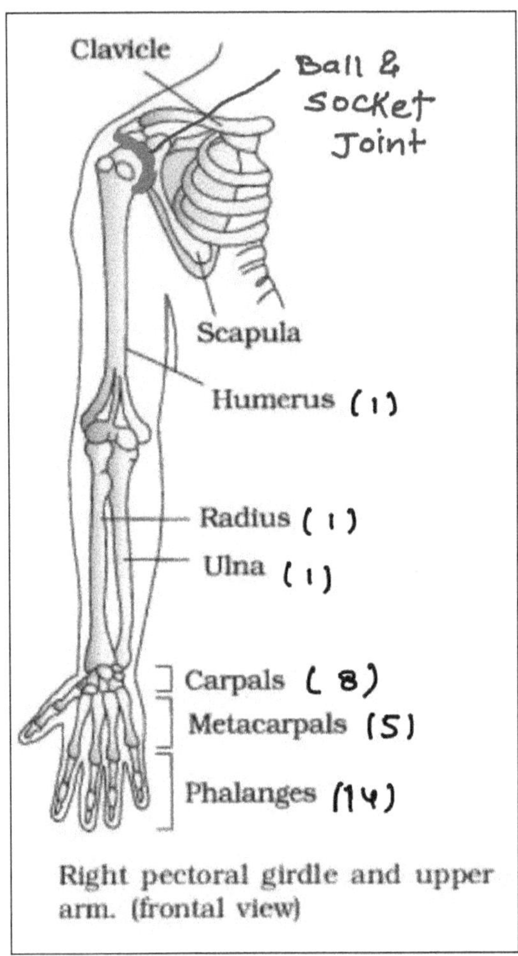

Right pectoral girdle and upper arm. (frontal view)

d. Pectoral (shoulder girdle)

- Each girdle is formed of **two halves.**
- Each half of pectoral girdle consists of a clavicle and a **scapula.**
- Scapula is a **large triangular flat bone** situated in the dorsal part of the thorax between the second and the seventh ribs.
- The **dorsal, flat, triangular body** of scapula has a slightly elevated ridge called the spine which projects as a flat, expanded process called **the acromion.**
- **The clavicle** articulates with sternum.
- Below the **acromion is a depression** called **the glenoid cavity** which articulates with the head of the humerus to form the shoulder joint.
- Each **clavicle is a long slender** bone with **two curvatures.**
- **Clavicle** bone is commonly called the **collar bone.**
- **Clavicle** also called **beauty** bone.

e. Pelvic girdle (Hip girdle)

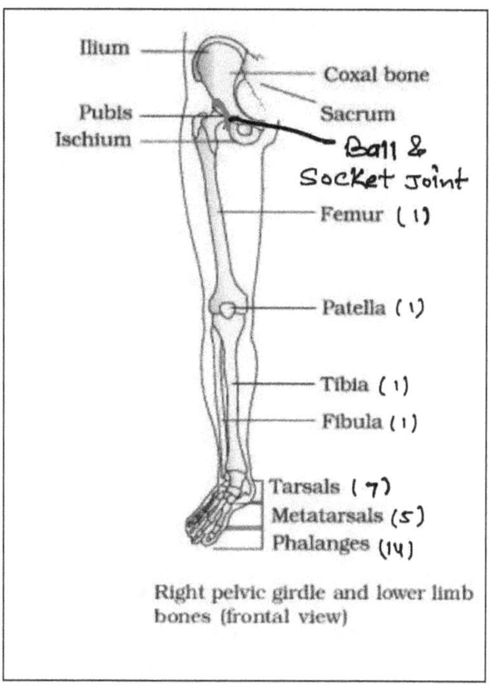

Right pelvic girdle and lower limb bones (frontal view)

- **Pelvic** girdle consists of two coxal bones.
- Each **coxal** bone is formed by the fusion of three bones – **ilium**, **ischium** and **pubis**.
- At the point of fusion of the above bones is a cavity called **acetabulum** to which the thigh bone articulates.
- The two halves of the **pelvic** girdle meet ventrally to form the pubic symphysis containing fibrous cartilage.

7.4 JOINTS

- Joints are essential for all types of **movements** involving the bony parts of the body.
- **Locomotory** movements are no exception to this.
- Joints are points of contact between bones, or between **bones** and **cartilages**.
- Force **generated** by the muscles is used to carry out **movement** through joints, where the joint acts as a fulcrum.
- The **movability** at these joints vary **depending** on different factors.
- Joints have been classified into **three major** structural forms, namely, fibrous, cartilaginous and synovial.

a. Fibrous joints

- **Fibrous joints** do not allow any movement.
- This type of joint is shown by the flat **skull bones** which fuse end-to-end with the help of dense fibrous **connective** tissues in the form of sutures, to form the cranium.

b. Cartilaginous joints

- In **cartilaginous joints,** the bones involved are joined together with the help of cartilages.
- The **joint** between the adjacent vertebrae in the **vertebral** column is of this pattern and it permits **limited** movements.

c. Synovial joints

- **Synovial joints** are characterised by the presence of a fluid filled synovial cavity between the articulating surfaces of the two bones.
- Such an **arrangement** allows considerable movement.
- These joints help in **locomotion** and many other movements.

  Some examples of Synovial joints-

  I. **Ball and socket joint** (between humerus and pectoral girdle)

  II. **Hinge joint** (knee joint)

  III. **Pivot joint** (between atlas and axis)

  IV. **Gliding joint** (between the carpals)

  V. **Saddle joint** (between carpal and metacarpal of thumb)

7.5 Disorders of Muscular and Skeletal System

I. **Myasthenia gravis:** Auto immune disorder affecting neuromuscular junction leading to fatigue, weakening and paralysis of skeletal muscle.

II. **Tetany:** Rapid spasms (wild contractions) in muscle due to low Ca^{++} in body fluid.

III. **Gout:** Inflammation of joints due to accumulation of uric acid crystals.

IV. **Arthritis:** Inflammation of joints.

V. **Muscular dystrophy:** Progressive degeneration of skeletal muscle mostly due to genetic disorder.

VI. **Osteoporosis:** Age-related disorder characterised by decreased bone mass and increased chances of fractures.Decreased levels of estrogen is a common cause.

VII. **Arthritis:** Inflammation of joints.

VIII. **Muscular dystrophy:** Progressive degeneration of skeletal muscle mostly due to genetic disorder.

1. Consider the following statements and find out the correct option-

A. Movement is one of the significant features of living beings. Animals and plants exhibit a wide range of movements.

B. Streaming of protoplasm in the unicellular organisms like *Amoeba* is a simple form of movement.

C. Movement of cilia, flagella and tentacles are shown by many organisms.

D. Human beings can move limbs, jaws, eyelids, tongue with the help of muscles.

Which of the above are correct with respect to movement-

1. A,B,C only
2. B,C only
3. D,B,A only
4. A,B,C,D

2. Match the list 1 and 2-

List 1   List 2

a. *Paramoecium*	j. tentacles
b. *Amoeba*	k. cilia
c. *Hydra*	l. pseudopodia
d. *Earthworm*	m. setae

Find out the correct option –

1. a.k, b.j, c.l, d.m
2. a.k,b.l,c.j,d.m
3. a.l,b.j,c.k,d.m
4. a.l,b.j,c.m,d.k

3. Consider the following statements-

I. Some of the movements result in a change of place or location.

II. Walking, running, climbing, flying, swimming are all some forms of locomotory movements.

III. Locomotory structures are different types.

IV. In *Paramoecium*, cilia helps in the movement of food through cytopharynx and in locomotion as well.

How many of them are/is correct -

1. one	2. two
3. three	4. four

4. Read the following statements carefully with respect to Locomtion and movement-

   I.   We use limbs for changes in body postures and locomotion as well.

   II.   The movements and locomotion cannot be studied separately.

   III.   The two may be linked by stating that all locomotions are movements but all movements are not locomotions.

   IV.   Methods of locomotion performed by animals vary with their habitats and the demand of the situation.

   V.   The locomotion is generally for search of food, shelter, mate, suitable breeding grounds, favourable climatic conditions or to escape from enemies/predators.

How many of them are usually correct -

1. three	2. four
3. five	4. two

5. Consider the following statements and find out the correct option-

STATEMENT 1. Some specialised cells in our body like macrophages and leucocytes in blood exhibit amoeboid movement.

STATEMENT 2. Amoeboid movement is effected by pseudopodia formed by the streaming of protoplasm (as in *Amoeba*).

1. Both are correct statements	2. Only statement 1 correct
3. Both are wrong statements	4. Only statement 2 correct

6. Go through the following statements-

ASSERTION(A). The contractile property of muscles are effectively used for locomotion and other movements by human beings and majority of multicellular organisms.

REASON(R). Locomotion requires a perfect coordinated activity of muscular, skeletal and neural systems.

1. A correct and R is correct explanation of A

2. A correct and R is also correct but R is not correct explanation of A

3. A correct but R incorrect

4. A and R both are incorrect

7. Which one is incorrect statement-

   1.   Ciliary movement occurs in most of our internal tubular organs which are lined by ciliated epithelium.

   2.   The coordinated movements of cilia in the trachea help us in removing dust particles and some of the foreign substances inhaled alongwith the atmospheric air.

3. Passage of ova through the female reproductive tract is also facilitated by the ciliary movement.

4. Movement of our limbs, jaws, tongue, etc, not require muscular movement.

8. Go through the following statements-

I. Muscle is a specialised tissue of mesodermal origin.

II. About 40-50 per cent of the body weight of a human adult is contributed by muscles.

III. Muscles have special properties like excitability, contractility, extensibility and elasticity.

IV. Muscles have been classified using different criteria, namely location, appearance and nature of regulation of their activities.

V. Based on their location, three types of muscles are identified.

How many of them are correct-

1. two

2. three

3. four

4. five

9. Match the list 1 and 2-

List 1   List 2

a. **Sternum**	j. 24
b. **Ribs**	k. 30
c. **Each limb**	l. 1
d. **Ear Ossicles**	m. 6

Find out the correct option –

1. a.k, b.j, c.l, d.m

2. a.k,b.l,c.j,d.m

3. a.l,b.j,c.k,d.m

4. a.l,b.j,c.m,d.k

10. Consider the following statements and find out the correct option-

STATEMENT 1. Each vertebra has a central hollow portion (neural canal) through which the spinal cord passes.

STATEMENT 2 First vertebra is the atlas and it articulates with the occipital condyles.

1. Both are wrong statements

2. Only statement 1 correct

3. Both are correct statements

4. Only statement 2 correct

11. Read the following statements very carefully and find out the incorrect-

a) Each middle ear contains three tiny bones – Malleus, Incus and Stapes, collectively called **Ear Ossicles**.

b) The skull region articulates with the superior region of the vertebral column with the help of two occipital condyles (dicondylic skull).

c) Our **vertebral column** is formed by 20 serially arranged units called vertebrae and is dorsally placed.

d) **Vertebral column** extends from the base of the skull and constitutes the main framework of the trunk.

Which above statement are/is incorrect?

1. a and c both

2. a,b,c,d

3. c only

4. b and c both

12. Go through the following statement-

ASSERTION(A). Axial skeleton comprises 80 bones distributed along the main axis of the body.

REASON(R). The skull, vertebral column, sternum and ribs constitute axial skeleton.

1. A correct and R is correct explanation of A

2. A correct and R is also correct but R is not correct explanation of A

3. A correct but R incorrect

4. A and R both are incorrect

13. Find out incorrect statement with respect to Humans-

1. The vertebral column is differentiated into cervical (7), thoracic (12), lumbar (5), sacral (1-fused) and coccygeal (1-fused) regions starting from the skull.

2. The number of cervical vertebrae are seven in almost all mammals including human beings.

3. The vertebral column protects the spinal cord, supports the head and serves as the point of attachment for the ribs and musculature of the back.

4. **Sternum** is a flat bone on the dorsal midline of thorax.

14. Read the following statements and find out correct option-

I. Skeletal system consists of a framework of bones and a few cartilages.

II. Skeletal system has a significant role in movement shown by the body.

III. Total 80 limb bones found in humans.

IV. Bone and cartilage are specialised connective tissue.

How many of them is/are correct-

1. four

2. one

3. two

4. three

15. Consider the following statements and find out the correct option

STATEMENT 1. The vertebral column protects the spinal cord, supports the head and serves as the point of attachment for the ribs and musculature of the back.

STATEMENT 2. Dorsally, false ribs are attached to the thoracic vertebrae and ventrally connected to the sternum with the help of hyaline cartilage.

1. Both are wrong statements

2. Only statement 1 correct

3. Both are correct statements

4. Only statement 2 correct

16. Match the list 1 and 2

List 1   List 2

a. cervical vertebra	7 in number
b. thoracic vertebra	12 in number
c. lumbar vertebra	5 in number

Which of the above are correctly matched-

1. a and b
2. b and c
3. c and a
4. a, b, c

17. Consider the following statements w.r.t. humans-

a) First seven pairs of ribs are called true ribs.

b) Dorsally, true ribs are attached to the thoracic vertebrae and ventrally connected to the sternum with the help of hyaline cartilage.

c) The 8th, 9th and 10th pairs of ribs do not articulate directly with the sternum but join the seventh rib with the help of hyaline cartilage.

d) True ribs are also called vertebra chondral ribs.

Which of the above statement are correct?

1. a and d only
2. c and b only
3. a,b,c only
4. a,b,c,d

18. Consider the following statements-

a) The number of cervical vertebrae are seven in almost all mammals including human beings.

b) The vertebral column protects the spinal cord, supports the head and serves as the point of attachment for the ribs and musculature of the back.

c) **Sternum** is a flat bone on the ventral midline of thorax.

d) There are 12 pairs of **ribs.**

e) Each rib is a thin flat bone connected dorsally to the vertebral column and ventrally to the sternum.

Which of the above statements are correct w.r.t. humans?

1. a and d only
2. c and a only
3. a,b,c,d only
4. a,b,c,d,e

19. Consider the following statements and find out the incorrect one w.r.t. Humans-

1. The Human **skull** is composed of two sets of bones – cranial and facial, that totals to 22 bones.

2. Cranial bones are 8 in number.

3. The facial region is made up of 24 skeletal elements which form the front part of the skull.

4. A single U-shaped bone called hyoid is present at the base of the buccal cavity and it is also included in the skull.

20. Read the following statements-

   I. The bone has a very hard matrix due to calcium salts in it.

   II. In human skeletal system is made up of 190 bones and a few cartilages.

   III. Human skeletal system is grouped into two principal divisions – the axial and the appendicular skeleton.

   IV. **Axial skeleton** comprises 80 bones distributed along the main axis of the body.

   V. The skull, vertebral column, sternum and ribs constitute axial skeleton.

How many of them are correct **statements-**

1. two   2. three

3. four   4. five

21. Consider the following statements and find out the correct option for humans-

STATEMENT 1. Based on appearance, cardiac muscles are striated.

STATEMENT 2. They are involuntary in nature as the nervous system does not control their activities directly.

1. Both are wrong statements   2. Only statement 1 correct

3. Both are correct statements   4. Only statement 2 correct

22. Go through the following statement and find out the correct option-

ASSERTION(A). Visceral muscles do not exhibit any striation and are smooth in appearance.

REASON(R). A and I bands are absent in these muscles.

1. A correct and R is correct explanation of A

2. A correct and R is also correct but R is not correct explanation of A

3. A correct but R incorrect

4. A and R both are incorrect

23. Go through the following statements and find out the correct option-

   A. Skeletal muscles are closely associated with the skeletal components of the body.

   B. Skeletal muscles have a striped appearance under the microscope and hence are called **striated muscles**.

   C. Visceral muscles are located in the inner walls of hollow visceral organs of the body like the alimentary canal, reproductive tract, etc.

   D. Visceral muscles do not exhibit any striations and are smooth in appearance.

Which of the above statements are correct -

1. A and C only   2. C and D only

3. A,B,C only   4. A,B,C,D

24. Read the statements given below-

G. Each organised skeletal muscle in our body is made of a number of **muscle bundles** or **fascicles** held together by a common collagenous connective tissue layer called **fascia**.

H. Each muscle bundle contains a number of muscle fibres.

I. Each muscle fibre is lined by the plasma membrane called sarcolemma enclosing the sarcoplasm. Muscle fibre is a syncitium as the sarcoplasm contains many nuclei.

J. The endoplasmic reticulum, i.e., sarcoplasmic reticulum of the muscle fibres is the store house of calcium ions.

Which of the above statements are/is correct?

1. A and C only

2. B only

3. D and B only

4. A,B,C,D

25. Consider the following statements-

A. A characteristic feature of the muscle fibre is the presence of a large number of parallelly arranged filaments in the sarcoplasm called myofilaments or **myofibrils**.

B. Each myofibril has alternate dark and light bands on it. A detailed study of the myofibril has established that the striated appearance is due to the distribution pattern of two important proteins – **Actin** and **Myosin**.

C. The light bands contain actins and called as I-band or Isotropic band,

D. The dark band called 'A' or Anisotropic band and they contains myosin.

Which of the above statements are/is correct?

1. A and C only

2. A and D only

3. D and C only

4. A,B,C,D

26. Consider the following statements-

I. Actin filaments are thinner as compared to the myosin filaments, hence are commonly called thin and thick filaments respectively.

II. In the centre of each 'I' band is an elastic fibre called 'Z' line which bisects it. The thin filaments are firmly attached to the 'Z' line.

III. The thick filaments in the 'A' band are also held together by a thin fibrous membrane called 'M' line.

IV. The 'A' and 'I' bands are arranged alternately throughout the length of the myofibrils.

How many of them are correct-

1. one

2. two

3. three

4. four

27. Match the list 1 and 2-

List 1   List 2(per Hand or leg)

a. palm bones	5 in number
b. wrist bones	8 in number
c. ankle bones	7 in number
d. bone in digits	14 in number

How many of them are correctly matched –

1. one   2. two

3. three   4. four

28. Consider the following statements-

a) A cup shaped bone called patella cover the knee ventrally (knee cap).

b) **Pectoral** and **Pelvic girdle** bones help in the articulation of the upper and the lower limbs respectively with the axial skeleton.

c) Each girdle is formed of two halves.

d) Each half of pectoral girdle consists of a clavicle and a scapula.

e) Scapula is a large triangular flat bone.

Which of the above statements is/are correct-

1. a and c only   2. a,b,c,d only

3. d and c only   4. all are correct

29. Consider the following statements and find out incorrect one-

1. The ventral, flat, triangular body of scapula has a slightly elevated ridge called the spine which projects as a flat, expanded process called the acromion.

2. The clavicle articulates with sternum.

3. Each clavicle is a long slender bone with two curvatures.

4. The clavicle bone is commonly called the collar bone.

30. Read the following points -

a) Pelvic girdle consists of two coxal bones.

b) Each coxal bone is formed by the fusion of three bones – ilium, ischium and pubis.

c) At the point of fusion of the above bones is a cavity called acetabulum to which the thigh bone articulates.

d) The two halves of the pelvic girdle meet ventrally to form the pubic symphysis containing fibrous cartilage.

How many of them are/is correct –

1. four   2. two

3. three   4. one

31. Read the following statements and find out the correct option

STATEMENT 1. Thoracic vertebrae, ribs and sternum together form the rib cage.

STATEMENT 2. The bones of the limbs alongwith their girdles constitute the **appendicular skeleton.**

1. Both are wrong statements

2. Both are correct statements

3. Only statement 1 correct

4. Only statement 2 correct

32. Go through the following statements and find out the correct option-

ASSERTION(A). The facial region is made up of 14 skeletal elements which form the front part of the skull.

REASON(R). A single U-shaped bone called hyoid is present at the base of the buccal cavity and it is also included in the skull.

1. A correct and R is correct explanation of A

2. A correct and R is also correct but R is not correct explanation of A

3. A correct but R incorrect

4. A and R both are incorrect

33. Find out the incorrect option-

1. Myoglobin content is low in some of the muscles which gives them a reddish appearance, such muscles are called the Red fibres.

2. Red muscle fibers also contain plenty of mitochondria which can utilise the large amount of oxygen stored in them for ATP production.

3. The red muscle fibres also called as aerobic muscles.

4. The number of mitochondria are also few in white muscle fibres, but the amount of sarcoplasmic reticulum is high.

34. Consider the following statements-

I. Repeated activation of the muscles can lead to the accumulation of lactic acid due to anaerobic breakdown of glycogen in them, causing fatigue.

II. Muscle contains a white coloured oxygen storing pigment called myoglobin.

III. Myoglobin content is high in some of the muscles which gives a reddish appearance. Such muscles are called the Red fibres.

IV. Red muscles also contain plenty of mitochondria which can utilise the large amount of oxygen stored in them for ATP production.

How many of above is/are incorrect-

1. three

2. four

3. two

4. one

35. Which of the following is incorrect statement-

1. Each actin (thin) filament is made of two 'F' (filamentous) actins helically wound to each other. Each 'F' actin is a polymer of monomeric 'G' (Globular) actins.

2. Two filaments of another protein, tropomyosin also run close to the 'F' actins throughout its length.

3. A complex protein Troponin is distributed at regular intervals on the myosin.

4. In the resting state a subunit of troponin masks the active binding sites for myosin on the actin filaments.

36. Consider the following statements –

i. Each myosin (thick) filament is also a polymerised protein.

ii. Many monomeric proteins called Meromyosins constitute one thick filament.

iii. Each meromyosin has two important parts, a globular head with a short arm and a tail, the former being called the heavy meromyosin (HMM) and the latter, the light meromyosin (LMM).

iv. The HMM component, i.e.; the head and short arm projects outwards at regular distance and angle from each other from the surface of a polymerised myosin filament and is known as cross arm.

Which of the above statements are correct-

1. i,ii only

2. i, iii,iv only

3. i,ii,iii only

4 all are correct

37. Read the following statements-

i. Cells of the human body exhibit three main types of movements, namely, amoeboid, ciliary and muscular.

ii. Some specialised cells in our body like macrophages and leucocytes in blood exhibit amoeboid movement.

iii. It is effected by pseudopodia formed by the streaming of protoplasm (as in *Amoeba*).

iv. Cytoskeletal elements like microfilaments are also involved in amoeboid movement.

v. Ciliary movement occurs in most of our internal tubular organs which are lined by ciliated epithelium.

Which of the above statements is/are correct-

1. i and ii only

2. iii And ii only

3. iv and iii only

4. All are correct

38. Consider the following statements-

I. The coordinated movements of cilia in the trachea help us in removing dust particles and some of the foreign substances inhaled alongwith the atmospheric air.

II. Passage of ova through the female reproductive tract is also facilitated by the ciliary movement.

III. Movement of our limbs, jaws, tongue, etc, require muscular movement.

IV. The contractile property of muscles are effectively used for locomotion and other movements by human beings and majority of multicellular organisms.

How many of above is/are correct-

1. three

2. four

3. two

4. one

39. Read the following statements and find out the correct option-

STATEMENT 1. The skull region articulates with the superior region of the vertebral column with the help of two occipital condyles (dicondylic skull).

STATEMENT 2. Our **vertebral column** is formed by 26 serially arranged units called vertebrae and is dorsally placed.

1. Both are wrong statements

2. Both are correct statements

3. Only statement 1 correct

4. Only statement 2 correct

40. Read the following statements-

a) The **skull** is composed of two sets of bones – cranial and facial, that totals to 22 bones.

b) Cranial bones are 14 in number.

c) Cranial bones form the hard protective outer covering, cranium for the brain.

d) The facial region is made up of 8 skeletal elements which form the front part of the skull.

e) A single U-shaped bone called hyoid is present at the base of the buccal cavity and it is also included in the skull.

Which of the following are incorrect?

1. a and b only

2. b and c only

3. b and d only

4. All are correct

41. Go through the following statements and find out the correct option-

ASSERTION(A). First vertebra is the atlas and it articulates with the occipital condyles.

REASON(R). The vertebral column is differentiated into cervical (7), thoracic (12), lumbar (5), sacral (1-fused) and coccygeal (1-fused) regions starting from the skull.

1. A correct and R is correct explanation of A

2. A correct and R is also correct but R is not correct explanation of A

3. A correct but R incorrect

4. A and R both are incorrect

42. Find out the incorrect statement w.r.t. voluntary muscle contraction-

1. The 'I' bands get reduced.

2. A band remains constant.

3. Z-lines comes closer.

4. H-Zone increases.

43. Consider the following statements w.r.t. muscle contraction-

A. The junction between a motor neuron and the sarcolemma of the muscle fibre is called the neuromuscular junction or motor-end plate.

B. A neural signal reaching at neuromuscular junction releases a neurotransmitter (Acetyl choline) which generates an action potential in the sarcolemma.

C. This spreads through the muscle fibre and causes the release of calcium ions into the sarcoplasm.

D. Increase in Ca^{++} level leads to the binding of calcium with a subunit of troponin on actin filaments and thereby remove the masking of active sites for myosin.

E. Utilising the energy from ATP hydrolysis, the myosin head now binds to the exposed active sites on actin to form a cross bridge.

F. The above events pulls the attached actin filaments towards the centre of 'A' band.

How many of them are correct-

1. five
2. three
3. four
4. six

44. Read the following statements and find out the correct option –

STATEMENT 1. A neural signal reaching neuro-muscular junction releases a neurotransmitter (Acetyl choline) which generates an action potential in the sarcolemma.

STATEMENT 2. The action potential spreads through the muscle fibre and causes the release of calcium ions into the sarcoplasm from SR.

1. Both are correct statements
2. Both are wrong statements
3. Only statement 1 correct
4. Only statement 2 correct

45. Find out the incorrect statement-

1. Mechanism of muscle contraction is best explained by the sliding filament theory which states that contraction of a muscle fibre takes place by the sliding of the thin filaments over the thick filaments.

2. Muscle contraction is initiated by a signal sent by the central nervous system (CNS) via a motor neuron.

3. A motor neuron along with the muscle fibres connected to it constitute a motor unit.

4. The junction between a motor neuron and the sarcolemma of the muscle fibre is called the synaptic knob.

46. Read the following statements and find out the correct option

STATEMENT 1. Last 2 pairs (11th and 12th) of ribs are not connected ventrally and are therefore, called floating ribs.

STATEMENT 2. First seven pairs of ribs are called floting ribs,they are attached dorsally to the thoracic vertebrae and ventrally connected to the sternum with the help of hyaline cartilage.

1. Both are correct statements
2. Both are wrong statements.
3. Only statement 1 correct
4. Only statement 2 correct

47. Go through the following statements and find out the correct option-

ASSERTION(A). The 8th, 9th and 10thpairs of ribs are called vertebra-chondral ribs.

REASON(R). The 8th, 9th and 10thpairs of ribs articulate directly with the sternum but join the seventh rib with the help of hyaline cartilage.

1. A correct and R is correct explanation of A

2. A correct and R is also correct but R is not correct explanation of A

3. A but R incorrect

4. A and R both are incorrect

48. Find out the incorrect statement w.r.t. human ribs–

1. There are 12 pairs of **ribs.**

2. Each rib is a thin flat bone connected dorsally to the vertebral column and ventrally to the sternum.

3. It has two articulation surfaces on its dorsal end and is hence called monocephalic.

4. First seven pairs of ribs are called true ribs.

49. Consider the following statements -

A. Each vertebra has a central hollow portion (neural canal) through which the spinal cord passes.

B. First vertebra is the atlas and it articulates with the occipital condyles.

C. The vertebral column is differentiated into cervical (7), thoracic (12), lumbar (5), sacral (1-fused) and coccygeal (1-fused) regions starting from the skull.

D. The number of cervical vertebrae are seven in almost all mammals including human beings.

Which of the above statements are correct-

1. A and C only

2. D and B only

3. B and C only

4. All are correct

50. Read the following statements -

A. Bone and cartilage are specialised connective tissues.

B. The bone has a very hard matrix due to calcium salts in it and the cartilage has slightly pliable matrix due to chondroitin salts.

C. In human beings, this system is made up of 206 bones and a few cartilages.

D. It is grouped into two principal divisions – the axial and the appendicular skeleton.

E. **Axial skeleton** comprises 80 bones distributed along the main axis of the body.

Which of the above statements are correct-

1. A and C only

2. D and A only

3. B and D only

4. All are correct

NEURAL CONTROL AND COORDINATION

8.1 Neural System

8.2 Human Neural System

8.3 Neuron as Structural and Functional Unit of NeuralSystem

8.4 Central Neural System

8.5 Reflex Action and Reflex Arc

- The functions of the organs/organ systems in our body must be coordinated to maintain **homeostasis.**

- **Coordination** is the process through which two or more organs interact and supports the functions of one another.

- When we do **physical exercises**, the energy demand is increased for maintaining an increased muscular activity.

- So supply of oxygen is also **increased.**

- The increased supply of oxygen cause increase in the rate of respiration, heart beat and increased blood flow via **blood vessels.**

- When **physical exercise** is stopped, the activities of nerves, lungs, heart and kidney gradually return to their normal conditions.

- So, the functions of **muscles, lungs, heart, blood vessels, kidney and other organs** are coordinated while performing physical exercises.

- The neural system and the endocrine system jointly coordinate and integrate all the activities of the organs so that they function in a **synchronised** fashion.

- The neural system provides an organised network of point-to-point connections for a quick **coordination.**

- The endocrine system provides chemical integration through hormones.

8.1 NEURAL SYSTEM

- **Neural system** consist of neuron and neuroglial cells.

- The neural system of animals is composed of highly specialised cells called **neurons.**

- **Neurons are** structural and functional unit of neural system.
- Neuron can detect, receive and transmit different kinds of stimuli.
- The neural organisation is very simple in lower invertebrates.
- In *Hydra* neural organisation is composed of a network of neurons.
- The neural system is **better organised** in insects.
- In insects brain is present along with a number of ganglia and neural tissues.
- The vertebrates have a more developed neural system.

8.2 HUMAN NEURAL SYSTEM

- The human neural system is divided into two parts:

(i) the **central neural system** (CNS)

(ii) the **peripheral neural system** (PNS)

- The CNS includes the **brain** and the **spinal cord.**
- CNS is the site of information processing and control.
- The PNS comprises of all the nerves of the body associated with the CNS (brain and spinal cord).
- PNS has two types of nerve fibers:

(a) **afferent fibres**

(b) **efferent fibres**

- The afferent nerve fibres transmit impulses from tissues/organs to the CNS.
- The efferent fibres transmit regulatory impulses from the CNS to the concerned peripheral tissues/organs.
- The PNS is divided into two divisions called **somatic neural system** and **autonomic neural system.**
- The somatic neural system relays impulses from the CNS to skeletal muscles.
- The autonomic neural system transmits impulses from the CNS to the involuntary organs and smooth muscles of the body.
- The autonomic neural system is further divided into **sympathetic neural system** and **parasympathetic neural system.**

8.3 NEURON AS STRUCTURAL AND FUNCTIONAL UNIT OF NEURAL SYSTEM

- A neuron is a microscopic structure composed of three major parts, **cyton, dendrites** and **axon.**
- The cell body/cyton contains cytoplasm with typical cell organelles and certain granular bodies called **Nissl's granules.**
- **Nissl's granules** are made by ribosome and RER.
- **Nissl's granules** helps in protein synthesis.
- Short fibres which branch repeatedly and project out of the cell body also contain Nissl's granules and are called dendrites.

- **Dendrites** transmit impulses towards the cell body.

- The axon is a long fibre, the distal end of which is **branched.**

- Each branch of axon terminates as a bulb-like structure called **synaptic knob** which possess synaptic vesicles containing chemicals called **neurotransmitters.**

- The axons transmit nerve impulses away from the cell body to a synapse or to a neuro-muscular junction.

A. Based on the number of axon and dendrites, types of Neuron -

On basis the number of axon and dendrites, the neurons are divided into three types, -

I. **Multipolar** (with one axon and two or more dendrites; found in the cerebral cortex)

II. **Bipolar** (with one axon and one dendrite, found in the retina of eye)

III. **Unipolar** (cell body with one axon only; found usually in the embryonic stage).

B. Myelinated and non-myelinated nerve fibres

- There are two types of axons, namely, **myelinated** and **nonmyelinated.**

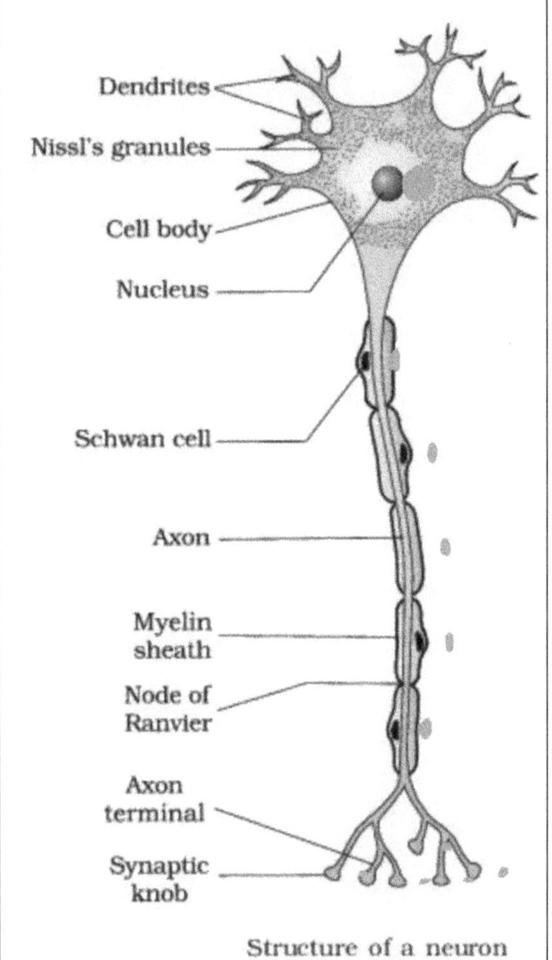

Structure of a neuron

I. Myelinated nerve fibres

- The myelinated nerve fibres are enveloped with **Schwann cells,** which form a myelin sheath around the axon.

- Speed of nerve impulse conduction is high.

- The gaps between two adjacent myelin sheaths are called **nodes of Ranvier.**

- Myelinated nerve fibres are found in spinal and cranial nerves.

- Speed of nerve impulse conduction is low.

II. Un-myelinated nerve fibre

- Unmyelinated nerve fibre is enclosed by a **Schwann cell** that does not form a myelin sheath around the axon, and is commonly found in autonomous and the somatic neural systems.

8.3.1 Generation and Conduction of Nerve Impulse

During this three stages found-

1.Polarisation, 2. Depolarisation, 3. Repolarisation

1.Polarisation

- Neurons are excitable cells because their membranes are in a polarized state.

- Different types of ion channels are present on the neural membrane.

- These ion channels are selectively permeable to different ions.

- When a neuron is not conducting any impulse, i.e., resting stage, the axonal membrane is comparatively more permeable to potassium ions (K^+) and nearly impermeable to sodium ions (Na^+). Similarly, the membrane is impermeable to negatively charged proteins present in the axoplasm.

- The axoplasm inside the axon contains high concentration of K^+ and negatively charged proteins and low concentration of Na^+.

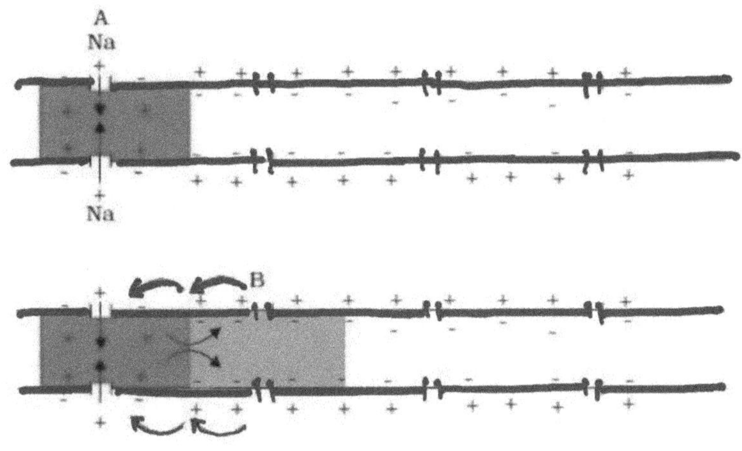

Diagrammatic representation of impulse conduction through an axon (at points A and B)

- The fluid outside the axon contains a **low concentration of K^+**, a high concentration of Na+ and thus form a **concentration** gradient.

- These ionic gradients across the resting membrane are maintained by the active transport of ions by the sodium-potassium pump which transports **3 Na^+ outwards** for **2 K^+ into** the cell.

- So the outer surface of the **axonal** membrane possesses a positive charge while its inner surface becomes negatively charged and therefore is polarised.

- The **electrical potential** difference across the resting **plasma membrane** is called as the **resting potential**.

- The value of resting potential is −70mv.

2. **Depolarisation**

- When a stimulus is applied on the **polarised membrane**, the membrane becomes freely permeable to Na^+.

- So **rapid influx of Na^+** followed by the reversal of the polarity at that site, i.e., the outer surface of the membrane becomes negatively charged and the inner side becomes positively charged.

- The **polarity** of the membrane is now reversed and so **depolarization occur.**

- The **electrical** potential difference across the plasma membrane now called the **action potential**, which creates a **nerve impulse**.

- The value of action potential is **+30mv.**

- At sites immediately ahead, the **axon membrane** has a positive charge on the outer surface and a negative charge on its inner surface.

- As a result, a **current** flows on the inner surface of axon.

- The sequence is **repeated** along the length of the axon and consequently the impulse is conducted.

- The rise in the stimulus-induced **permeability** to **Na⁺ is extremely** short lived (takes place in mili seconds)

3. Repolarisation

- It is quickly followed by a rise in **permeability** to **K⁺**.

- Within a fraction of a second, **K⁺ diffuses** outside the membrane and restores the resting potential of the **membrane** at the site of excitation.

- So the fibre becomes once more responsive to further **stimulation**.

8.3.2 Transmission of Impulses

- A nerve impulse is transmitted from one neuron to another through junctions called synapses.

- A **synapse** is formed by the membranes of a pre-synaptic neuron and a post-synaptic neuron, which may or may not be separated by a gap called **synaptic cleft**.

- There are two types of synapses, namely, **electrical synapses and chemical synapses**.

a. Electrical synapses

- At **electrical** synapses, the membranes of pre- and post-synaptic neurons are in very close proximity.

- **Electrical** current can flow directly from one neuron into the other across these synapses.

- **Transmission** of an impulse across electrical synapses is very similar to impulse conduction along a single axon.

- Impulse **transmission** across an electrical synapse is always faster than that across a chemical synapse.

- **Electrical** synapses are rare in our system.

b. Chemical synapses.

- **At a chemical synapse**, the membranes of the pre- and post-synaptic neurons are separated by a fluid-filled space called synaptic cleft.

- Chemicals called **neurotransmitters** are involved in the transmission of impulses at these synapses.

- The axon terminals contain vesicles filled with these neurotransmitters.

- When an **impulse (action potential)** arrives at the axon terminal, it stimulates the movement of the synaptic vesicles

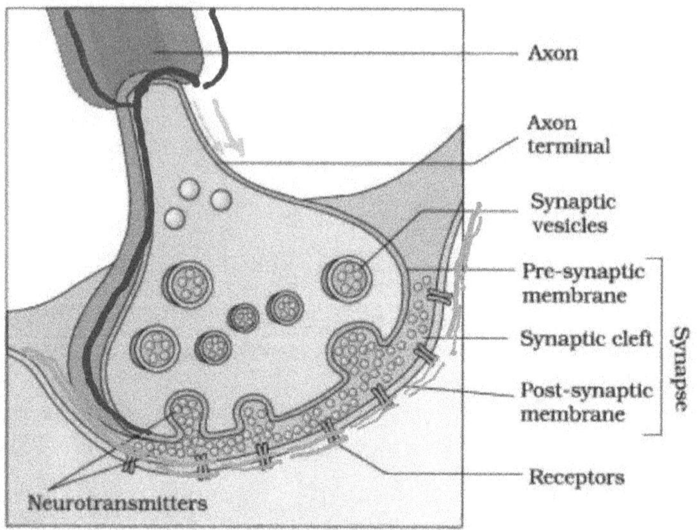

Diagram showing axon terminal and synapse

towards the membrane where they fuse with the plasma membrane and release their neurotransmitters in the synaptic cleft.

- The released neurotransmitters bind to their specific **receptors**, present on the post-synaptic membrane.

- This binding opens ion channels allowing the entry of ions which can generate a new potential in the **post-synaptic** neuron.

- The new potential developed may be either excitatory or inhibitory.

8.4 CENTRAL NEURAL SYSTEM

- **The brain** is the central information processing organ of our body.

- **The brain** acts as the 'command and control system'.

- **The brain** controls the voluntary movements, balance of the body, functioning of vital involuntary organs (e.g., lungs, heart, kidneys, etc.), thermoregulation, hunger, thirst, circadian (24-hour) rhythms of our body, activities of several endocrine glands and human behaviour.

- It is also the site for processing of **vision, hearing, speech, memory, intelligence, emotions** and **thoughts**.

- The human brain is **well protected by the skull**.

- Inside the skull, the brain is covered by **cranial meninges** consisting of an outer layer called **dura mater**, a very thin middle layer called **arachnoid** and an inner layer (which is in contact with the brain tissue) called **pia mater**.

- The brain can be divided into three major parts: (i) **forebrain**, (ii) **midbrain**, and (iii) **hindbrain**

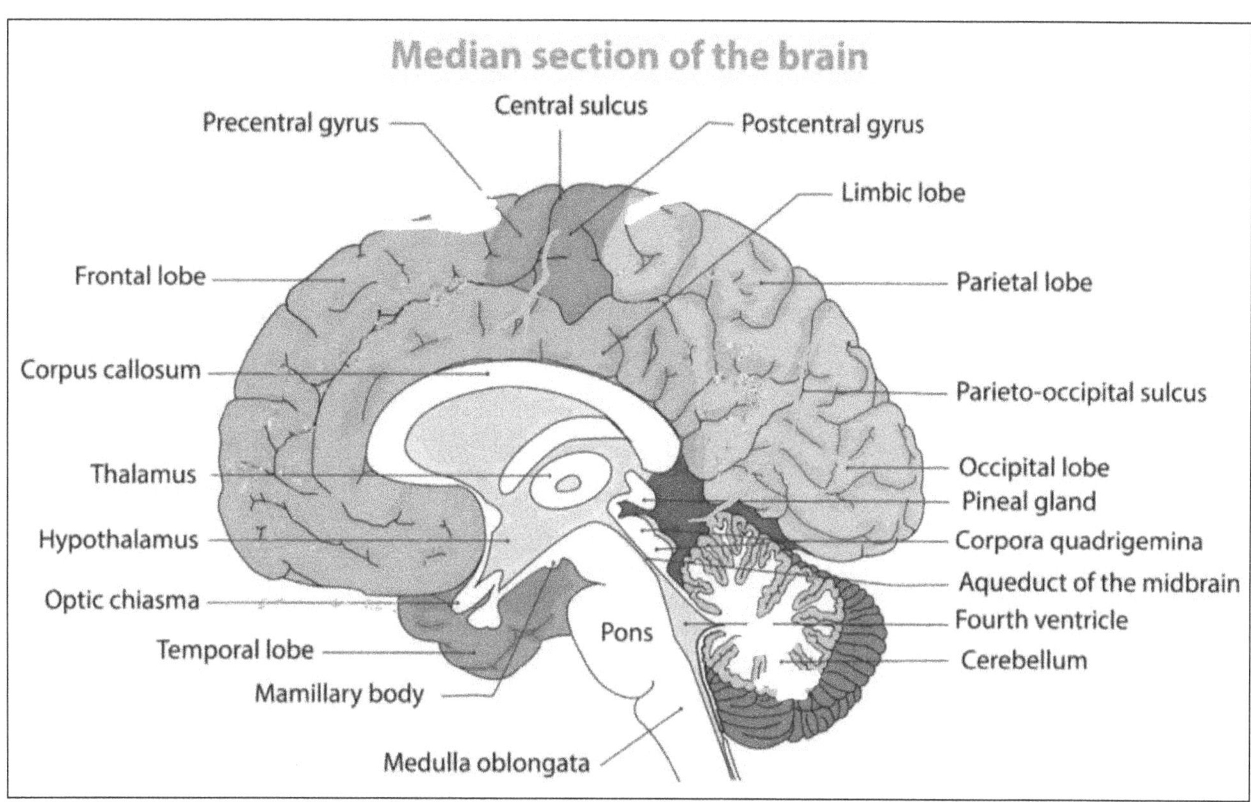

8.4.1 Forebrain

- The forebrain consists of **cerebrum, thalamus** and **hypothalamus.**

a. Cerebrum

- Cerebrum forms the major part of the human brain.
- A deep cleft divides the cerebrum longitudinally into two halves, which are termed as the left and right **cerebral hemispheres.**
- The hemispheres are connected by a tract of nerve fibres called **corpus callosum.**
- The layer of cells which covers the cerebral hemisphere is called cerebral cortex and is thrown into prominent folds.
- **The cerebral cortex** is referred to as the grey matter due to its greyish appearance.
- **The neuron cell bodies** are concentrated here **giving the colour.**
- The cerebral cortex contains **motor areas, sensory areas and large regions** that are neither clearly sensory nor motor in function.
- These regions called as the **association areas** are responsible for complex functions like intersensory associations, memory and **communication.**
- Fibres of the tracts are covered with the myelin sheath, which constitute the inner part of cerebral hemisphere.
- They give an opaque white appearance to the layer and, hence, is called the white matter.

b. Thalamus

- The cerebrum wraps around a structure called thalamus, which is a major coordinating centre for sensory and motor signaling.

c. Hypothalamus

- The **hypothalamus** lies at the base of the thalamus.
- The **hypothalamus** contains a number of centres to control body temperature, urge for eating and drinking.
- It also contains several groups of **neurosecretory** cells.
- Neurosecretory cells secrete hormones called hypothalamic hormones.

Points to remember-

- The inner parts of cerebral hemispheres and a group of associated deep structures like amygdala, hippocampus, etc., form a complex structure called **the limbic lobe or limbic system.**
- Along with the hypothalamus, it is involved in the regulation of sexual behaviour, expression of emotional reactions (e.g., **excitement, pleasure, rage and fear**), and **motivation.**

8.4.2 Midbrain

- The midbrain is located between the thalamus/hypothalamus of the forebrain and pons of the hindbrain.

a. Cerebral aqueduct

- A canal called the **cerebral aqueduct** passess through the midbrain.

b. Corpora quadrigemina.

- **The dorsal portion of the midbrain** consists mainly of four round swellings (lobes) called **corpora quadrigemina**.

c. Brain stem

- Midbrain and hindbrain form the brain stem.

8.4.3 Hindbrain

- The hindbrain comprises **pons, cerebellum** and **medulla** (also called the medulla oblongata).

a. Pons

- Pons consists of fibre tracts that **interconnect** different regions of the brain.

b. Cerebellum

- Cerebellum has very **convoluted** surface in order to provide the additional space for many more neurons.

c. Medulla

- The medulla of the brain is connected to the spinal cord.

- The medulla contains centres which control respiration, cardiovascular reflexes and gastric secretions.

8.5 Reflex Action and Reflex Arc

- A sudden **withdrawal** of a body part which comes in contact with objects that are extremely hot, cold pointed or animals that are scary or poisonous.

- The entire process of **response** to a peripheral nervous stimulation, that occurs involuntarily, i.e., without **conscious** effort or thought and requires the involvement of a part of the central nervous system is called a **reflex action**.

- Reflex actions are quick, involuntary, fast.

- The reflex pathway **comprises** at least one afferent neuron (receptor) and one efferent (effector or exciter) neuron appropriately arranged in a series.

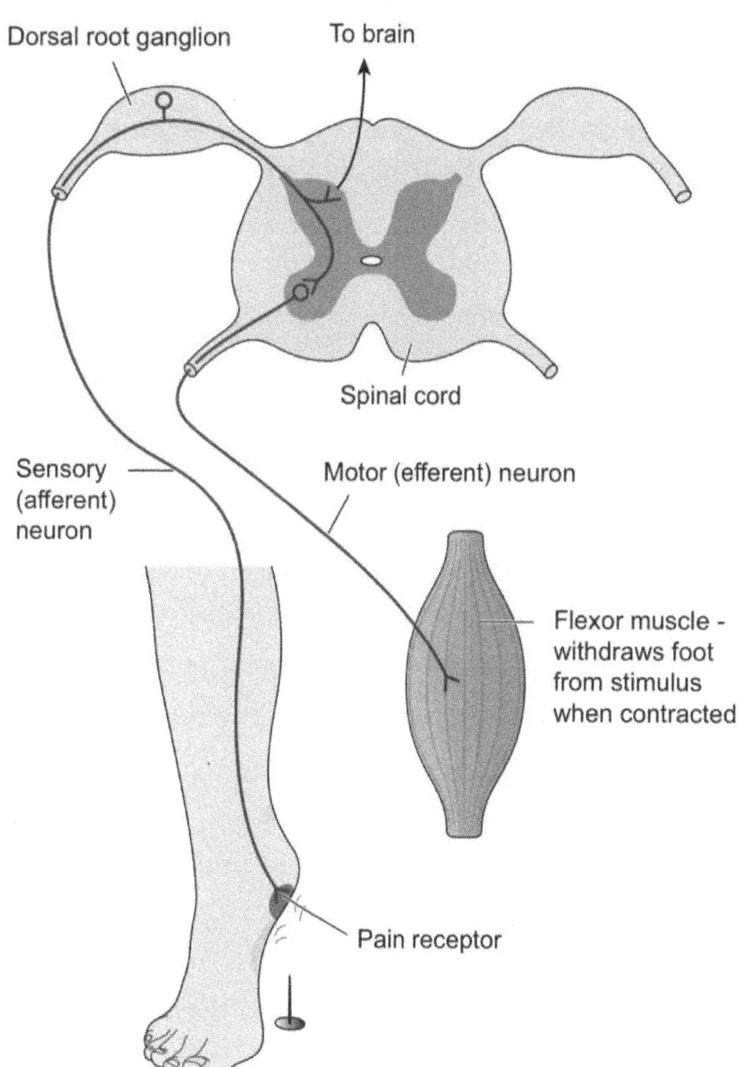

- The afferent neuron **receives** signal from a sensory organ and transmits the impulse via a dorsal nerve root into the **CNS** (at the level of spinal cord).
- The efferent neuron then carries signals from CNS to the **effector**.

ADDITIONAL IMPORTANT CONTENT

Eye

- Our paired eyes present.
- Eyes are located in sockets of the skull called **orbits**.

a. Parts of an eye

- The eye ball is nearly a spherical structure.
- The wall of the eye ball is composed of three layers.

b. The external layer of eye ball

- **The external layer** is composed of a dense connective tissue and is called the **sclera**.
- The anterior portion of this layer is called the **cornea**.

c. The middle layer of eye ball

- **The middle layer, choroid**, contains many blood vessels and looks bluish in colour.
- The choroid layer is thin over the posterior two-thirds of the eye ball, but it becomes thick s in the anterior part to form the **ciliary body**.
- **The ciliary body** itself continues forward to form a pigmented and opaque structure called the **iris** which is the visible coloured portion of the eye.
- The eye ball contains a transparent crystalline **lens** which is held in place by ligaments attached to the ciliary body.
- In front of the lens, the aperture surrounded by the iris is called the **pupil**.
- The diameter of the pupil is regulated by the muscle fibres of iris.

d. The inner layer of eye ball

- **The inner layer is the retina** and it contains three layers of cells – from inside to outside – ganglion cells, bipolar cells and photoreceptor cells
- There are two types of photoreceptor cells, namely, **rods** and **cones**.
- These cells contain the light-sensitive proteins called the **photopigments**.
- The daylight (photopic) vision and colour vision are functions of cones and the **twilight** (scotopic) vision is the function of the rods.
- The rods contain a purplish-red protein called the **rhodopsin** or visual purple, which contains a derivative of **Vitamin A**.

Points to remember-

- The **optic nerves** leave the eye and the retinal blood vessels enter it at a point medial to and slightly above the posterior pole of the eye ball.

- Photoreceptor cells are not present in that region and hence it is called the **blind spot**.
- At the posterior pole of the eye lateral to the blind spot, there is a yellowish pigmented spot called macula lutea with a central pit called the **fovea**.
- **The fovea** is a thinned-out portion of the retina where only the cones are densely packed.
- It is the point where the visual acuity (resolution) is the greatest.

e. Chambers in eyes

- The space between the cornea and the lens is called the **aqueous chamber** and contains a thin watery fluid called aqueous humor.
- The space between the lens and the retina is called the **vitreous chamber** and is filled with a transparent gel called vitreous humor.

Points to remember-

- In the human eye, there are **three types of cones** which possess their own characteristic photopigments that respond to red, green and blue lights.
- The sensations of different colours are produced by various combinations of these cones and their photopigments.
- When these cones are stimulated equally, a sensation of white light is produced.

f. Mechanism of Vision

- The light rays in visible wavelength **focussed** on the retina.
- The potentials created (impulses) in rods and cones.
- The photosensitive compounds (photopigments) in the human eyes is composed of **opsin** (a protein) and **retinal** (an aldehyde of vitamin A).
- Due to light dissociation of the **retinal** from opsin resulting in changes in the structure of the opsin.
- So membrane **permeability** changes.
- Now potential differences are generated in the **photoreceptor** cells.
- Which produces a signal that generates action potentials in the ganglion cells through the bipolar cells.
- The action potentials (impulses) are **transmitted** by the optic nerves to the **visual cortex** area of the brain.
- The neural impulses are analysed by brain and the image formed on the retina is identified based on earlier memory and experience.

The Ear

- The ears perform two sensory functions, hearing and maintenance of **body balance**.
- Anatomically, the ear can be divided into three major sections called the **outer ear**, the **middle ear** and the **inner ear.**

a. The outer ear

- **The** outer ear consists of the **pinna** and **external auditory meatus** (canal).
- The pinna collects the vibrations in the air which produce sound.

- The external auditory meatus leads inwards and extends up to the **tympanic membrane** (the **ear drum**).
- There are very fine hairs and wax-secreting sebaceous glands in the skin of the pinna and the meatus.
- The tympanic membrane is composed of connective tissues covered with skin outside and with mucus membrane inside.

b. The middle ear

- The middle ear contains three ossicles called **malleus**, **incus** and **stapes** which are attached to one another in a chain-like fashion.
- The malleus is attached to the tympanic membrane and the stapes is attached to the **oval window** of the cochlea.
- The ear ossicles increase the efficiency of transmission of sound waves to the inner ear.
- An **Eustachian tube** connects the middle ear cavity with the pharynx.
- The Eustachian tube helps in equalising the pressures on either sides of the ear drum.

c. The inner ear

- The fluid-filled inner ear called **labyrinth** consists of two parts, the bony and the membranous labyrinths.
- The bony **labyrinth** is a series of channels.
- Inside these channels lies the membranous labyrinth, which is surrounded by a fluid called perilymph.
- The **membranous** labyrinth is filled with a fluid called **endolymph**.
- It contain cochlea and **vestibular** apparatus.

d. Cochlea

- The coiled portion of the labyrinth is called **cochlea**.
- The membranes constituting cochlea, the reissner's and basilar, divide the surounding perilymph filled bony labyrinth into an upper **scala vestibuli** and a lower scala tympani.
- The space within cochlea called **scala media** is filled with endolymph.
- At the base of the cochlea, the **scala vestibuli** ends at the oval window, while the scala tympani terminates at the round window which opens to the middle ear.
- The **organ of corti** is a structure located on the basilar membrane which contains **hair cells** that act as auditory receptors.
- The hair cells are present in rows on the **internal side** of the organ of corti.
- The basal end of the hair cell is in close contact with the afferent nerve fibres.
- A large number of processes called **stereo cilia** are projected from the apical part of each hair cell.
- Above the rows of the hair cells is a thin elastic membrane called **tectorial membrane**.

e. Vestibular apparatus,

- The inner ear also contains a complex system called **vestibular apparatus,** located above the cochlea.

- The vestibular apparatus is composed of three **semi-circular canals** and the **otolith organ** consisting of the saccule and utricle.

- Each **semi-circular** canal lies in a different plane at right angles to each other.

- The membranous canals are suspended in the **perilymph** of the bony canals.

- The base of canals is swollen and is called ampulla, which contains a projecting ridge called **crista ampullaris** which has hair cells.

- The saccule and utricle contain a projecting ridge called **macula**.

- The crista and macula are the specific receptors of the vestibular apparatus responsible for maintenance of balance of the body and posture.

d. Mechanism of Hearing

Takes place in following steps-

a) The external ear **receives** sound waves and directs them to the ear drum.

b) The ear drum vibrates in response to the sound waves and these vibrations are transmitted through the ear **ossicles** (malleus, incus and stapes) to the oval window.

c) The **vibrations** are passed through the oval window on to the fluid of the cochlea, which generate waves in the lymphs.

d) The waves in the lymphs induce a **ripple** in the **basilar** membrane.

e) These movements of the basilar membrane **bend** the hair cells, **pressing** them against the tectorial membrane.

f) So nerve impulses are **generated** in the **associated** afferent neurons.

g) These impulses are transmitted by the afferent fibres via auditory nerves to the auditory cortex of the brain, where the impulses are analysed and the sound is identified by **auditory system**.

1. Consider the following statements and find out the correct option-

    A. The neural organisation is very simple in lower invertebrates.

    B. *Hydra* it is composed of a bipolar of neurons.

    C. The neural system is better organised in insects, where a brain is present along with a number of ganglia and neural tissues.

    D. The vertebrates have a more developed neural system.

    Which of the above are correct -

    1. A,B,C   2. B,C

    3. A,D,C   4. A,B,C,D

2. Match the list 1 and 2-

    List 1   List 2

List 1	List 2
a. A neuron is a microscopic structure	composed of three major parts, namely, **cell body**, **dendrites** and **axon**
b. The cell body contains	cytoplasm with typical cell organelles and certain granular bodies called **Nissl's granules.**
c. Each branch of axon	terminates as a bulb-like structure called **synaptic knob** which possess synaptic vesicles containing chemicals called **neurotransmitters.**
d. The gaps	between two adjacent myelin sheaths are called **nodes of Ranvier.**

    How many of them are correctly matched –

    1. one   2. two

    3. three   4. four

3. Consider the following statements-

I. There are two types of axons, namely, **myelinated** and **nonmyelinated.**

II. The myelinated nerve fibres are enveloped with **Schwann cells,** which form a myelin sheath around the axon.

III. The gaps between two adjacent myelin sheaths are called **nodes of Ranvier.**

IV. **Myelinated** nerve fibres are found in spinal and cranial nerves.

How many of them are/is correct -

1. one   2. two

3. three   4. four

4. Read the following statement carefully with respect to Humans-

A. Neurons are excitable cells because their membranes are in a polarized state.

B. **synapse** is formed by the membranes of a pre-synaptic neuron and a post-synaptic neuron, which never separated by a gap called **synaptic cleft.**

C. There are two types of synapses found namely, electrical synapses and chemical synapses.

D. At electrical synapses, the membranes of pre- and post-synaptic neurons are in very close proximity.

How many of them are/is correct -

1. three   2. four

3. one   4. two

5. Consider the following statements and find out the correct option

STATEMENT 1. Unmyelinated nerve fibre is enclosed by a Schwann cell that does not form a myelin sheath around the axon, and is commonly found in autonomous and the somatic neural systems.

STATEMENT 2. The axons transmit nerve impulses away from the cell body to a synapse or to a neuro-muscular junction.

1. Both are correct statements   2. Only Statement 1 correct

3. Both are wrong statements   4. Only statement 2 correct

6. Go through the following statement-

ASSERTION(A). Neurons are excitable cells because their membranes are in a polarized state.

REASON(R). Different types of ion channels are present on the neural membrane and these ion channels are selectively permeable to different ions so polarization arises.

1. A correct and R is correct explanation of A

2. A correct and R is also correct but R is not correct explanation of A

3. A. correct but R incorrect

4. A and R both are incorrect

7. Find out the incorrect statement-

1. A nerve impulse is transmitted from one neuron to another through junctions called synapses.

2. A **synapse** is formed by the membranes of a pre-synaptic neuron and a post-synaptic neuron, which not separated by a gap called **synaptic cleft**.

3. There are two types of synapses, namely, electrical synapses and chemical synapses.

4. At electrical synapses, the membranes of pre- and post-synaptic neurons are in very close proximity.

8. Go through the following statements-

I. The axon terminals contain vesicles filled with neurotransmitters.

II. When an impulse (action potential) arrives at the axon terminal, it stimulates the movement of the synaptic vesicles towards the membrane where they fuse with the plasma membrane and release their neurotransmitters in the synaptic cleft.

III. The released neurotransmitters bind to their specific **receptors**, present on the post-synaptic membrane.

IV. This binding opens ion channels allowing the entry of ions which can generate a new potential in the post-synaptic neuron.

V. The new potential developed only excitatory type.

How many of them are correct-

1. two

2. three

3. four

4. five

9. Match the list 1 and 2-

List 1   List 2

a. **RMP**	j. + 30mv
b. **Action potential**	k.-90mv
c. **Hyperpolarization**	l. -70mv
d. **Spike potential**	m. -70 to +30mv

Find out the correct option –

1. a.k, b.j, c.l, d.m

2. a.k,b.l,c.j,d.m

3. a.l,b.j,c.k,d.m

4. a.l,b.j,c.m,d.k

10. Consider the following statements and find out the correct option-

STATEMENT 1. When a neuron is not conducting any impulse, i.e., resting, the axonal membrane is comparatively more permeable to potassium ions and nearly impermeable to sodium ions.

STATEMENT 2. In resting stage the membrane is impermeable to negatively charged proteins present in the axoplasm.

1. Both are wrong statements

2. Only Statement 1 correct

3. Both are correct statements

4. Only statement 2 correct

11. Read the following statements very carefully and find out the incorrect-

a) There are two types of axons, namely, **myelinated** and **nonmyelinated**.

b) The myelinated nerve fibres are enveloped with **Schwann cells,** which form a myelin sheath around the axon.

c) The gaps between two adjacent myelin sheaths are called **nodes of Bartholin.**

d) Myelinated nerve fibres are found in spinal and cranial nerves.

Which of the above statement are correct?

1. a and c both

2. a,b,c,d

3. a,b,c

4. a,b,d

12. Go through the following statements-

ASSERTION(A). The cell body of neuron contains cytoplasm with typical cell organelles and certain granular bodies called **Nissl's granules.**

REASON(R). Short fibres which branch repeatedly and project out of the cell body also contain Nissl's granules and are called dendrites.

1. A correct and R is correct explanation of A

2. A correct and R is also correct but R is not correct explanation of A

3. A. correct but R incorrect

4. A and R both are incorrect

13. Find out incorrect statement with respect to neurotransmitters -

1. Chemicals called neurotransmitters are involved in the transmission of impulses at these synapses.

2. The axon terminals contain vesicles filled with these neurotransmitters.

3. When an impulse (action potential) arrives at the axon terminal, it stimulates the movement of the synaptic vesicles towards the membrane where they fuse with the plasma membrane and release their neurotransmitters in the synaptic cleft.

4. The released neurotransmitters bind to their specific **receptors**, present on the pre-synaptic membrane.

14. Read the following statements and find out correct option-

I. At electrical synapses, the membranes of pre- and post-synaptic neurons are in very close proximity.

II. Electrical current can flow directly from one neuron into the other across these synapses.

III. Transmission of an impulse across electrical synapses is very similar to impulse conduction along a single axon.

IV. Impulse transmission across an electrical synapse is always faster than that across a chemical synapse.

How many of them is/are correct-

1. four

2. one

3. two

4. three

15. Consider the following statements and find out the correct option-

STATEMENT 1. The brain is the central information processing organ of our body, and acts as the 'command and control system'.

STATEMENT 2. Brain controls the voluntary movements, balance of the body, functioning of vital involuntary organs (e.g., lungs, heart, kidneys, etc.), thermoregulation, hunger and thirst, circadian (24-hour) rhythms of our body, activities of several endocrine glands and human behaviour.

1. Both are wrong statements

2. Only Statement 1 correct

3. Both are correct statements

4. Only statement 2 correct

16. Match the list 1 and 2 -

List 1

List 2

a. The forebrain consists of	cerebrum, thalamus and hypothalamus
b. A deep cleft divides the cerebrum longitudinally into two halves, which are termed as	the left and right cerebral hemispheres.
c. The cerebral cortex is referred to as the grey matter due to	its greyish appearance.

Which of the above are correctly matched-

1 a and b

2 b and c

3 c and a

4 a, b, c

17. Consider the following -

a) Cerebrum forms the major part of the human brain.

b) A deep cleft divides the cerebrum longitudinally into two halves, which are termed as the left and right **cerebral hemispheres.**

c) The hemispheres are connected by a tract of nerve fibres called **corpus callosum.**

d) The layer of cells which covers the cerebral hemisphere is called cerebral cortex and is thrown into prominent folds.

Which of the above statement/s is/are correct?

1. a and d only

2. a,b,c only

3. d and c only

4. a,b,c,d

18. Consider the following -

a) The cerebral cortex contains motor areas, sensory areas and large regions that are neither clearly sensory nor motor in function.

b) These regions called as the **association areas** are responsible for complex functions like intersensory associations, memory and communication.

c) Fibers of the tracts are covered with the myelin sheath, which constitute the inner part of cerebral hemisphere.

d) Myelin sheath give an opaque white appearance to the layer and, hence, is called the white matter.

Which of the above statement are correct?

1. a and d only

2. c and a only

3. d and b only

4. a,b,c,d

19. Consider the following statements and find out the incorrect one-

1. The cerebral cortex contains motor areas and sensory areas.

2. The **association areas** are also found in cerebral cortex, which responsible for complex functions like intersensory associations, memory and communication.

3. Cerebral hemisphere is a part of hind brain.

4. Pons is a part of hind brain.

20. Read the following statements-

I. The hypothalamus contains a number of centres which control body temperature, urge for eating and drinking.

II. Hypothalamus also contains several groups of neurosecretory cells, which secrete hormones called hypothalamic hormones.

III. The inner parts of cerebral hemispheres and a group of associated deep structures like amygdala, hippocampus, etc., form a complex structure called the limbic lobe or limbic system.

IV. Along with the hypothalamus, limbic system is involved in the regulation of sexual behaviour, expression of emotional reactions (e.g., excitement, pleasure, rage and fear), and motivation.

How many of them are/is correct **statements-**

1. two

2. three

3. four

4. one

21. Consider the following statements and find out the correct option for humans-

STATEMENT 1. The midbrain is located between the thalamus/hypothalamus of the forebrain and pons of the hindbrain.

STATEMENT 2. A canal called the **cerebral aqueduct** passess through the midbrain.

1. Both are wrong statements

2. Only Statement 1 correct

3. Both are correct statements

4. Only statement 2 correct

22. Go through the following statement and find out the correct option-

ASSERTION(A). Midbrain and hindbrain form the brain stem.

REASON(R). The hindbrain comprises **pons** and **medulla** only.

1. A correct and R is correct explanation of A

2. A correct and R is also correct but R is not correct explanation of A

3. A correct but R incorrect

4. A and R both are incorrect

23. Go through the following statement and find out the correct option-

   A. Pons consists of fibre tracts that interconnect different regions of the brain.

   B. Cerebellum has very convoluted surface in order to provide the additional space for many more neurons.

   C. Midbrain and hindbrain form the brain stem.

   D. The hypothalamus do not contains a number of centres which control body temperature, urge for eating and drinking.

Which of the above statement are correct -

1. A and C only

2. C and D only

3. A,B,C only

4. A,B,C,D

24. Read the statements given below-

A. Pons contain pneumotaxic centre.

B. Cerebellum has very convoluted surface in order to provide the additional space for many more neurons.

C. The medulla of the brain is connected to the spinal cord.

D. The medulla contains centres which control respiration, cardiovascular reflexes and gastric secretions.

Which of the above statement are correct?

1. A and C only

2. C and D only

3. A,B,C only

4. A,B,C,D

25. Consider the following-

   A. You must have experienced a sudden withdrawal of a body part which comes in contact with objects that are extremely hot, cold pointed or animals that are scary or poisonous.

   B. The entire process of response to a peripheral nervous stimulation, that occurs involuntarily, i.e., without conscious effort or thought and requires the involvement of a part of the central nervous system is called a **reflex action**.

   C. The reflex pathway comprises at least one afferent neuron (receptor) and one efferent (effector or exciter) neuron appropriately arranged in a series.

   D. The afferent neuron receives signal from a sensory organ and transmits the impulse via a dorsal nerve root into the CNS (at the level of spinal cord).

Which of the above statement are correct?

1. A and C only

2. A only

3. D and C only

4. A,B,C,D

26. Consider the following statements-

A. The sensory organs detect all types of changes in the environment and send appropriate signals to the CNS, where all the inputs are processed and analysed.

B. Signals are then sent to different parts/ centres of the brain.

C. Sense organ can sense changes in the environment.

D. The ear is a sensory organ for hearing and balancing.

How many of them are correct-

1. one   2. two

3. three   4. four

27. Match the list 1 and 2-

List 1   List 2

a. The choroid layer is thin over the posterior two-thirds of the eye ball, but it becomes thick s in the anterior part to form the	ciliary body
b. In front of the lens, the aperture surrounded by the iris is called the	**pupil**
c. Photoreceptor cells are not present in that region and hence it is called the	**blind spot**
d. At the posterior pole of the eye lateral to the blind spot, there is a yellowish pigmented spot called macula lutea with a central pit called the	**fovea**

How many of them are correctly matched –

1. one   2. two

3. three   4. four

28. Consider the following-

a) The adult human eye ball is nearly a spherical structure.

b) The wall of the eye ball is composed of three layers.

c) The external layer is composed of a dense connective tissue and is called the **sclera**.

d) The anterior portion of this layer is called the **cornea**.

e) The middle layer, **choroid**, contains many blood vessels and looks bluish in colour.

Which of the above statements are correct-

1. a and c only   2. a only

3. d and c only   4. all are correct

29. Consider the following statements and find out incorrect one-

1. There are two types of photoreceptor cells, namely, **rods** and **cones**.

2. These cells contain the light-sensitive proteins called the photopigments.

3. The daylight (photopic) vision and colour vision are functions of cones and the twilight (scotopic) vision is the function of the rods.

4. The rods contain a purplish-red protein called the rhodopsin or visual purple, which contains a derivative of Vitamin D.

30. Read the following points -

a) In the human eye, there are three types of cones which possess their own characteristic photopigments that respond to red, green and blue lights.

b) The sensations of different colours are produced by various combinations of these cones and their photopigments.

c) When these cones are stimulated equally, a sensation of white light is produced.

d) The **optic nerves** leave the eye and the retinal blood vessels enter it at a point medial to and slightly above the posterior pole of the eye ball.

How many of them are/is correct –

1. four

2. two

3. three

4. one

31. Read the following statements and find out the correct option

STATEMENT 1. The **optic nerves** leave the eye and the retinal blood vessels enter it at a point medial to and slightly above the posterior pole of the eye ball.

STATEMENT 2. Photoreceptor cells are not present in that region and hence it is called the **blind spot**.

1. Both are wrong statements

2. Both are correct statements

3. Only statement 1 correct

4. Only statement 2 correct

32. Go through the following statement and find out the correct option-

ASSERTION(A). The fovea is a thinned-out portion of the retina where only the cones are densely packed.

REASON(R). It is the point where the visual acuity (resolution) is the greatest.

1. A correct and R is correct explanation of A

2. A correct and R is also correct but R is not correct explanation of A

3. A correct but R incorrect

4. A and R both are incorrect

33. Find out the incorrect option w.r.t. retina-

1. The **retina** and it contains two layers of cells only – from inside to outside – ganglion cells and photoreceptor cells

2. There are two types of photoreceptor cells, namely, **rods** and **cones**.

3. These cells contain the light-sensitive proteins called the photopigments.

4. The daylight (photopic) vision and colour vision are functions of cones and the twilight (scotopic) vision is the function of the rods.

34. Read the following statements

I. The light rays in visible wavelength focussed on the retina through the cornea and lens generate potentials (impulses) in rods and cones.

II. The photosensitive compounds (photopigments) in the human eyes is composed of **opsin** (a protein) and **retinal** (an aldehyde of vitamin A).

III. Light induces dissociation of the retinal from opsin resulting in changes in the structure of the opsin.

IV. The changes in the structure of the opsin causes membrane permeability changes.

How many of above is/are correct-

1. three

2. four

3. two

4. one

35. Which of the following is an incorrect statement-

1. The reflex pathway comprises at least one afferent neuron (receptor) and one efferent (effector or exciter) neuron appropriately arranged in a series.

2. The afferent neuron receives signal from a sensory organ and transmits the impulse via a dorsal nerve root into the CNS (at the level of spinal cord).

3. The efferent neuron then carries signals from effector to the CNS.

4. The knee jerk reflex is an example of monosynaptic reflex.

36. Consider the following statements –

i. The space between the cornea and the lens is called the **aqueous chamber** and contains a thin watery fluid called aqueous humor.

ii. The space between the lens and the retina is called the **vitreous chamber** and is filled with a transparent gel called vitreous humor.

iii. The eye ball contains a transparent crystalline **lens** which is held in place by ligaments attached to the ciliary body.

iv. In front of the lens, the aperture surrounded by the iris is called the **pupil**.

Which of the above statements are correct-

1. i,ii only

2. i,iii,iv only

3. i,ii,iii only

4. all are correct

37. Read the following statements-

i. Cerebellum has very convoluted surface in order to provide the additional space for many more neurons.

ii. The medulla of the brain is connected to the spinal cord.

iii. The medulla contains centres which control respiration, cardiovascular reflexes and gastric secretions.

iv. The inner parts of cerebral hemispheres and a group of associated deep structures like amygdala, hippocampus, etc., form a complex structure called the limbic lobe or limbic system.

v. Along with the hypothalamus, it is involved in the regulation of sexual behaviour, expression of emotional reactions (e.g., excitement, pleasure, rage and fear), and motivation.

Which of the above statements is/are correct-

1. i and ii only

2. iii And ii only

3. iv and iii only

4. All are correct

38. Consider the following statements-

I. Cerebrum forms the major part of the human brain.

II. A deep cleft divides the cerebrum longitudinally into two halves, which are termed as the left and right **cerebral hemispheres**.

III. The hemispheres are connected by a tract of nerve fibres called **corpus callosum**.

IV. The layer of cells which covers the cerebral hemisphere is called cerebral cortex and is thrown into prominent folds.

V. The cerebral cortex is referred to as the grey matter due to its greyish appearance.

How many of above are correct-

1. three

2 .four

3. two

4. five

39. Read the following statements and find out the correct option-

STATEMENT 1. The cerebral cortex contains motor areas, sensory areas and large regions that are neither clearly sensory nor motor in function.

STATEMENT 2. These regions called as the **association areas** are responsible for complex functions like intersensory associations, memory and communication.

1. Both are wrong statements

2. Both are correct statements

3. Only statement 1 correct

4. Only statement 2 correct

40. Read the following statements-

a. The ear can be divided into the outer ear, the middle ear and the inner ear.

b. The middle ear contains three ossicles called malleus, incus and stapes.

c. The fluid filled inner ear is called the labyrinth, and the coiled portion of the labyrinth is called cochlea.

d. The organ of corti is a structure which contains hair cells that act as auditory receptors and is located on the basilar membrane.

e. The vibrations produced in the ear drum are transmitted through the ear ossicles and oval window to the fluid-filled inner ear.

Which of the following are correct?

1. a and b only

2. b and c only

3. a,b,c,d only

4. All are correct

41. Go through the following statement and find out the correct option-

ASSERTION(A). Nerve impulses are generated and transmitted by the afferent fibres to the auditory cortex of the brain.

REASON(R). The inner ear contains a simple system located above the cochlea called vestibular apparatus.

1. A correct and R is correct explanation of A

2. A correct and R is also correct but R is not correct explanation of A

3. A. correct but R incorrect

4. A and R both are incorrect

42. Find out the incorrect statement-

1. The external ear receives sound waves and directs them to the ear drum.

2. The ear drum vibrates in response to the sound waves and these vibrations are transmitted through the ear ossicles (malleus, incus and stapes) to the oval window.

3. The vibrations are passed through the oval window on to the fluid of the cochlea, where they generate waves in the lymphs.

4. Firstly these waves comes in scala media and induce a ripple in the tectorial membrane.

43. Consider the following statements-

A. The inner ear also contains a complex system called **vestibular apparatus**, located above the cochlea.

B. The vestibular apparatus is composed of three **semi-circular canals** and the **otolith organ** consisting of the saccule and utricle.

C. Each semi-circular canal lies in a different plane at right angles to each other.

D. The membranous canals are suspended in the perilymph of the bony canals.

E. The base of canals is swollen and is called ampulla, which contains a projecting ridge called **crista ampullaris** which has hair cells.

F. The saccule and utricle contain a projecting ridge called **macula**.

How many of them are correct-

1. five   2. three

3. four   4. six

44. Read the following statements and find out the correct option –

STATEMENT 1. The base of semicircular canals is swollen and is called ampulla, which contains a projecting ridge called **crista ampullaris** which has hair cells.

STATEMENT 2. The saccule and utricle contain a projecting ridge called **crista**.

1. Both are correct statements   2. Both are wrong statements

3. Only statement 1 correct   4. Only statement 2 correct

45. Find out the incorrect statement-

1. In organ of corti the basal end of the hair cell is in close contact with the afferent nerve fibres.

2. In organ of corti a large number of processes called stereo cilia are projected from the apical part of each hair cell.

3. In organ of corti below the rows of the hair cells is a thin elastic membrane called **tectorial membrane**.

4. The inner ear also contains a complex system called **vestibular apparatus**, located above the cochlea.

46. Read the following statements and find out the correct optios-

STATEMENT 1. The vestibular apparatus is composed of three **semi-circular canals** and the **otolith organ** consisting of the saccule and utricle.

STATEMENT 2. Each semi-circular canal lies in a different plane at right angles to each other

1. Both are correct statements

2. Both are wrong statements.

3. Only statement 1 correct

4. Only statement 2 correct

47. Go through the following statement and find out the correct option-

ASSERTION(A). The **organ of corti** is a structure located on the basilar membrane which contains **hair cells** that act as auditory receptors.

REASON(R). The hair cells are not present in rows on the internal side of the organ of corti.

1. A correct and R is correct explanation of A

2. A correct and R is also correct but R is not correct explanation of A

3. A. correct but R incorrect

4. A and R both are incorrect

48. Find out the incorrect statement –

1. The ear ossicles increase the efficiency of transmission of sound waves to the inner ear.

2. An **Eustachian tube** connects the middle ear cavity with the cochlea.

3. The Eustachian tube helps in equalising the pressures on either sides of the ear drum.

4. The fluid-filled inner ear called **labyrinth** consists of two parts, the bony and the membranous labyrinths. The bony labyrinth is a series of channels

49. Consider the following statements -

A. There are very fine hairs and wax-secreting sebaceous glands in the skin of the pinna and the meatus.

B. The tympanic membrane is composed of connective tissues covered with skin outside and with mucus membrane inside.

C. The middle ear contains three ossicles called **malleus, incus** and **stapes** which are attached to one another in a chain-like fashion.

D. The malleus is attached to the tympanic membrane and the stapes is attached to the **oval window** of the cochlea.

Which of the above statements are correct-

1. A and C only

2. D and B only

3. A,B,C only

4. All are correct

50. Read the following -

A. The ears perform two sensory functions, hearing and maintenance of body balance.

B. Anatomically, the ear can be divided into three major sections called the **outer ear**, the **middle ear** and the **inner ear**.

C. The outer ear consists of the **pinna** and **external auditory meatus** (canal).

D. The pinna collects the vibrations in the air which produce sound.

E. The external auditory meatus leads inwards and extends up to the **tympanic membrane** (the **ear drum**).

Which of the above statements are correct-

1. A and C only

2. A,B,C only

3. A,B,C.D only

4. All are correct

Chemical Coordination and Integration

- **The neural system** provides a point-to-point rapid coordination among organs.

- The neural coordination **is fast but short-lived.**

- The nerve fibres do not innervate **all cells of the body** and the cellular functions need to be continuously regulated; a special kind of coordination and integration has to be provided.

- The function is carried out by hormones.

- **The neural system** and **the endocrine system** jointly coordinate and regulate the physiological functions in the body.

9.1 Endocrine Glands and Hormones

- Endocrine glands lack ducts so called **ductless glands.**

- Endocrine glands secretes **hormones.**

- Study of Endocrine glands called **Endocrinology.**

- Father of Endocrinology **Thomas Edison.**

- First hormone was **secretin.**

- **The classical definition** of hormone as a chemical produced by endocrine glands and released into the blood and transported to a distantly located target organ.

- **The current scientific definition** of hormone: Hormones are non-nutrient chemicals which act as intercellular messengers and are produced in trace amounts.

- The new definition covers a number of new molecules in addition to the hormones secreted by the **organised** endocrine glands.

- Invertebrates have very simple endocrine systems with few hormones.

- But a large number of chemicals which can act as hormones found in vertebrates to help coordination of body **functions.**

9.2 HUMAN ENDOCRINE SYSTEM

- The endocrine glands and hormones are **constitute** of the endocrine system.
- Pituitary, **pineal**, thyroid, adrenal, pancreas, **parathyroid**, thymus and gonads (testis in males and ovary in females) are the organized endocrine bodies in our body.

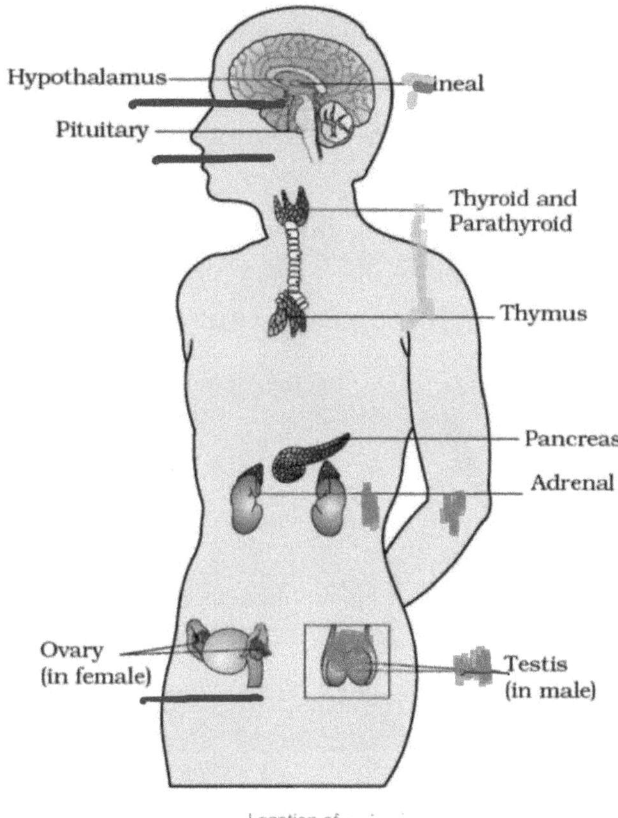

- Some other organs which act as **endocrine** glands are, gastrointestinal tract, liver, kidney, heart, placenta etc.

9.2.1 The Hypothalamus

- The hypothalamus is the **basal part** of diencephalon, forebrain and it regulates a wide spectrum of body functions.
- Also called **masters** of **master** gland.
- Connect neurons to **endocrine** system.
- Origin **ectodermal**.
- The hypothalamus **contains** several groups of **neurosecretory** cells called nuclei which produce hormones.
- These hormones regulate the **synthesis** and secretion of **pituitary** hormones.

- The hormones produced by **hypothalamus** are of two types, the **releasing hormones** (which stimulate secretion of pituitary hormones) and the **inhibiting hormones** (which inhibit secretions of pituitary hormones).

a. Gonadotrophin releasing hormone (GnRH)

- A hypothalamic hormone called Gonadotrophin releasing hormone (GnRH) stimulates the pituitary synthesis and release of gonadotrophins.

b. Somatostatin

- Somatostatin from the **hypothalamus** inhibits the release of growth hormone from the pituitary.

c. Path of hormones - Hypothalamic hormone.

- Hypothalmic hormones originating in the **hypothalamic** neurons, pass through axons and are released from their nerve endings.

- These hormones reach the **pituitary** gland through a portal circulatory system and regulate the functions of the anterior pituitary.

- The posterior pituitary is under the direct neural regulation of the **hypothalamus**.

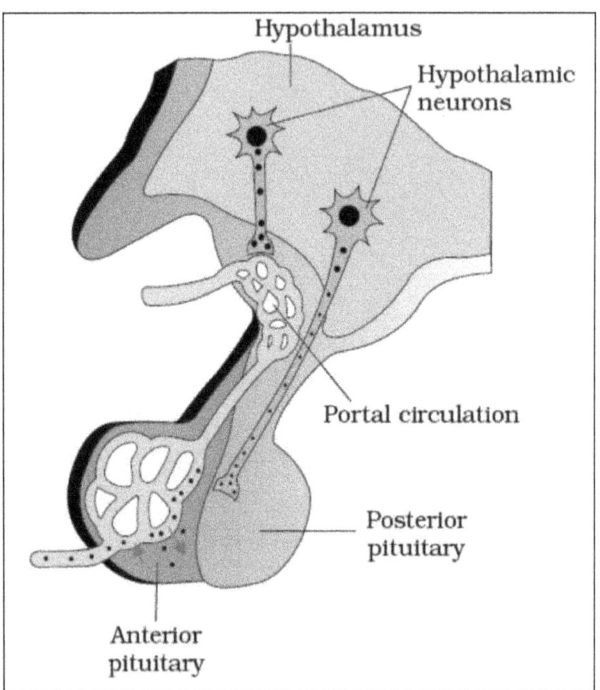

9.2.2 The Pituitary Gland

- The pituitary gland is located in a bony cavity called **sella tursica.**
- The pituitary gland is attached to hypothalamus by a **stalk.**
- Origin of this gland is **Ectodermal.**
- Also called as **Band master of endocrine orchestra.**
- The pituitary gland is divided anatomically into an **adenohypophysis** and a **neurohypophysis.**

Adenohypophysis

- Adenohypophysis has two portions, **pars distalis** and **pars intermedia**.
- The pars distalis region of pituitary, commonly called anterior pituitary, produces **growth hormone** (GH), **prolactin** (PRL), **thyroid stimulating hormone** (TSH), **adrenocorticotrophic hormone** (ACTH), **luteinizing hormone** (LH) and **follicle stimulating hormone** (FSH).
- Pars intermedia secretes only one hormone called **melanocyte stimulating hormone** (MSH).
- In humans, the pars intermedia is almost merged with pars distalis.

a. Growth Hormone

- Over-secretion of GH **stimulates** abnormal growth of the body leading to gigantism and low secretion of GH results in **stunted** growth resulting in pituitary dwarfism.

b. Prolactin

- Prolactin **regulates** the growth of the mammary glands and formation of milk in them.

c. TSH

- TSH stimulates the **synthesis** and secretion of thyroid hormones from the thyroid gland

d. ACTH

- ACTH stimulates the **synthesis** and secretion of steroid hormones called **glucocorticoids** from the adrenal cortex.

e. FSH & LH

- **LH** and **FSH** stimulate gonadal activity and hence are called **gonadotrophins**.
- In males, **LH** stimulates the synthesis and secretion of hormones called **androgens** from testis.
- In males, **FSH** and androgens regulate spermatogenesis.
- In females, **LH** induces ovulation of fully mature follicles (graafian follicles) and maintains the corpus luteum, formed from the remnants of the graafian follicles after ovulation.
- **FSH** stimulates growth and development of the ovarian follicles in females.

f. MSH

- **MSH** acts on the melanocytes (melanin containing cells) and regulates pigmentation of the skin.

Neurohypophysis

- **Neurohypophysis** (pars nervosa) also known as posterior pituitary, stores and releases two hormones called **oxytocin** and **vasopressin,** which are actually synthesised by the hypothalamus and are transported axonally to neurohypophysis.

a. Oxytocin

- **Oxytocin** acts on the smooth muscles of our body and stimulates their contraction.
- In females, **Oxytocin** stimulates a vigorous contraction of uterus at the time of child birth.
- **Oxytocin** also helps in milk ejection from the mammary gland.

b. Vasopressin

- **Vasopressin** acts mainly at the kidney.

- **Vasopressin** stimulates resorption of water and electrolytes by the distal tubules so reduces loss of water through urine.
- **Vasopressin** reduces loss of water through urine it is called diuresis.
- **Vasopressin** is also called as **anti-diuretic hormone** (ADH).

9.2.3 The Pineal Gland

- The **pineal** gland is located on the dorsal side of forebrain.
- Origin of Pineal, Pituitary and hypothalamus is ectodermal.
- Pineal secretes a hormone called **melatonin**.
- **Melatonin** is a tryptophan derivative.

Functions of Melatonin

- **Melatonin** plays a very important role in the regulation of a 24-hour (diurnal) rhythm of our body.
- **Melatonin** helps in maintaining the normal rhythms of sleep-wake cycle, body temperature.
- **The melatonin** also influences metabolism, pigmentation, the menstrual cycle as well as our defense capability.

9.2.4 Thyroid Gland

- The thyroid gland is **bilobed** in mammals and birds.
- Both the lobes are connected by a thin flap of connective tissue called **isthmus.**
- This gland located on either side of the **trachea.**
- Origin **endodermal.**
- **H-shaped** or Butterfly shaped.
- The thyroid gland is composed of **follicles** and **stromal tissues.**
- Each thyroid follicle is composed of follicular cells, enclosing a cavity.
- These follicular cells synthesise two hormones, **tetraiodothyronine** or **thyroxine** (T4) and **triiodothyronine** (T3).
- T_3 is more active than T_4.
- **Iodine** is essential for the normal rate of hormone synthesis in the thyroid.

Hypothyroidism

- Deficiency of iodine in our diet results in **hypothyroidism** and enlargement of the thyroid gland, commonly called **goitre.**
- **Hypothyroidism** during pregnancy causes-

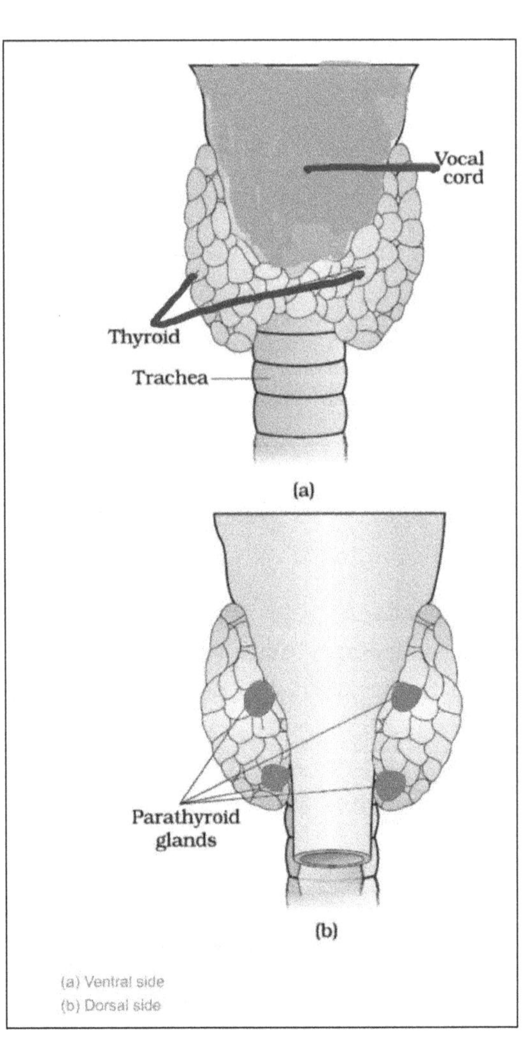

(a) Ventral side
(b) Dorsal side

- ➢ defective development and maturation of the growing baby
- ➢ stunted growth (cretinism)
- ➢ mental retardation
- ➢ low intelligence quotient
- ➢ abnormal skin
- ➢ deaf-mutism
- In adult women, **hypothyroidism** may cause menstrual cycle to become irregular.

Hyperthyroidism

- Due to cancer of the thyroid gland or due to development of nodules of the thyroid glands **hyperthyroidism occur.**
- In **hyperthyroidism** the rate of synthesis and secretion of the thyroid hormones is increased.
- The abnormal high levels of thyroid hormone called as **hyperthyroidism** which adversely affects our physiology.
- Grave and Plummer diseases are examples of **hyperthyroidism.**

Functions of thyroid hormones

- **Thyroid hormones** play an important role in the regulation of the basal metabolic rate.
- **These hormones** also support the process of red blood cell formation.
- **Thyroid hormones** control the metabolism of carbohydrates, proteins and fats.
- Maintenance of water and electrolyte balance is also influenced by **thyroid hormones**.
- Thyroid gland **also secretes** a protein hormone called **thyrocalcitonin (TCT)** which regulates the blood calcium levels.
- **Thyrocalcitonin (TCT)** do not contain iodine.

9.2.5 Parathyroid Gland

- In humans, **four parathyroid glands** are present.
- These glands are present on the **back side of the thyroid gland,** one pair each in the two lobes of the thyroid gland.
- **Endodermal** in origin.
- Structurally and functionally not connected to **thyroid** gland.
- The parathyroid glands secrete a peptide hormone called **parathyroid hormone** (PTH).

Functions of parathyroid hormones

- The secretion of **PTH** is regulated by the circulating levels of calcium ions.
- Parathyroid hormone (**PTH**) increases the Ca^{2+} levels in the blood. PTH on bones and stimulates the process of bone resorption (dissolution/ demineralisation).
- PTH also stimulates reabsorption of Ca^{2+} by the renal tubules and increases Ca^{2+} absorption from the digested food.

- PTH is a **hypercalcemic** hormone, i.e., it increases the blood **Ca²⁺** levels.
- Along with TCT, it plays a **significant** role in **calcium balance** in the body.

9.2.6 Thymus

- The **thymus** gland is a lobular structure located on the dorsal side of the heart and the aorta.
- The **thymus** plays a major role in the development of the immune system.
- The **thymus** gland secretes the peptide hormones called **thymosins**.
- The **thymus** gland has 2 portion cortex and medulla.

Functions of Thymosin

- Thymosins play a major role in the differentiation of **T lymphocytes**, which provide **cell-mediated immunity**.
- Thymosins also promote production of antibodies to provide **humoral immunity**.
- Thymus is degenerated in old individuals resulting in a decreased production of **thymosins**.
- So the immune responses of old **persons** become weak.

9.2.7 Adrenal Gland

- Our body has one pair of adrenal glands, one at the anterior part of each kidney.
- Origin **ecto-mesodermal**.
- Also called **4 S** gland.
- **Helps to control sex, salt, stress and sugar.**
- This gland **secretes** life saving hormones.

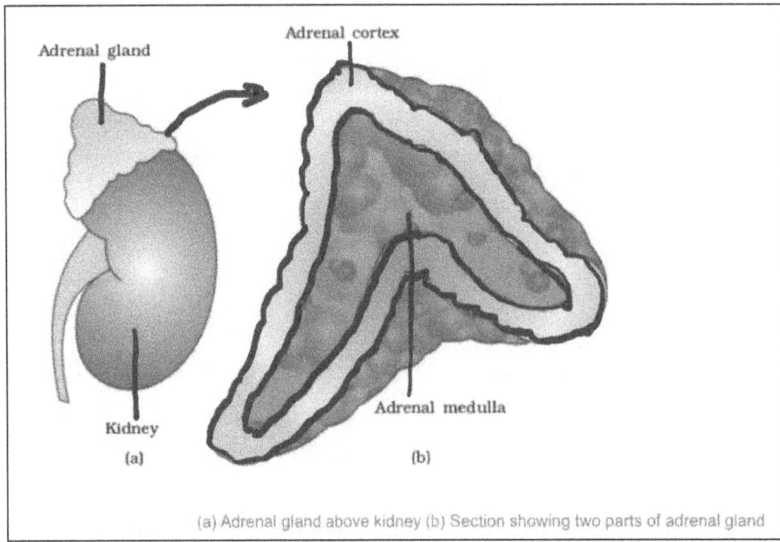

(a) Adrenal gland above kidney (b) Section showing two parts of adrenal gland

- The gland is composed of **two** types of tissues.
- The centrally located tissue is called the **adrenal medulla**, and outside this lies the **adrenal cortex**.

a. Adrenal medulla

- Origin - ectodermal.
- Also known as 3 F gland- Fear, Fight, Flight
- The adrenal medulla secretes two hormones called **adrenaline** or **epinephrine** and **noradrenaline** or **norepinephrine**.
- These are commonly called as **catecholamines**.
- Adrenaline and noradrenaline are rapidly secreted in response to stress of any kind and during emergency situations and are called **emergency hormones** or **hormones of Fight or Flight**.
- These **hormones** increase alertness, pupilary dilation, piloerection (raising of hairs), sweating etc.
- Both the **hormones** increase the heart beat, the strength of heart contraction and the rate of respiration.
- **Catecholamines** also stimulate the breakdown of glycogen resulting in an increased concentration of glucose in blood.
- They also stimulate the breakdown of lipids and proteins.

b. Adrenal cortex

- Origin-ectodermal.
- The adrenal cortex can be divided into three layers, called **zona reticularis** (inner layer), **zona fasciculata** (middle layer) and **zona glomerulosa** (outer layer).
- The adrenal cortex secretes many hormones, commonly called as **corticoids**.

c. Glucocorticoids.

- The corticoids, which are involved in carbohydrate metabolism are called glucocorticoids.
- In our body, cortisol is the main glucocorticoid.
- Glucocorticoids stimulate, gluconeogenesis, lipolysis and proteolysis; and inhibit cellular uptake and utilisation of amino acids.
- Cortisol is also involved in maintaining the cardio-vascular system as well as the kidney functions.
- Glucocorticoids, particularly cortisol, produces antiinflamatory reactions and suppresses the immune response.
- Cortisol stimulates the RBC production.
- Given after transplantation surgery.

d. Mineralocorticoid

- Main examples are aldosterone and deoxy-corticosterone.
- Aldosterone is the main mineralocorticoid in our body.
- Corticoids, which regulate the balance of water and electrolytes in our body are called mineralocorticoids.
- Aldosterone acts mainly at the renal tubules and stimulates the reabsorption of Na+ and water and excretion of K^+ and phosphate ions.
- Thus, aldosterone helps in the maintenance of electrolytes, body fluid volume, osmotic pressure and blood pressure.

e. Sex corticoids

- Small amounts of androgenic steroids are also secreted by the adrenal cortex which play a role in the growth of axial hair, pubic hair and facial hair during puberty.

9.2.8 Pancreas

- Origin endodermal.
- Pancreas is a composite gland/ Heterocrine/ Mixed gland.
- Pancreas acts as both exocrine and endocrine gland.
- The endocrine pancreas known as 'Islets of Langerhans'.
- There are about 1 to 2 million Islets of Langerhans in a normal human pancreas representing only 1 to 2 per cent of the pancreatic tissue.
- The two main types of cells in the Islet of Langerhans are called α **cells** and β **cells**.
- The α cells secrete a hormone called **glucagon**.
- The β cells secrete **insulin**.

a. Glucagon

- Glucagon is a peptide hormone, and plays an important role in maintaining the normal blood glucose levels.
- Glucagon made by 29 amino acids.
- Glucagon acts mainly on the liver cells (hepatocytes) and stimulates glycogenolysis resulting in an increased blood sugar (**hyperglycemia**).
- In addition, this hormone stimulates the process of gluconeogenesis which also contributes to hyperglycemia.
- Glucagon reduces the cellular glucose uptake and utilisation.
- Thus, glucagon is a **hyperglycemic hormone**.

b. Insulin

- Insulin is a peptide hormone, which plays a major role in the regulation of glucose homeostasis.
- Insulin acts mainly on hepatocytes and adipocytes (cells of adipose tissue), and enhances cellular glucose uptake and utilisation.
- As a result, there is a rapid movement of glucose from blood to hepatocytes and adipocytes resulting in decreased blood glucose levels (**hypoglycemia**).
- Insulin also stimulates conversion of glucose to glycogen (**glycogenesis**) in the target cells.
- The glucose homeostasis in blood is thus maintained jointly by the two – insulin and glucagons.
- Prolonged hyperglycemia leads to a complex disorder called **diabetes mellitus** which is associated with loss of glucose through urine and formation of harmful compounds known as ketone bodies.
- Diabetic patients are successfully treated with insulin therapy.
- Mature Insulin made by **51** amino acids.

9.2.9 Testis

- A pair of testis is present in the scrotal sac (outside abdomen) of male individuals.
- Testis can act as a primary sex organ as well as an endocrine gland.
- Testis is composed of **seminiferous tubules** and **stromal or interstitial tissue.**
- The **Leydig cells** or **interstitial cells**, which are present in the intertubular spaces produce a group of hormones called **androgens** mainly **testosterone.**

a. Functions of Androgens

- **Androgens** regulate the development, maturation and functions of the male accessory sex organs like epididymis, vas deferens, seminal vesicles, prostate gland, urethra etc.
- **Androgens** stimulate muscular growth, growth of facial and axillary hair, aggressiveness, low pitch of voice etc.
- **Androgens** play a major stimulatory role in the process of spermatogenesis (formation of spermatozoa).
- **Androgens** act on the central neural system and influence the male sexual behaviour (libido).
- **Androgens** hormones produce anabolic (synthetic) effects on protein and carbohydrate metabolism.

9.2.10 Ovary

- **Females** have a pair of ovaries located in the abdomen.
- Ovary is the primary female sex organ which produces one ovum during each menstrual cycle.
- In addition, ovary also produces two groups of steroid hormones called **estrogen** and **progesterone**.
- **Estrogen** and **Progesterone** chemically steroid hormones.
- Ovary is composed of ovarian follicles and stromal tissues.
- The estrogen is synthesised and secreted mainly by the growing ovarian follicles.

a. Estrogens

- **Estrogens** produce wide ranging actions such as-
  - ➢ stimulation of growth and activities of female secondary sex organs
  - ➢ development of growing ovarian follicles
  - ➢ appearance of female secondary sex characters (e.g., high pitch of voice, etc.)
  - ➢ mammary gland development.
- **Estrogens** also regulate female sexual behavior.
- The **estrogen** is synthesised and secreted mainly by the growing ovarian follicles.

b. Progesterone

- After ovulation, the ruptured follicle is converted to a structure called **corpus luteum**, which secretes mainly **progesterone.**
- **Progesterone** supports pregnancy.
- **Progesterone** also acts on the mammary glands and stimulates the formation of alveoli (sac-like structures which store milk) and milk secretion.
- **Progesterone** also called anti-abortion hormone.

9.3 HORMONES OF HEART, KIDNEY AND GASTROINTESTINAL TRACT

a. Atrial natriuretic factor (ANF)

- The atrial wall of our heart secretes a very important peptide hormone called **atrial natriuretic factor** (ANF), which decreases blood pressure.

- When blood pressure is increased, ANF is secreted which causes dilation of the blood vessels.

- **ANF** reduces the blood pressure.

- **ANF works opposite to RAAS.**

b. Erythropoietin

- The juxtaglomerular cells of kidney produce a peptide hormone called **erythropoietin.**

- **Erythropoietin** stimulates erythropoiesis (i.e. formation of RBC).

c. Hormones from gastro-intestinal tract

- Endocrine cells present in different parts of the gastro-intestinal tract secrete four major peptide hormones, namely **gastrin**, **secretin**, **cholecystokinin** (CCK) and **gastric inhibitory peptide** (GIP).

d. Gastrin

- Gastrin acts on the gastric glands and stimulates the secretion of hydrochloric acid and pepsinogen.

e. Secretin

- Secretin acts on the exocrine pancreas and stimulates secretion of water and bicarbonate ions.

f. Cholecystokinin (CCK)

- CCK acts on both pancreas and gall bladder and stimulates the secretion of pancreatic enzymes and bile juice, respectively.

g. GIP

- GIP inhibits gastric secretion and motility.

Points to remember-

- Several other non-endocrine tissues secrete hormones called **growth factors.**

- These factors are essential for the normal growth of tissues and their repairing/regeneration.

9.4 MECHANISM OF HORMONE ACTION

- Hormones produce their effects on target tissues by binding to specific proteins called **hormone receptors** located in the target tissues only.

- Hormone receptors present on the cell membrane of the target cells are called membrane-bound receptors called extra cellular receptor.

- **Peptide, polypeptide, protein hormones** (e.g., insulin, glucagon, pituitary hormones, hypothalamic hormones, etc. shows extra cellular receptor based mechanism.

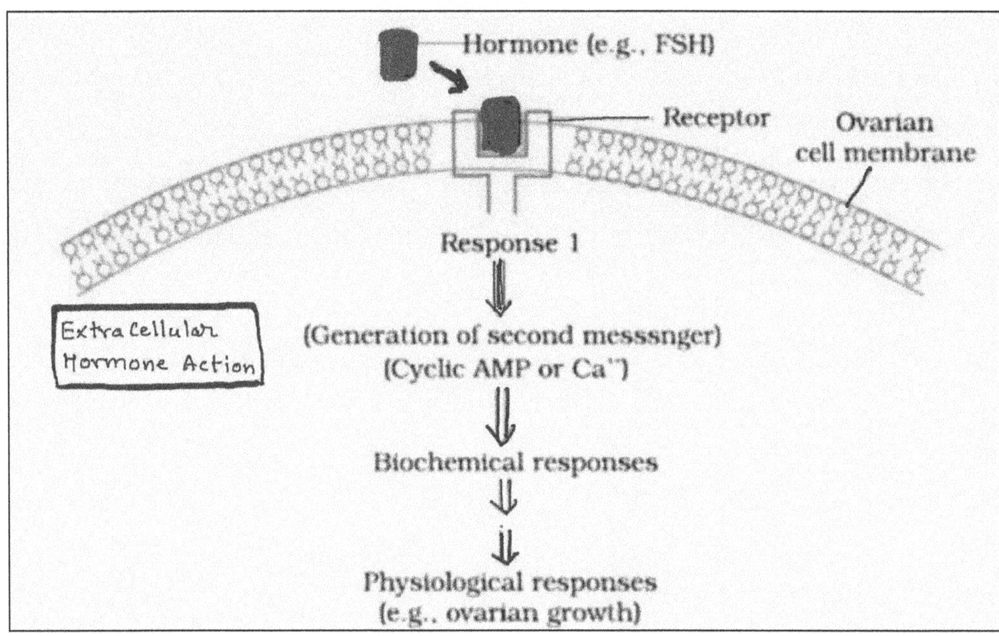

- The receptors present inside the target cell are called intracellular receptors, mostly nuclear receptors (present in the nucleus).

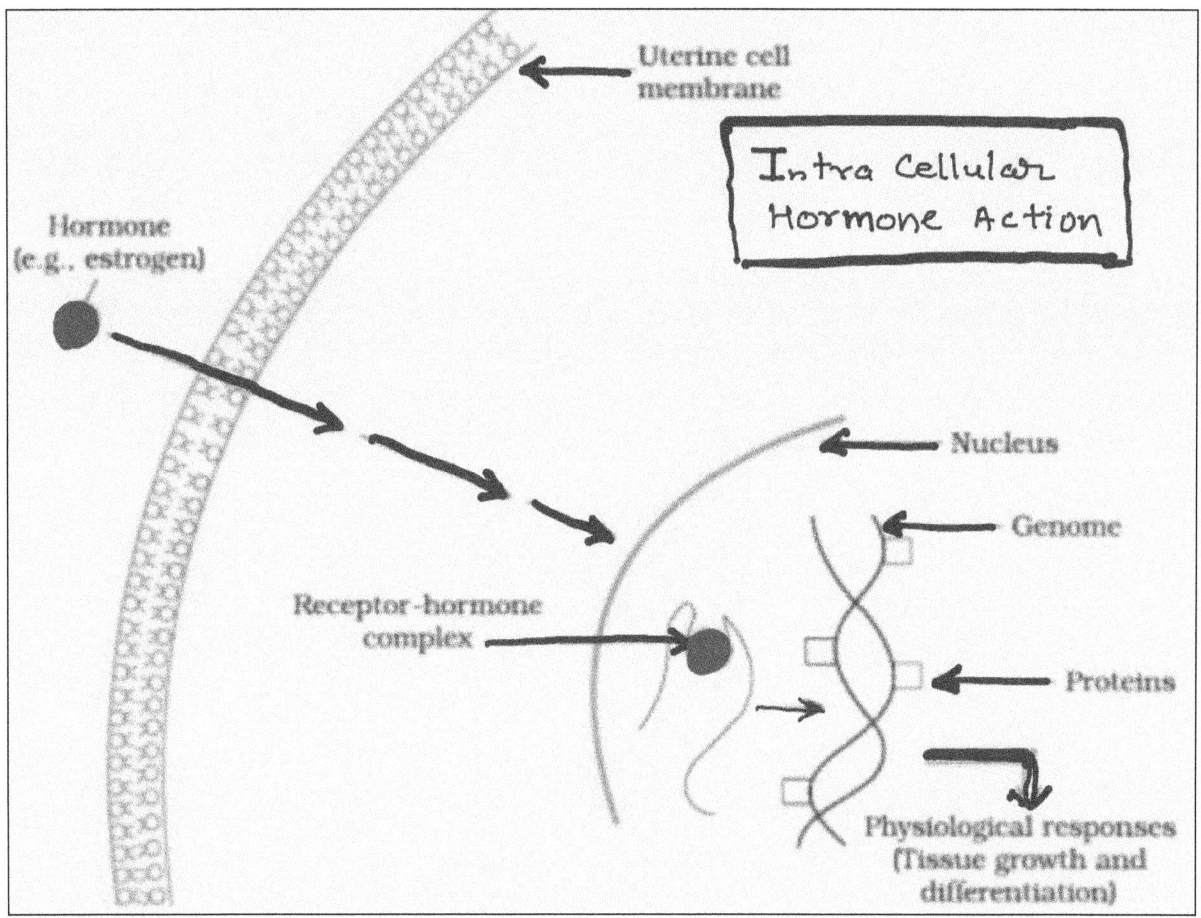

Hormone-receptor complex

- Binding of a hormone to its receptor leads to the formation of a **hormone-receptor complex.**
- **Each receptor is specific** to one hormone only and hence receptors are specific.
- **Hormone-Receptor complex** formation leads to certain biochemical changes in the target tissue.
- **Target tissue metabolism** and hence physiological functions are regulated by hormones.

Chemical nature of hormones

On the basis of their chemical nature, hormones can be divided into groups:

(i) **peptide, polypeptide, protein hormones** (e.g., insulin, glucagon, pituitary hormones, hypothalamic hormones, etc.)

(ii) **steroids** (e.g., cortisol, testosterone, estradiol and progesterone)

(iii) **iodothyronines** (thyroid hormones)

(iv) **amino-acid derivatives** (e.g., epinephrine).

Points to remember-

- Hormones which interact with membrane-bound receptors normally do not enter the target cell, but generate second messengers **(e.g., cyclic AMP, IP3, Ca^{++} etc)** which in turn regulate cellular metabolism.
- Hormones which interact with **intracellular receptors (e.g., steroid hormones, iodothyronines, etc.)** mostly regulate gene expression or chromosome function by the interaction of hormone-receptor complex with the genome.
- **Cumulative biochemical** actions result in physiological and developmental effects.

1. Consider the following statements and find out the correct option-

A. The endocrine glands and hormone producing diffused tissues/cells located in different parts of our body constitute the endocrine system.

B. Pituitary, pineal, thyroid, adrenal, pancreas, parathyroid, thymus and gonads (testis in males and ovary in females) are the organized endocrine bodies in our body.

C. Some other organs, e.g., gastrointestinal tract, liver, kidney, heart also produce hormones.

D. The hypothalamus is the basal part of diencephalon, forebrain and it regulates a wide spectrum of body functions.

E. Hypothalamus contains several groups of neurosecretory cells called nuclei which produce hormones.

Which of the above are correct with respect to humans-

1. A,E,C

2. B,C

3. A,B,D,E

4. A,B,C,D,E

2. Match the list 1 and 2-

List 1   List 2

a. The pars distalis region of pituitary	**follicle stimulating hormone** (FSH)
b. Pars intermedia secretes	**melanocyte stimulating hormone** (MSH)
c. Neurohypophysis (pars nervosa) also known as posterior pituitary, stores and releases	**oxytocin** and **vasopressin**
d. The pineal gland	**melatonin.**

How many of them are/is correctly matched –

1. one

2. two

3. three

4. four

3. Consider the following statements-

I. The hormones produced by hypothalamus are of two types, the releasing hormones (which stimulate secretion of pituitary hormones) and the inhibiting hormones (which inhibit secretions of pituitary hormones).

II. A hypothalamic hormone called Gonadotrophin releasing hormone (GnRH) stimulates the pituitary synthesis and release of gonadotrophins.

III. Somatostatin from the hypothalamus inhibits the release of growth hormone from the pituitary.

IV. ADH and Oxytocin hormones originating in the hypothlamic neurons, pass through axons and are released from their nerve endings.

How many of them are/is correct -

1. one

2. two

3. three

4. four

4. **Read the following statement carefully with respect to Humans-**

I. The pituitary gland is located in a bony cavity called sella tursica and is attached to hypothalamus by a stalk.

II. The pituitary gland is divided anatomically into an **adenohypophysis** and a **neurohypophysis**.

III. Adenohypophysis consists of two portions, pars distalis and pars intermedia.

IV. The pars distalis region of pituitary, commonly called anterior pituitary, produces **growth hormone (GH)**, **prolactin (PRL)**, **thyroid stimulating hormone (TSH)**, **adrenocorticotrophic hormone (ACTH)**, **luteinizing hormone** (LH) and **follicle stimulating hormone** (FSH).

V. Pars intermedia secretes only one hormone called **ADH**.

How many of them are usually correct -

1. three

2. four

3. five

4. two

5. **Consider the following statements and find out the correct option-**

STATEMENT 1. Neurohypophysis (pars nervosa) also known as posterior pituitary, stores and releases two hormones called **oxytocin** and **vasopressin,** which are actually synthesised by the hypothalamus and are transported axonally to neurohypophysis.

STATEMENT 2. Over-secretion of GH stimulates abnormal growth of the body leading to gigantism and low secretion of GH results in stunted growth resulting in pituitary dwarfism.

1. Both are correct statements

2. Only Statement 1 correct

3. Both are wrong statements

4. Only statement 2 correct

6. **Go through the following statements-**

ASSERTION(A). Prolactin regulates the growth of the mammary glands and formation of milk in them.

REASON(R). TSH stimulates the synthesis and secretion of thyroid hormones from the thyroid gland.

1. A correct and R is correct explanation of A

2. A correct and R is also correct but R is not correct explanation of A

3. A correct but R incorrect

4. A and R both are incorrect

7. Which one is an incorrect statement

1. ACTH stimulates the synthesis and secretion of steroid hormones called **glucocorticoids** from the adrenal cortex.

2. LH and FSH stimulate gonadal activity and hence are called **gonadotrophins**.

3. In males, LH stimulates the synthesis and secretion of hormones called **androgens** from testis.

4. In males, FSH and androgens not regulate spermatogenesis.

8. Go through the following statements-

I. In females, LH induces ovulation of fully mature follicles (graafian follicles) and maintains the corpus luteum, formed from the remnants of the graafian follicles after ovulation.

II. FSH stimulates growth and development of the ovarian follicles in females.

III. LH acts on the smooth muscles of our body and stimulates their contraction.

IV. In females, LH stimulates a vigorous contraction of uterus at the time of child birth, and milk ejection from the mammary gland.

V. FSH acts mainly at the kidney and stimulates resorption of water and electrolytes by the distal tubules and thereby reduces loss of water through urine (diuresis).

How many of them are correct-

1. two
2. three
3. four
4. five

9. Match the list 1 and 2-

List 1   List 2

a. Melatonin	j. diuresis
b. Vasopressin	k. development of the ovarian follicles
c. FSH	l. 24-hour (diurnal) rhythm of our body
d. MSH	m. regulates pigmentation of the skin

Find out the correct option –

1. a.k, b.j, c.l, d.m

2. a.k, b.l, c.j, d.m

3. a.l, b.j, c.k, d.m

4. a.l, b.j, c.m, d.k

10. Consider the following statements and find out the correct option

STATEMENT 1. The pineal gland is located on the dorsal side of forebrain.

STATEMENT 2. Pineal secretes a hormone called **melatonin.**

1. Both are wrong statements

2. Only Statement 1 correct

3. Both are correct statements

4. Only statement 2 correct

11. Read the following statements very carefully -

a) The thyroid gland is composed of two lobes which are located on either side of the trachea

b) Both the lobes of the thyroid gland are interconnected with a thin flap of connective tissue called isthmus.

c) The thyroid gland is composed of **follicles** and **stromal tissues.**

d) Each thyroid follicle is composed of follicular cells, enclosing a cavity.

Which of the above statement are correct?

1. a and c both

2. a,b,c,d

3. c only

4. b and c both

12. Go through the following statements-

ASSERTION(A). Iodine is essential for the normal rate of hormone synthesis in the thyroid.

REASON(R). Deficiency of iodine in our diet results in **hypothyroidism** and enlargement of the thyroid gland, commonly called **goitre.**

1. A correct and R is correct explanation of A

2. A correct and R is also correct but R is not correct explanation of A

3. A correct but R incorrect

4. A and R both are incorrect

13. Find out incorrect with respect to Hypothyroidism –

1. cretinism

2. mental retardation

3. high intelligence quotient

4. abnormal skin

14. Read the following statements and find out correct option-

a) In adult women, hypothyroidism may cause menstrual cycle to become irregular.

b) Due to cancer of the thyroid gland or due to development of nodules of the thyroid glands, the rate of synthesis and secretion of the thyroid hormones is increased to abnormal high levels leading to a condition called **hyperthyroidism** which adversely affects the body physiology.

c) Thyroid hormones play an important role in the regulation of the basal metabolic rate.

d) Thyroid hormones also support the process of red blood cell formation.

How many of them is/are correct-

1. four

2. one

3. two

4. three

15. Consider the following statements and find out the correct option-

STATEMENT 1. Thyroid hormones control the metabolism of carbohydrates, proteins and fats.

STATEMENT 2. Thyroid hormones controls the voluntary movements, balance of the body, functioning of vital involuntary organs (e.g., lungs, heart, kidneys, etc.), thermoregulation, hunger and thirst, circadian (24-hour) rhythms of our body, activities of several endocrine glands and human behaviour.

1. Both are wrong statements

2. Only Statement 1 correct

3. Both are correct statements

4. Only statement 2 correct

16. Consider the following statements-

a) Pars intermedia secretes only one hormone called **melanocyte stimulating hormone** (MSH).

b) In humans, the pars intermedia is almost merged with pars distalis.

c) Neurohypophysis (pars nervosa) also known as posterior pituitary, stores and releases two hormones called **oxytocin** and **vasopressin,** which are actually synthesised by the hypothalamus and are transported axonally to neurohypophysis.

d) Over-secretion of GH stimulates abnormal growth of the body leading to gigantism and low secretion

Which of the above are/is correct-

1. a and b

2. a,b,c only

3. c and a

4. a, b, c,d

17. Consider the following statements -

a) There are special chemicals which act as hormones and provide chemical coordination, integration and regulation in the human body.

b) These hormones regulate metabolism, growth and development of our organs, the endocrine glands or certain cells.

c) The endocrine system is composed of hypothalamus, pituitary and pineal, thyroid, adrenal, pancreas, parathyroid, thymus and gonads (testis and ovary).

d) Some other organs, e.g., gastrointestinal tract, kidney, heart etc., also produce hormones.

Which of the above statements are correct?

1. a and d only

2. c and b only

3. a,b,c only

4. a,b,c,d

18. Consider the following statements -

a) The pituitary gland is divided into three major parts, which are called as pars distalis, pars intermedia and pars nervosa.

b) Pars distalis produces six trophic hormones. Pars intermedia secretes only one hormone, while pars nervosa (neurohypophysis) secretes two hormones.

c) The pituitary hormones regulate the growth and development of somatic tissues and activities of peripheral endocrine glands.

d) Pineal gland secretes MSH, which plays a very important role in the regulation of 24-hour (diurnal) rhythms of our body (e.g., rhythms of sleep and state of being awake, body temperature,etc.).

Which of the above statement are correct?

1. a and d only

2. c and a only

3. a,b,c only

4. a,b,c,d

19. **Consider the following statements and find out the incorrect one for thyroid gland-**

1. Help to play an important role in the regulation of the basal metabolic rat

2. Help to development and maturation of the central neural system

3. Do not play any role in erythropoiesis.

4. Help to regulate menstrual cycle.

20. **Read the following statements-**

a) Due to cancer of the thyroid gland or due to development of nodules of the thyroid glands, the rate of synthesis and secretion of the thyroid hormones is increased to abnormal high levels leading to a condition called **hyperthyroidism** which adversely affects the body physiology.

b) Maintenance of water and electrolyte balance is also influenced by thyroid hormones.

c) Thyroid gland also secretes a protein hormone called thyrocalcitonin (TCT) which regulates the blood calcium levels.

d) The thyroid gland is composed of **follicles** and **stromal tissues**.

How many of them are/is correct **statements-**

1. two

2. three

3. four

4. one

21. **Consider the following statements and find out the correct option for humans-**

STATEMENT 1. Prolactin regulates the growth of the mammary glands and formation of milk in them.

STATEMENT 2. ACTH stimulates the synthesis and secretion of steroid hormones called **glucocorticoids** from the adrenal cortex.

1. Both are wrong statements

2. Only Statement 1 correct

3. Both are correct statements

4. Only statement 2 correct

22. **Go through the following statements and find out the correct option-**

ASSERTION(A). Melatonin plays a very important role in the regulation of a 24-hour (diurnal) rhythm of our body.

REASON(R). it helps in maintaining the normal rhythms of sleep-wake cycle, body temperature.

1.A correct and R is correct explanation of A

2. A correct and R is also correct but R is not correct explanation of A

3. A correct but R incorrect

4. A and R both are incorrect

23. Go through the following statements and find out the correct option-

A. The thyroid gland is composed of two lobes which are located on either side of the trachea.

B. Both the lobes of thyroid are interconnected with a thin flap of connective tissue called isthmus.

C. The thyroid gland is composed of **follicles** and **stromal tissues**.

D. Each thyroid follicle is composed of follicular cells, enclosing a cavity.

E. These follicular cells synthesise **tetraiodothyronine** or **thyroxine** (T4) only.

Which of the above statement are correct -

1. A and C only
2. A,B,C,D only
3. D and A only
4. A,B,C,D,E

24. Read the statements given below-

A. Thyroid hormones play an important role in the regulation of the basal metabolic rate.

B. These hormones also support the process of red blood cell formation.

C. Thyroid hormones control the metabolism of carbohydrates, proteins and fats.

D. Maintenance of water and electrolyte balance is also influenced by thyroid hormones.

E. Thyroid gland also secretes a steroid hormone called thyrocalcitonin (TCT) which regulates the blood calcium levels.

Which of the above statement are/is incorrect?

1. A and C only
2. E only
3. D and E only
4. A,B,C,D

25. Read the following-

A. In humans, four parathyroid glands are present on the back side of the thyroid gland, one pair each in the two lobes of the thyroid gland.

B. The parathyroid glands secrete a peptide hormone called **parathyroid hormone** (PTH).

C. The secretion of PTH is regulated by the circulating levels of calcium ions.

D. Parathyroid hormone (PTH) increases the Ca^{2+} levels in the blood. PTH on bones and stimulates the process of bone resorption (dissolution/ demineralisation).

Which of the above statement are correct?

1. A and C only
2. A only
3. D and C only
4. A,B,C,D

26. Consider the following statements-

A. The parathyroid glands secrete a peptide hormone called **parathyroid hormone** (PTH).

B. The secretion of PTH is regulated by the circulating levels of calcium ions.

C. Parathyroid hormone (PTH) increases the Ca^{2+} levels in the blood. PTH on bones and stimulates the process of bone resorption (dissolution/ demineralisation).

D. PTH also stimulates reabsorption of Ca^{2+} by the renal tubules and increases Ca^{2+} absorption from the digested food. It is, thus, clear that PTH is a hypercalcemic hormone, i.e., it increases the blood Ca^{2+} levels.

E. Along with TCT, PTH plays a significant role in calcium balance in the body.

How many of them are correct-

1. five

2. two

3. three

4. four

27. Match the list 1 and 2-

List 1   List 2

a. **steroid**	cortisol
b. **protein**	testosterone
c. **steroid**	estradiol
d. **steroid**	progesterone

How many of them are/is correctly matched –

1. one

2. two

3. three

4. four

28. Read the following-

a) Hormones produce their effects on target tissues by binding to specific proteins called **hormone receptors** located in the all tissues.

b) Hormone receptors present on the cell membrane of the target cells are called membrane-bound receptors and the receptors present inside the target cell are called intracellular receptors, mostly nuclear receptors (present in the nucleus).

c) Binding of a hormone to its receptor leads to the formation of a **hormone-receptor complex.**

d) Each receptor is specific to one hormone only and hence receptors are specific.

e) Hormone-Receptor complex formation leads to certain biochemical changes in the target tissue.

Which of the above statements is/are correct-

1. a and c only

2. a only

3. d and c only

4. all are correct

29. Consider the following statements and find out incorrect one-

1. CCK acts on both pancreas and gall bladder and stimulates the secretion of pancreatic enzymes and bile juice, respectively.

2. GIP increases gastric secretion and motility.

3. Several other non-endocrine tissues secrete hormones called **growth factors.**

4. These growth factors are essential for the normal growth of tissues and their repairing/regeneration.

30. Read the following points -

a) The atrial wall of our heart secretes a very important steroid hormone called **atrial natriuretic factor** (ANF), which increases blood pressure.

b) When blood pressure is increased, ANF is secreted which causes dilation of the blood vessels. The juxtaglomerular cells of kidney produce a peptide hormone called **erythropoietin.**

c) The **erythropoietin** stimulates erythropoiesis (formation of RBC).

How many of them are/is correct –

1. four   2. two

3. three   4. one

31. Read the following statements and find out the correct option

STATEMENT 1. Endocrine cells present in different parts of the gastro-intestinal tract secrete four major peptide hormones, namely **gastrin, secretin, cholecystokinin** (CCK) and **gastric inhibitory peptide** (GIP).

STATEMENT 2. Gastrin acts on the gastric glands and stimulates the secretion of hydrochloric acid and pepsinogen.

1. Both are wrong statements   2. Both are correct statements

3. Only statement 1 correct   4. Only statement 2 correct

32. Go through the following statement and find out the correct option-

ASSERTION(A). Binding of a hormone to its receptor leads to the formation of a **hormone-receptor complex.**

REASON(R). Each receptor is non-specific to one hormone and hence receptors are non-specific.

1. A correct and R is correct explanation of A

2. A correct and R is also correct but R is not correct explanation of A

3. A correct but R incorrect

4. A and R both are incorrect

33. Find out the incorrect option-

1. Ovary is the secondary female sex organ which produces one ovum during each menstrual cycle.

2. In addition, ovary also produces two groups of steroid hormones called **estrogen** and **progesterone**.

3. Ovary is composed of ovarian follicles and stromal tissues.

4. The estrogen is synthesised and secreted mainly by the growing ovarian follicles.

34. Read the following –

I. After ovulation, the ruptured follicle is converted to a structure called **corpus luteum**, which secretes mainly **progesterone**.

II. Estrogens produce wide ranging actions such as stimulation of growth and activities of female secondary sex organs, development of growing ovarian follicles, appearance of female secondary sex characters (e.g., high pitch of voice, etc.), mammary gland development.

III. Estrogens also regulate female sexual behaviour.

IV. Progesterone do not supports pregnancy.

V. Progesterone also acts on the mammary glands and stimulates the formation of alveoli (sac-like structures which store milk) and milk secretion.

How many of above is/are incorrect-

1. three

2. four

3. two

4. one

35. Which of the following is incorrect statement-

1. Androgens regulate the development, maturation and functions of the male accessory sex organs like epididymis, vas deferens, seminal vesicles, prostate gland, urethra etc.

2. These hormones stimulate muscular growth, growth of facial and axillary hair, aggressiveness, low pitch of voice etc.

3. Androgens play a major stimulatory role in the process of spermatogenesis (formation of spermatozoa).

4. Androgens do not act on the central neural system and not influence the male sexual behaviour (libido).

36. Consider the following statements –

i. A pair of testis is present in the scrotal sac (outside abdomen) of male individuals.

ii. Testis performs dual functions as a primary sex organ as well as an endocrine gland.

iii. Testis is composed of **seminiferous tubules** and **stromal or interstitial tissue.**

iv. The **Leydig cells** or **interstitial cells**, which are present in the intertubular spaces produce a group of hormones called **androgens** mainly **progesterone.**

Which of the above statements are correct-

1. i,ii only

2. i, iii,iv only

3. i,ii,iii only

4. all are correct

37. Read the following statements-

i. Pancreas is a composite gland which acts as both exocrine and endocrine gland.

ii. The endocrine pancreas consists of 'Islets of Langerhans'.

iii. Pancreas contain about 1 to 2 million Islets of Langerhans in a normal human pancreas representing only 1 to 2 per cent of the pancreatic tissue

iv. Glucagon is a peptide hormone, and plays an important role in maintaining the normal blood glucose levels.

v. Glucagon acts mainly on the liver cells (hepatocytes) and stimulates glycogenolysis resulting in an increased blood sugar (**hyperglycemia**).

Which above statements is/are correct-

1. i and ii only

2. iii And ii only

3. iv,ii,i, iii only

4. All are correct

38. Consider the following statements-

A. Glucagon reduces the cellular glucose uptake and utilisation.

B. The glucagon is a **hyperglycemic hormone**.

C. Insulin is a steroid hormone, which plays a major role in the regulation of glucose homeostasis.

D. Insulin acts mainly on hepatocytes and adipocytes (cells of adipose tissue), and enhances cellular glucose uptake and utilisation.

How many of above are/is incorrect-

1. three   2. four

3. two   4. one

39. Read the following statements and find out the correct option-

STATEMENT 1. Diabetic patients are successfully treated with insulin therapy.

STATEMENT 2. The glucose homeostasis in blood is maintained jointly by the two – insulin and glucagons.

1. Both are wrong statements   2. Both are correct statements

3. Only statement 1 correct   4. Only statement 2 correct

40. Read the following statements-

a) Glucagon is a peptide hormone, and plays an important role in maintaining the normal blood glucose levels.

b) Glucagon acts mainly on the liver cells (hepatocytes) and stimulates glycogenolysis resulting in an increased blood sugar (**hyperglycemia**).

c) In addition, this hormone stimulates the process of gluconeogenesis which also contributes to hyperglycemia.

d) Glucagon reduces the cellular glucose uptake and utilisation.

e) The glucagon is a **hyperglycemic hormone**.

Which of the above are correct?

1. a and b only   2. b and c only

3. c and d only   4. All are correct

41. Go through the following statements and find out the correct option-

ASSERTION(A). Insulin acts mainly on hepatocytes and adipocytes (cells of adipose tissue), and enhances cellular glucose uptake and utilisation.

REASON(R). As a result, there is a rapid movement of glucose from blood to hepatocytes and adipocytes resulting in decreased blood glucose levels (**hypoglycemia**).

1. A correct and R is correct explanation of A

2. A correct and R is also correct but R is not correct explanation of A

3. A correct but R incorrect

4. A and R both are incorrect

42. Find out the incorrect statement-

1. Our body has one pair of adrenal glands, one at the anterior part of each kidney.

2. The gland is composed of two types of tissues.

3. The outside located tissue is called the **adrenal medulla**, and centrally this lies the **adrenal cortex.**

4. The adrenal medulla secretes two hormones called **adrenaline** or **epinephrine** and **noradrenaline** or **norepinephrine.** These are commonly called as **catecholamines.**

43. Consider the following statements-

A. Adrenaline and noradrenaline are rapidly secreted in response to stress of any kind and during emergency situations and are called **emergency hormones** or **hormones of Fight or Flight.**

B. These hormones increase alertness, pupilary dilation, piloerection (raising of hairs), sweating etc.

C. Both the hormones increase the heart beat, the strength of heart contraction and the rate of respiration.

D. Catecholamines also stimulate the breakdown of glycogen resulting in an increased concentration of glucose in blood.

E. Catecholamines they also stimulate the breakdown of lipids and proteins.

F. The adrenal cortex can be divided into three layers, called **zona reticularis** (inner layer), **zona fasciculata** (middle layer) and **zona glomerulosa** (outer layer).

G. The adrenal cortex secretes many hormones, commonly called as **corticoids**.

How many of them are correct-

1. five   2. three

3. four   4. six

44. Read the following statements and find out the correct option –

STATEMENT 1. The corticoids, which are involved in carbohydrate metabolism are called glucocorticoids.

STATEMENT 2. Corticoids, which regulate the balance of water and electrolytes in our body are called mineralocorticoids.

1. Both are correct statements   2. Both are wrong statements

3. Only statement 1 correct   4. Only statement 2 correct

45. Which statements is incorrect -

1. Catecholamines also stimulate the breakdown of glycogen resulting in an increased concentration of glucose in blood.

2. In addition, they also stimulate the breakdown of lipids and proteins.

3. The adrenal cortex can be divided into two layers only, called **zona fasciculata** (outer layer) and **zona reticularis** (outer layer).

4. The adrenal cortex secretes many hormones, commonly called as **corticoids**.

46. Read the following statements and find out the correct option

STATEMENT 1. Cortisol is also involved in maintaining the cardio-vascular system as well as the kidney functions.

STATEMENT 2. Glucocorticoids, like insulin, produces antiinflamatory reactions and suppresses the immune response.

1. Both are correct statements

2. Both are wrong statements.

3. Only statement 1 correct

4. Only statement 2 correct

47. Go through the following statements and find out the correct option-

ASSERTION(A). Cortisol not stimulates the RBC production.

REASON(R). Aldosterone do not helps in the maintenance of electrolytes, body fluid volume, osmotic pressure and blood pressure

1. A correct and R is correct explanation of A

2. A correct and R is also correct but R is not correct explanation of A

3. A correct but R incorrect

4. A and R both are incorrect

48. Find out the incorrect statement –

1. Parathyroid hormone (PTH) increases the Ca^{2+} levels in the blood.

2. PTH do not stimulates reabsorption of Ca^{2+} by the renal tubules but increases Ca^{2+} absorption from the digested food.

3. Cortisol stimulates the RBC production.

4. Aldosterone acts mainly at the renal tubules and stimulates the reabsorption of Na^+ and water and excretion of K^+ and phosphate ions.

49. Consider the following statements -

A. The thymus gland secretes thymosins which play a major role in the differentiation of T-lymphocytes, which provide cell-mediated immunity.

B. Thymosins also increase the production of antibodies to provide humoral immunity.

C. The adrenal gland is composed of the centrally located adrenal medulla and the outer adrenal cortex.

D. The adrenal medulla secretes epinephrine and norepinephrine.

E. These hormones increase alertness, pupilary dilation, piloerection, sweating, heart beat, strength of heart contraction, rate of respiration, glycogenolysis, lipolysis, proteolysis.

Which of the above statements are correct-

1. A and C only

2. D and B only

3. A,B,C,D only

4. All are correct

50. Read the following statements -

A. The adrenal cortex secretes glucocorticoids and mineralocorticoids.

B. Glucocorticoids stimulate gluconeogenesis, lipolysis, proteolysis, erythropoiesis, cardio-vascular system, blood pressure, and glomerular filtration rate and inhibit inflammatory reactions by suppressing the immune response.

C. Mineralocorticoids regulate water and electrolyte contents of the body.

D. The endocrine pancreas secretes glucagon and insulin.

E. Glucagon stimulates glycogenolysis and gluconeogenesis resulting in hyperglycemia.

F.   Insulin stimulates cellular glucose uptake and utilisation, and glycogenesis resulting in hypoglycemia.

G.   Insulin deficiency and/or insulin resistance result in a disease called diabetes mellitus.

Which of the above statements are correct-

1. A and C only

2. A,B,C,E only

3. A,B,C,D,E only

4. All are correct

HUMAN REPRODUCTION

- **Humans are sexually reproducing and viviparous.**
- The reproductive events in humans include-
    - formation of gametes (**gametogenesis**), i.e., sperms in males and ovum in females.
    - transfer of sperms into the female genital tract (**insemination**).
    - fusion of male and female gametes (**fertilisation**) leading to formation of zygote.
    - formation and development of blastocyst and its attachment to the uterine wall (**implantation**).
    - embryonic development (**gestation**).
    - delivery of the baby (**parturition**).
- The reproductive events occur after **puberty**.
- There are remarkable differences between the **reproductive** events in the male and in the female.
- Sperm formation continues even in old men, but **formation** of ovum ceases in women around the age of **fifty** years.

10.1 THE MALE REPRODUCTIVE SYSTEM

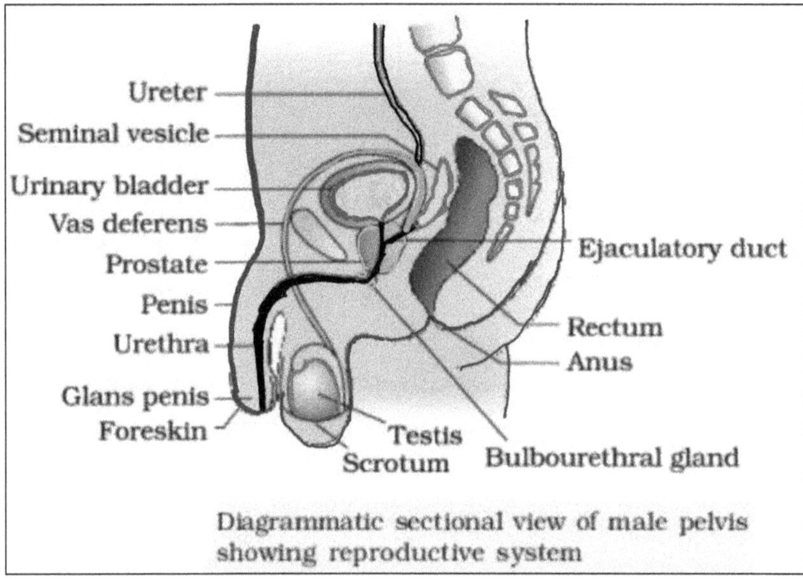

Diagrammatic sectional view of male pelvis showing reproductive system

- The male reproductive system is **composed** of a pair of **testes**, the male sex accessory ducts and the **accessory** glands and **external** genitalia.

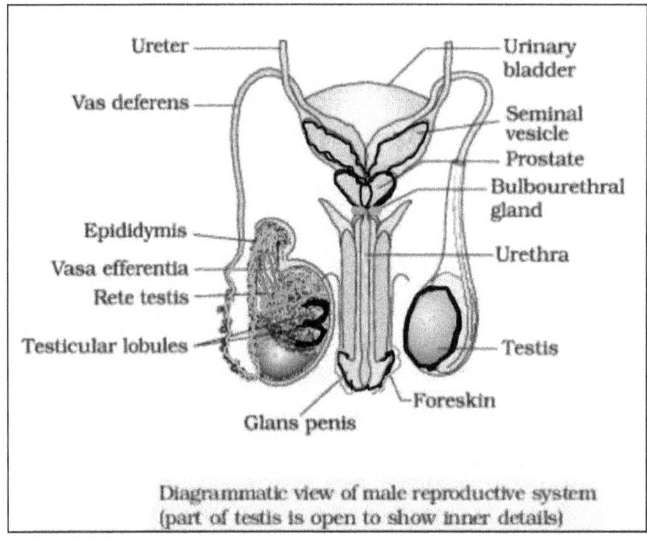

Diagrammatic view of male reproductive system (part of testis is open to show inner details)

a. Testes

- The testes are situated outside the abdominal cavity within a pouch called scrotum.
- The scrotum helps in maintaining the low **temperature** of the testes (2–2.5° C lower than the normal internal body temperature) **necessary** for spermatogenesis.
- Testes are **primary** sex organ.
- In adults, each testis is **oval** in shape.
- In adults, each testis - **length** of about 4 to 5 cm and a **width** of about 2 to 3 cm.
- The testis is covered by a **dense** covering.
- This dense covering known as **tunica albuginea**.
- Tunica albuginea made by **WFCT**.

- Each testis has about 250 compartments called **testicular lobules**.

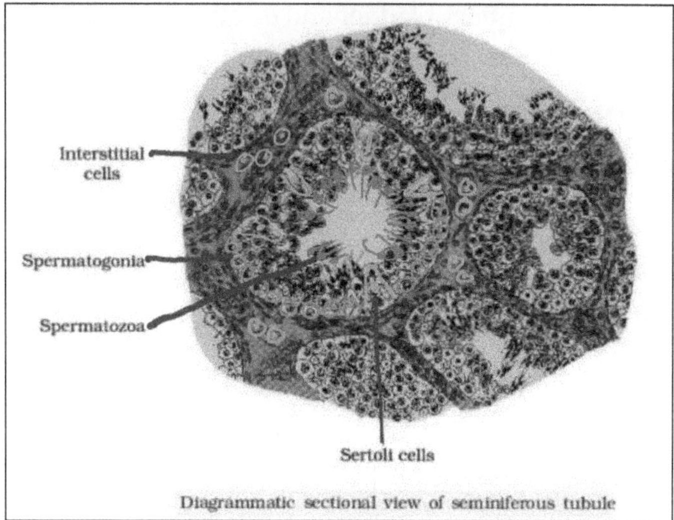

Diagrammatic sectional view of seminiferous tubule

- Each testicular lobule contains one to three highly coiled **seminiferous tubules.**

- In testicular lobule sperms are produced.

- Each seminiferous tubule is lined on its inside by two types of cells called **male germ cells** (*spermatogonia*) and **Sertoli cells.**

Sertoli cells and male germ cells

- The male germ cells undergo **meiotic** divisions finally leading to sperm formation.

- The Sertoli cells provide **nutrition** to the germ cells.

- Sertoli cells also release **AMF** and **ABP**.

Leydig cells

- The regions outside the **seminiferous** tubules called interstitial spaces.

- Interstitial spaces contain small blood vessels and **interstitial cells** or **Leydig cells.**

- Leydig cells synthesise and secrete **testicular** hormones called androgens.

Point to remember-

- Other **immunologically** competent cells are also present in testes.

- Origin of Gonads **endodermal.**

b. The male sex accessory duct system

- The male sex accessory ducts include **rete testis, vasa efferentia, epididymis** and **vas deferens.**

- The seminiferous tubules of the testis open into tubuli recti which open into rete testis.

- From rete testis, vasa efferentia arises.

- The **vasa efferentia** leave the testis and open into epididymis located along the posterior surface of each testis.

- The **epididymis** leads to vas deferens that ascends to the abdomen and loops over the urinary bladder.

- It receives a duct from **seminal vesicle** and opens into urethra as the **ejaculatory duct.**

- These **ducts store** and **transport the sperms** from the testis to the outside through urethra.
- The urethra originates from the urinary bladder and extends through the penis to its external opening called **urethral meatus.**

c. Penis (The external genitalia of Male)

- The penis is the **male external genitalia.**
- It is made up of special tissue that **helps in erection** of the penis to facilitate insemination.
- Penis contain **3 cords of erectile tissues** – 2 dorsal corpora covernosa and 1 ventral corpora spongiosa.
- The enlarged end of penis called the **glans penis.**
- **Glans penis** is covered by a loose fold of skin called **foreskin.**

d. The male accessory glands

- The male accessory glands include paired **seminal vesicles**, a **prostate** and paired **bulbourethral** glands.
- Prostate gland **chestnut** shaped.
- **Bulbourethral gland** is small pea grain shape.
- Secretions of these glands constitute **the seminal plasma** which is rich in fructose, calcium and certain enzymes.
- The secretions of bulbourethral glands also helps in the **lubrication of the penis.**

10.2 THE FEMALE REPRODUCTIVE SYSTEM

- The female reproductive system consists of a pair of **ovaries** alongwith a pair of **oviducts, uterus, cervix, vagina** and the **external genitalia.**
- The female reproductive system located in pelvic region.

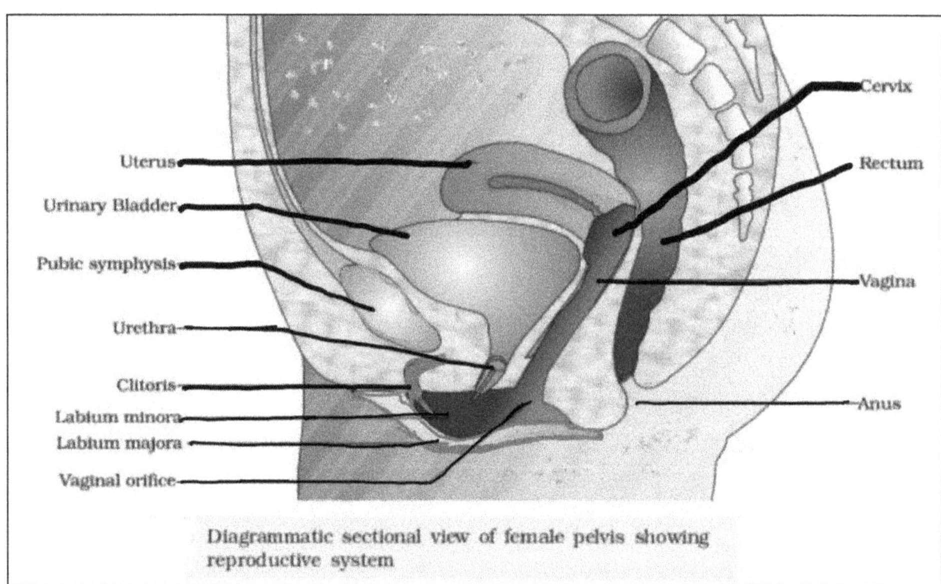

Diagrammatic sectional view of female pelvis showing reproductive system

- These parts of the system alongwith a pair of the **mammary glands** are integrated structurally and functionally to support the processes of ovulation, fertilisation, pregnancy, birth and child care.

a. Ovaries

- **Ovaries** are the primary female sex organs that produce the female gamete (ovum) and several steroid hormones (ovarian hormones).
- The ovaries are located one on each side of the lower abdomen.
- Each ovary is about **2 to 4** cm in length.
- Ovary is connected to the **pelvic wall** and uterus by **ligaments.**
- Each ovary is covered by a **thin epithelium.**
- This thin epithelium covers the ovarian stroma.
- The ovarian stroma is divided into two zones – **a peripheral cortex** and an **inner medulla**.

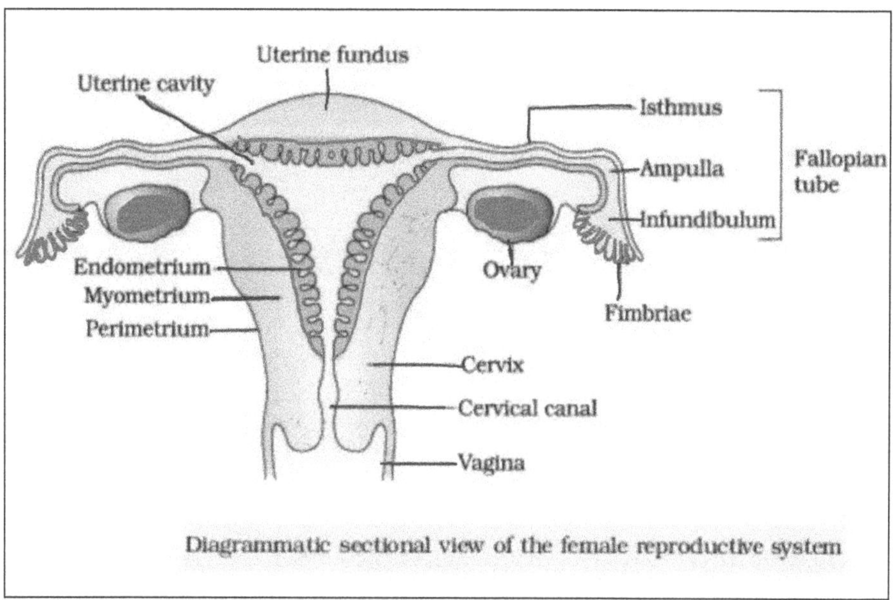

Diagrammatic sectional view of the female reproductive system

b. Oviducts (fallopian tubes)

- The **oviducts (fallopian tubes), uterus and vagina** constitute the female accessory ducts.
- Each fallopian tube is about **10-12 cm** long.
- It extends from the **periphery** of each ovary to the uterus.
- The part of Fallopian tube closer to the ovary is the funnel-shaped called as **infundibulum.**
- The edges of the infundibulum possess finger-like projections called **fimbriae.**
- **Fimbriae** helps in collection of the ovum after ovulation.
- The infundibulum leads to a wider part of the oviduct called **ampulla.**
- **Ampulla** is the site of fertilization.
- The last part of the oviduct, **isthmus** has a narrow lumen and it joins the uterus.

c. Utreus/Metra/Womb

- The uterus is single and it is also called **womb.**
- Uterus is an **inverted pear** shaped.
- It is supported by **ligaments** attached to the pelvic wall.

- The uterus opens into vagina through a **narrow cervix.**
- The cavity of the cervix is called **cervical canal** which along with vagina forms the birth canal.
- The wall of the uterus has **three layers** of tissue-
    - The external thin membranous **perimetrium**
    - Middle thick layer of smooth muscle **myometrium**
    - Inner glandular layer called **endometrium** that lines the uterine cavity.
- **The endometrium** undergoes cyclical changes during menstrual cycle.
- **The endometrium** maintained by progesterone.
- **The myometrium** exhibits strong contraction during delivery of the baby.

d. The female external genitalia

- **The female external genitalia** include mons pubis, labia majora, labia minora, hymen and clitoris.

i. Mons pubis

- **Mons pubis** is a cushion of fatty tissue covered by **skin and pubic hair.**

ii. Labia majora

- The **labia majora** are fleshy folds of tissue, which extend down from the mons pubis and surround the vaginal opening.

iii. Labia minora

- The **labia minora** are paired folds of tissue under the labia majora.

iv. Clitoris

- The **clitoris** is a tiny finger-like structure which lies at the upper junction of the two labia minora above the urethral opening.

v. Hymen

- The opening of the vagina is often covered partially by a membrane called **hymen.**
- The hymen is often torn during the **first coitus (intercourse).**
- The hymen can also be broken by a sudden **fall or jolt,** insertion of a **vaginal tampon,** active participation in some sports like horseback riding, cycling, etc.
- In some women the **hymen** persists even after coitus.
- In fact, the presence or absence of **hymen is not a reliable indicator** of virginity or sexual experience.

e. Mammary gland

- **A functional mammary gland** is characteristic of all female mammals.
- **Mammary gland** modified sweat gland.
- The mammary glands are **paired structures (breasts)** that contain glandular tissue and variable amount of fat.
- The glandular tissue of each breast is divided into 15-20 **mammary lobes** containing clusters of cells called alveoli.

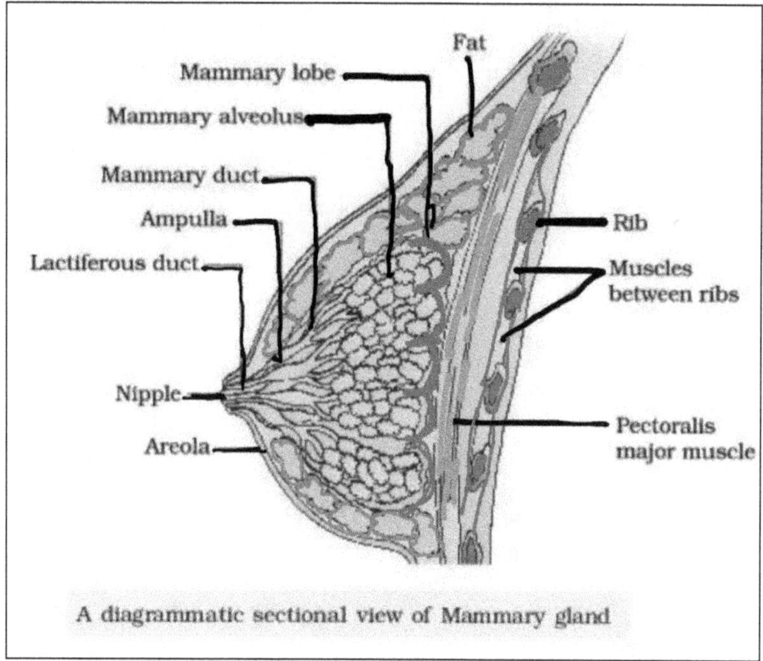

A diagrammatic sectional view of Mammary gland

- The cells of **alveoli secrete milk,** which is stored in the cavities (lumens) of alveoli.

- The **alveoli** open into mammary tubules.

- The tubules of each lobe join to form a **mammary duct**.

- Many mammary ducts join to form a wider **mammary** ampulla which is connected to **lactiferous duct** through which milk is sucked out.

- **Progesterone** and **estrogen** helps in development of mammary gland.

- **Estrogen** helps to develop duct system.

- **Progesterone** helps to develop alveolar system.

10.3 GAMETOGENESIS

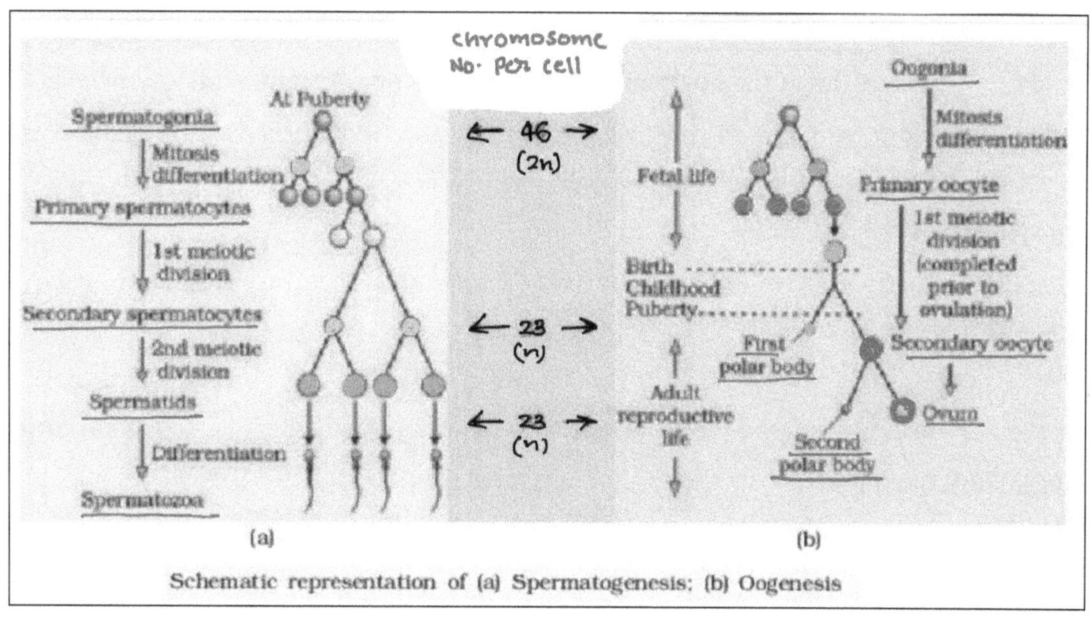

Schematic representation of (a) Spermatogenesis: (b) Oogenesis

- **The primary sex organs** – the testis in the males and the ovaries in the females – produce gametes, i.e, sperms and ovum, respectively, by the process called gametogenesis.

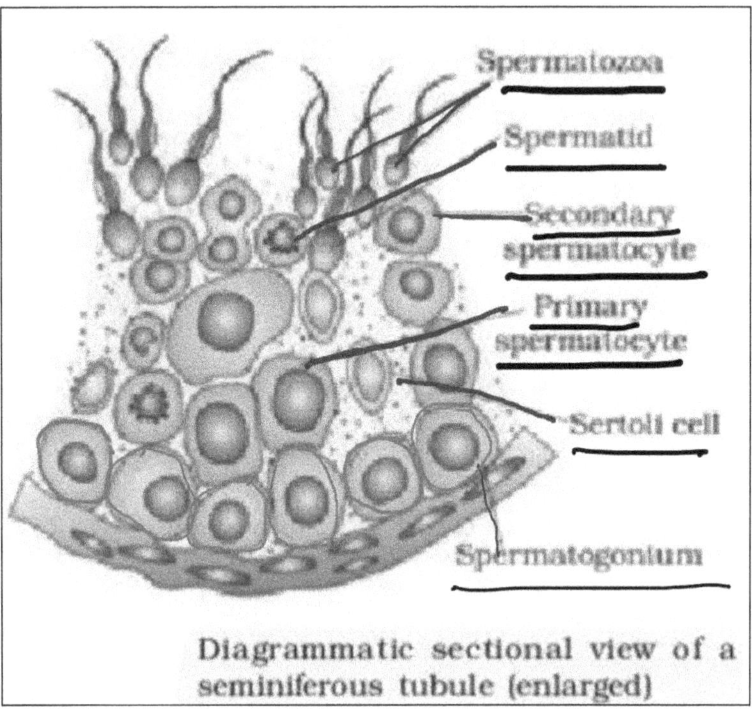

Diagrammatic sectional view of a seminiferous tubule (enlarged)

I. Spermatogenesis

- In testis, the immature male germ cells (spermatogonia) produce sperms by **spermatogenesis** that begins at puberty.

a. Spermatogonia

- The **spermatogonia** (sing. spermatogonium) present on the inside wall of seminiferous tubules multiply by mitotic division and increase in numbers.
- Each spermatogonium is diploid and contains 46 chromosomes.

b. Primary spermatocytes

- Some of the spermatogonia called **primary spermatocytes** periodically undergo meiosis.
- A primary spermatocyte completes the first meiotic division (reduction division) leading to formation of two equal, haploid cells called **secondary spermatocytes**, which have only 23 chromosomes each.

c. Secondary spermatocytes

- The secondary spermatocytes undergo the second meiotic division to produce four equal, haploid **spermatids.**

d. Spermatids

- The spermatids are transformed into **spermatozoa (sperms)** by the process called **spermiogenesis.**
- The spermatids are haploid.

e. Spermiation

- After **spermiogenesis,**sperm heads become embedded in the **Sertoli cells,** and are finally released from the seminiferous tubules by the process called **spermiation.**

II. Hormonal control of Spermatogenesis

- Spermatogenesis starts at the age of puberty due to significant increase in the secretion of gonadotropin releasing hormone**(GnRH).**
- **GnRH** is a hypothalamic hormone.
- The increased levels of GnRH then acts at the anterior pituitary gland and stimulates secretion of two gonadotropins – **Luteinising Hormone (LH)** and **Follicle Stimulating Hormone (FSH).**
- **LH** acts at the **Leydig** cells and **stimulates** synthesis and secretion of androgens.
- Androgens stimulate the process of **spermatogenesis.**
- FSH acts on the **Sertoli** cells and **stimulates** secretion of some factors which help in the process of spermiogenesis.

III. Structure of sperm

- It is a microscopic structure composed of a **head, neck,** a **middle piece** and a **tail.**
- In middle piece **mitochondria** spirally present called as nebenkern.
- **Manchette** is a kind of temporary collar sheath present around head of the sperm that serves for maintaining shape of developing sperm.
- A **plasma** membrane envelops the whole body of sperm.
- The **sperm** head contains an elongated haploid nucleus, the anterior portion of which is covered by a cap-like structure, **acrosome.**

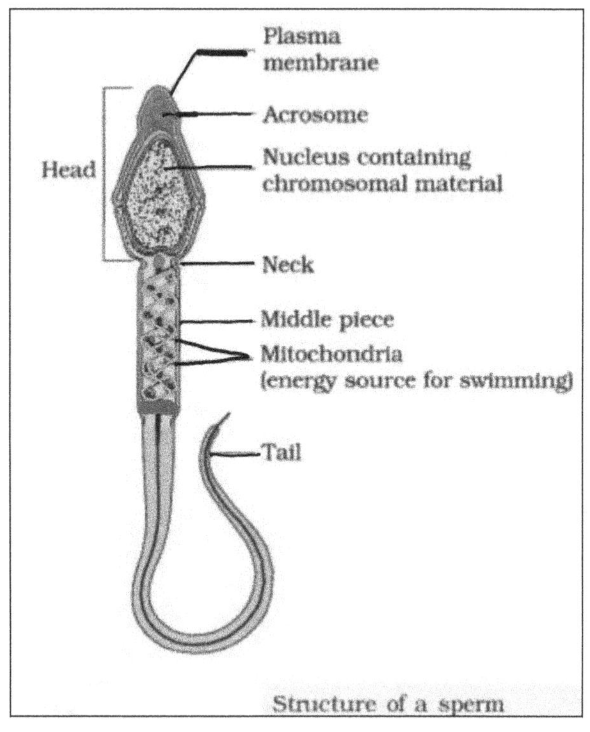

Structure of a sperm

- The acrosome is filled with enzymes that help **fertilisation** of the ovum.
- The middle piece possesses numerous **mitochondria,** which produce energy for the movement of tail that facilitate sperm motility essential for fertilisation.
- The human male ejaculates about **200** to **300** million sperms during a coitus of which, for normal fertility, at least **60** per cent sperms must have normal shape and size and for at least 40 per cent of them must show **vigorous** motility.
- Sperms released from the **seminiferous** tubules, are transported by the accessory ducts.
- Secretions of **epididymis, vas deferens, seminal vesicle** and **prostate** are essential for maturation and motility of sperms.
- The **seminal plasma** along with the sperms constitute the **semen.**
- The functions of male **sex accessory** ducts and glands are maintained by the testicular hormones (androgens).

I. Oogenesis

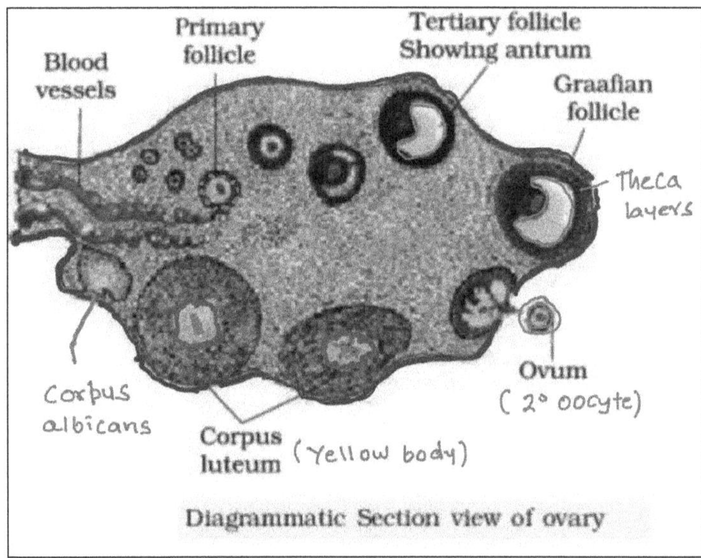

Diagrammatic Section view of ovary

- The process of formation of a mature female gamete is called **oogenesis.**
- **Oogenesis** is markedly different from spermatogenesis.

II. Oogonia

- Oogenesis is initiated during the embryonic development stage when a couple of million gamete mother cells (**oogonia**) are formed within each fetal ovary; no more oogonia are formed and added after birth.

III. Primary oocytes

- These cells start division and enter into prophase-I of the meiotic division and get temporarily arrested at that stage, called **primary oocytes.**
- Each primary oocyte then gets surrounded by a layer of granulosa cells and then called the **primary follicle.**
- A large number of these follicles degenerate during the phase from birth to puberty.

- Therefore, at puberty only **60,000-80,000** primary follicles are left in each ovary.
- The primary follicles get **surrounded** by more layers of granulosa cells and a new theca and called **secondary follicles.**
- The secondary follicle soon transforms into a tertiary follicle which is characterised by a fluid filled cavity called **antrum.**
- The theca layer is **organised** into an inner theca **interna** and an outer theca **externa.**
- At this stage the **primary oocyte** within the **tertiary follicle** grows in size and completes its first meiotic division.

IV. Secondary oocyte

- It is an unequal division **resulting** in the formation of a large **haploid secondary oocyte** and a tiny first polar body.
- The secondary oocyte retains bulk of the nutrient **rich** cytoplasm of the primary oocyte.
- The tertiary follicle further changes into the mature follicle or **Graafian follicle.**
- The secondary oocyte forms a new membrane called **zona pellucida** surrounding it.
- The Graafian follicle now ruptures to release the secondary oocyte (ovum) from the ovary by the process called **ovulation.**

10.4 MENSTRUAL CYCLE

- The reproductive cycle in the female primates (e.g. monkeys, apes and human beings) is called menstrual cycle.

I. Menarche

- The first menstruation begins at puberty and is called **menarche**.
- It start at the age of 10-12 year.

II. Menstrual cycle/Lunar cycle

- In human females, menstruation is repeated at an average interval of about 28/29 days, and the cycle of events starting from one **menstruation** till the next one is called the **menstrual cycle.**
- One ovum is released (ovulation) during the middle of each menstrual cycle.
- The major events of the **menstrual** cycle are shown in Figure-
- Menstrual cycle has three main stages-

a. Menstrual phase b. Follicular phase c. Luteal phase

a. Menstrual phase/Bleeding phase

- The cycle starts with the **menstrual** phase.
- The menstrual blood comes out by **vagina.**
- It lasts for 3-5 **days.**
- The menstrual flow results due to **breakdown** of endometrial lining of the uterus and its blood vessels.
- Menstruation only occurs if the released ovum is not **fertilised.**

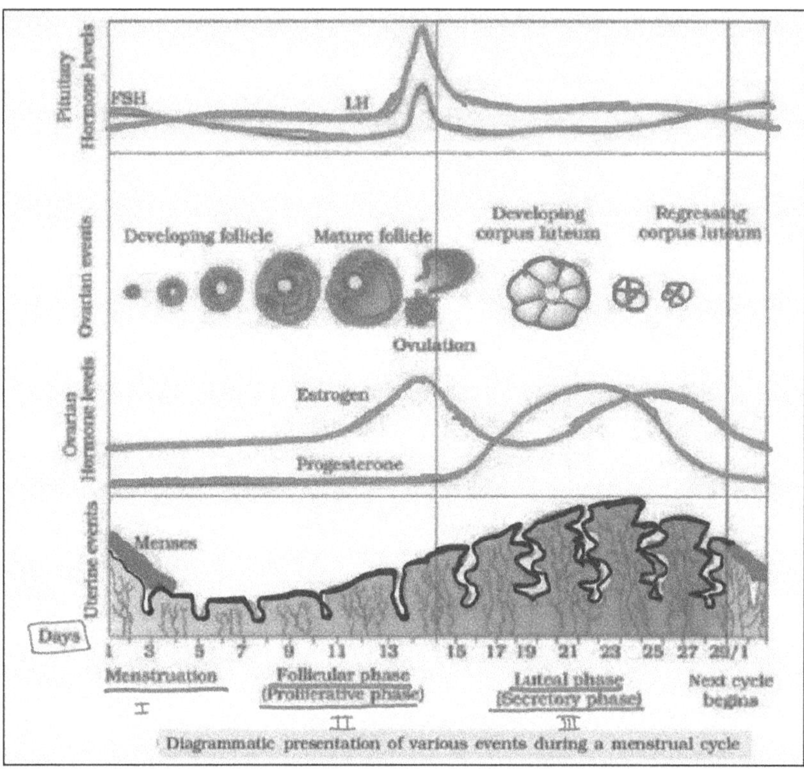

Diagrammatic presentation of various events during a menstrual cycle

- Lack of menstruation may be indicative of **pregnancy**.
- Lack of menstruation may also be caused due to some other underlying causes like **stress, poor** health etc.
- The menstrual phase is followed by the **follicular** phase.

b. Follicular phase/pre-ovulatory phase/ proliferative phase

- During this phase, the primary follicles in the ovary grow to become a fully mature **Graafian** follicle and simultaneously the **endometrium** of uterus regenerates through proliferation.
- These changes in the ovary and the uterus are induced by changes in the levels of pituitary and ovarian hormones.
- The secretion of **gonadotropins** (LH and FSH) increases gradually during the follicular phase, and stimulates follicular development as well as secretion of estrogens by the growing follicles.
- Both **LH** and **FSH** attain a peak level in the middle of cycle (about **14th** day).
- Rapid secretion of **LH** leading to its **maximum** level during the mid-cycle called LH surge induces rupture of Graafian follicle and thereby the release of ovum (**ovulation**).

c. Luteal phase/post-ovulatory/secretory phase

- The ovulation (ovulatory phase) is **followed** by the luteal phase during which the remaining parts of the Graafian follicle transform as the **corpus luteum**.
- The corpus luteum secretes large amounts of **progesterone** which is essential for maintenance of the endometrium.
- Such an **endometrium** is necessary for implantation of the fertilized ovum and other events of pregnancy.

- During pregnancy all events of the **menstrual** cycle stop and there is no menstruation.
- In the absence of fertilisation, the **corpus** luteum degenerates.
- This causes disintegration of the **endometrium** leading to menstruation, marking a new cycle.

Points to remember-

- In human beings, menstrual cycles ceases around **50** years of age; that is termed as **menopause**.
- Cyclic **menstruation** is an indicator of normal reproductive phase and extends between menarche and menopause.

10.5 FERTILISATION AND IMPLANTATION

- During **copulation** (coitus) semen is released by the penis into the vagina (insemination).
- The motile sperms swim rapidly.
- Speed of sperm 1.5-3.0 mm/minute.
- Sperm pass through the cervix, enter into the uterus and finally reach the junction of the **isthmus** and **ampulla** (ampullary-isthmic junction) of the fallopian tube.
- The **ovum** released by the ovary is also transported to the ampullary-isthmic junction where fertilisation takes place.
- Fertilisation can only occur if the ovum and sperms are transported simultaneously to the **Ampulla**(ampullary - isthmic) junction.
- This is the reason why not all copulations lead to **fertilisation** and pregnancy.
- The process of fusion of a sperm with an ovum is called **fertilisation**.
- During **fertilisation**, a sperm comes in contact with the **zona pellucida** layer of the secondary oocyte/ ovum and induces changes in the membrane that block the entry of additional sperms.
- Thus, it ensures that only one sperm can fertilise an ovum.

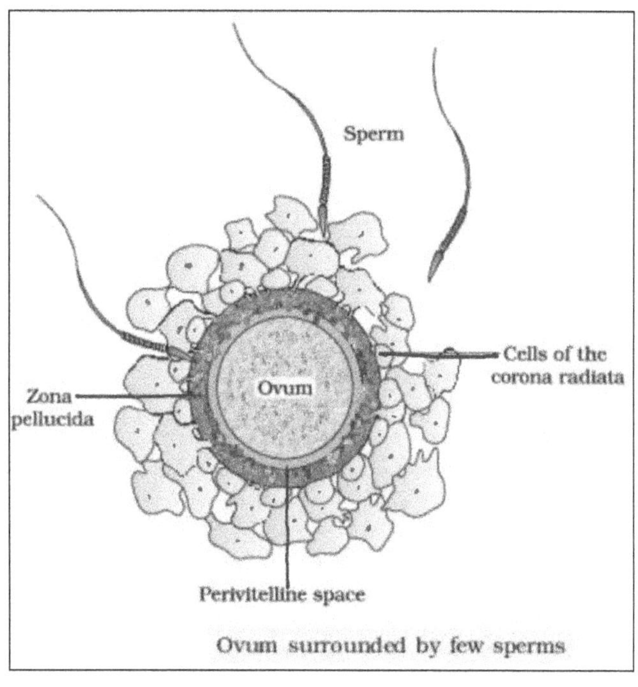

Ovum surrounded by few sperms

- The secretions of the acrosome help the sperm enter into the cytoplasm of the ovum through the **zona pellucida** and the plasma membrane.

- This induces the completion of the meiotic division of the secondary oocyte.

- The second meiotic division is also unequal and results in the formation of a **second polar body** and a haploid ovum (**ootid**).

- Soon the haploid nucleus of the sperms and that of the ovum fuse together to form a diploid **zygote**.

- The sex of the baby has been **decided** at this stage.

- The chromosome pattern in the human female is **XX** and that in the male is **XY**.

- All the haploid **gametes** produced by the female (ova) have the sex chromosome X whereas in the male gametes (sperms) the sex chromosome could be either X or Y, hence, **50** per cent of sperms carry the X chromosome while the other **50** per cent carry the Y.

- After fusion of the male and female gametes the zygote would carry either **XX** or **XY** depending on whether the sperm **carrying** X or Y fertilised the ovum.

- The zygote carrying XX would develop into a female baby and **XY** would form a male.

- **The sex of the baby is determined by the father and not by the mother.**

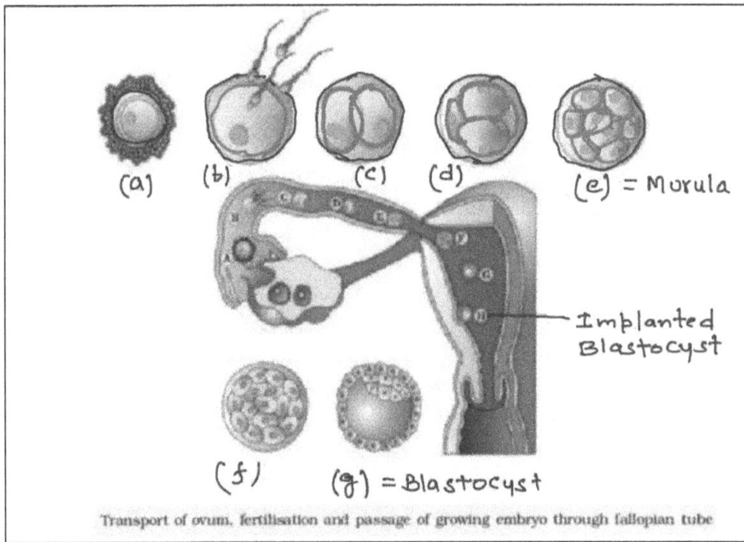

Transport of ovum, fertilisation and passage of growing embryo through fallopian tube

- The mitotic division starts as the zygote moves through the isthmus of the oviduct called **cleavage** towards the uterus and forms 2, 4, 8, 16 daughter cells called **blastomeres**.

- The embryo with **8 to 16** blastomeres is called a morula.

- The morula continues to divide and transforms into **blastocyst** as it moves further into the uterus.

- The blastomeres in the **blastocyst** are arranged into an outer layer called **trophoblast** and an inner group of cells attached to trophoblast called the **inner cell** mass.

- The trophoblast layer then gets attached to the endometrium and the inner cell mass gets differentiated as the embryo.

- After attachment, the uterine cells divide rapidly and covers the blastocyst.

- As a result, the blastocyst becomes embedded in the endometrium of the uterus.

- This is called **implantation** and it leads to pregnancy.

10.6 PREGNANCY AND EMBRYONIC DEVELOPMENT

Placenta

- After implantation, finger-like projections appear on the trophoblast called **chorionic villi** which are surrounded by the uterine tissue and maternal blood.

- The chorionic villi and uterine tissue become interdigitated with each other and jointly form a structural and functional unit between developing embryo (foetus) and maternal body called **placenta**.

- The placenta facilitate the supply of oxygen and nutrients to the embryo and also helps in removal of carbon dioxide and excretory/waste materials produced by the embryo.

- The placenta is connected to the embryo through an umbilical cord which helps in the transport of substances to and from the embryo.

Hormones from placenta

- Placenta also acts as an endocrine tissue and produces several hormones like **human chorionic gonadotropin** (hCG), **human placental lactogen** (hPL), **estrogens, progestogens,** etc.

- In the later phase of pregnancy, a hormone called **relaxin** is also secreted by the ovary.

- The hCG, hPL and relaxin are produced in women only during pregnancy.

- In addition, during pregnancy the levels of other hormones like **estrogens, progestogens, cortisol, prolactin, thyroxine,** etc., are increased several times in the maternal blood.

- Increased production of these hormones is **essential** for supporting the fetal growth, metabolic changes in the mother and **maintenance** of pregnancy.

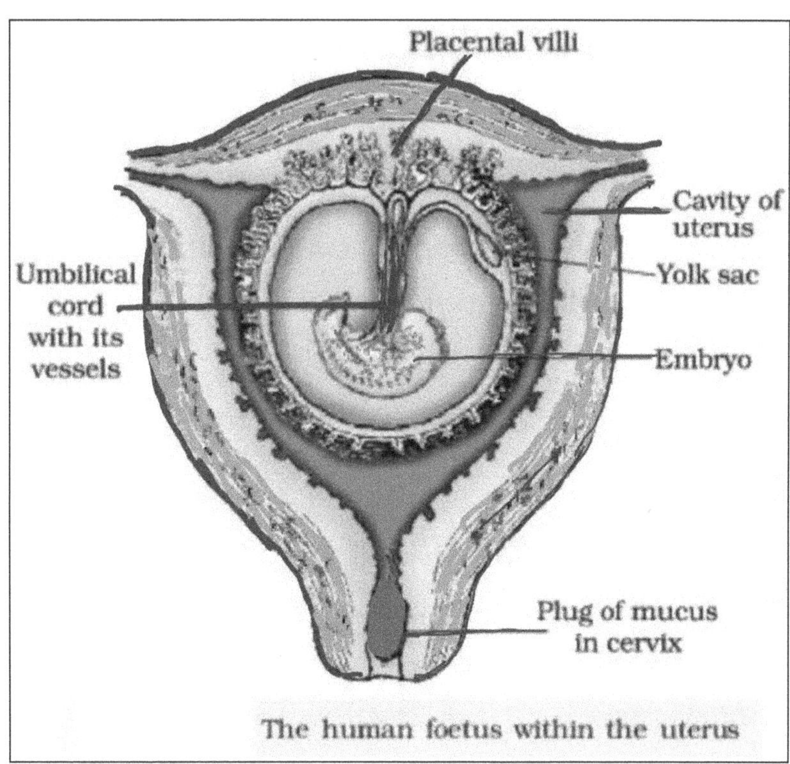

The human foetus within the uterus

Three germinal layers

- Immediately after implantation, the inner cell mass (embryo) differentiates into an outer layer called **ectoderm** and an inner layer called **endoderm**.
- A **mesoderm** soon appears between the ectoderm and the endoderm.
- These three layers give rise to all tissues (organs) in adults.

Organ Development

- The inner cell mass contains certain cells called **stem** cells which have the potency to give rise to all the tissues and organs.
- The human pregnancy lasts **9 months.**
- By the end of nine months of pregnancy, the foetus is fully developed and is ready for delivery.
- In human beings, **after one month of pregnancy,** the embryo's heart is formed.
- The first sign of growing foetus may be noticed by listening to the heart sound carefully through the stethoscope.
- By the **end of the second month of pregnancy**, the foetus develops limbs and digits.
- By the **end of 12 weeks (first trimester),** most of the major organ systems are formed, for example, the limbs and external genital organs are well-developed.
- The first movements of the foetus and appearance of hair on the head are usually observed during the fifth month.
- By the **end of 24 weeks (second trimester),** the body is covered with fine hair, eye-lids separate, and eyelashes are formed.

10.7 PARTURITION AND LACTATION

Parturition.

- The average duration of human pregnancy is **about 9 months** which is called the gestation period.
- Vigorous contraction of the uterus at the end of pregnancy causes expulsion/delivery of the foetus. This process of delivery of the foetus (childbirth) is called **parturition**.
- Parturition is induced by a **complex neuroendocrine mechanism.**
- Relaxin hormone is releases by placenta and ovary.
- Progesterone concentration decreases so placenta dissolves.

Foetal ejection reflex

- The signals for parturition originate from the **fully developed foetus and the placenta** which induce mild uterine contractions called **foetal ejection reflex.**
- **This triggers release** of oxytocin from the maternal pituitary.
- **Oxytocin** acts on the uterine muscle and causes stronger uterine contractions.
- As secretion of oxytocin increases the uterine contraction rate also increases.

- The **stimulatory reflex** between the uterine contraction and oxytocin secretion continues resulting in stronger and stronger contractions.
- This leads to **expulsion of the baby out** of the uterus through the birth canal – parturition.
- Soon after the infant is delivered, the placenta is also expelled out of the uterus.

Lactation

- The mammary glands of the female undergo differentiation during pregnancy and starts producing milk towards the end of pregnancy by the process called **lactation**.
- This helps the mother in feeding the newborn.
- Milk ejecting hormone **Oxytocin.**
- Milk forming hormone **Prolactin.**

Colostrum

- The milk produced during the initial few days of lactation is called **colostrum** which contains several antibodies absolutely essential to develop resistance for the new-born babies.
- Breast-feeding during the initial period of infant growth is recommended by doctors for bringing up a healthy baby.
- **Colostrum is rich in antibody IgA.**

1. Consider the following statements and find out the correct option-

A. In adults, each testis is oval in shape, with a length of about 4 to 5 cm.

B. Each testis has about 250 compartments called **testicular lobules**.

C. Each lobule contains one to three highly coiled **seminiferous tubules** in which sperms are produced.

D. Each seminiferous tubule is lined on its inside by two types of cells called **male germ cells** and **Sertoli cells.**

Which of the above are correct -

1. A,B,C only

2. B,C

3. D,B,A

4. A,B,C,D

2. Match the list 1 and 2

List 1	List 2
a. tertiary follicle	j. 60,000-80,000 primary follicles are left in each ovary
b. at puberty	k. zona pellucida
c. secondary oocyte forms a new membrane	l. antrum
d. primary follicle	m. surrounded by a layer of granulosa cells

Find out the correct option –

1. a.k, b.j, c.l, d.m

2. a.k,b.l,c.j,d.m

3. a.l,b.j,c.k,d.m

4. a.l,b.j,c.m,d.k

3. Consider the following features-

a) The testes are situated outside the abdominal cavity within a pouch called **scrotum**.

b) The scrotum helps in maintaining the low temperature of the testes (2–2.5o C lower than the normal internal body temperature) necessary for spermatogenesis.

c) The male germ cells undergo meiotic divisions finally leading to sperm formation, while Sertoli cells provide nutrition to the germ cells.

d) The regions outside the seminiferous tubules called interstitial spaces, contain small blood vessels and interstitial cells or Leydig cells.

e) Leydig cells synthesise and secrete testicular hormones called androgens.

Which of the above are/is correct -

1. only a and d

2. a,b,c,d,e

3. only c and d

4. a,e,c

4. The male sex accessory ducts include all, except -

a) rete testis

b) vasa efferentia

c) epididymis

d) vas deferens

e) prostate gland

1. a

2. a,b

3. b,d

4. e

5. Consider the following statements and find out the correct option-

STATEMENT 1. The seminiferous tubules of the testis open into the vasa efferentia directly.

STATEMENT 2. The vasa efferentia leave the testis and open into epididymis located along the posterior surface of each testis.

1. Both are correct statements

2. Only statement 1 correct

3. Both are wrong statements

4. Only statement 2 correct

6. Go through the following statements-

ASSERTION(A). The epididymis leads to vas deferens that ascends to the abdomen and loops over the urinary bladder.

REASON(R). It receives a duct from seminal vesicle and opens into urethra as the bartholin duct.

1. A correct and R is correct explanation of A

2. A correct and R is also correct but R is not correct explanation of A

3. A correct but R incorrect

4. A and R both are incorrect

7. Find out the incorrect statement -

1. The bartholin ducts store and transport the sperms from the testis to the outside through urethra.

2. The urethra originates from the urinary bladder and extends through the penis to its external opening called **urethral meatus.**

3. The penis is the male external genitalia

4. Penis is made up of special tissue that helps in erection of the penis to facilitate insemination.

8. Go through the following statements-

a) The enlarged end of penis called the glans penis is covered by a loose fold of skin called **foreskin**.

b) The male accessory glands include paired **seminal vesicles**, a **prostate** and paired **bulbourethral** glands.

c) Secretions of male accessory glands constitute the seminal plasma which is rich in fructose, calcium and certain enzymes.

d) The secretions of bulbourethral glands also helps in the lubrication of the penis.

How many of them are correct-

1. two

2. three

3. four

4. One

9. Match the list 1 and 2-

List 1   List 2

List 1	List 2
a. menstrual phase	j. 5th to 13th day
b. ovulation	k. 1st to 5th day
c. proliferative phase	l. 14th day
d. secretory phase	m. 15th to 28th day

Find out the correct option –

1. a.k, b.j, c.l, d.m

2. a.k,b.l,c.j,d.m

3. a.l,b.j,c.k,d.m

4. a.l,b.j,c.m,d.k

10. Consider the following statements and find out the correct option

STATEMENT 1. The testes are situated outside the abdominal cavity within a pouch called **scrotum**. **STATEMENT 2.** The scrotum helps in maintaining the high temperature of the testes (2–2.5° C higher than the normal internal body temperature) necessary for spermatogenesis.

1. Both are wrong statements

2. Only statement 1 correct

3. Both are correct statements

4. Only statement 2 correct

11. Read the following statements very carefully and find out the correct-

a) The female reproductive system consists of a pair of **ovaries** alongwith a pair of **oviducts, uterus, cervix, vagina** and the **external genitalia** located in pelvic region.

b) These parts of the system alongwith a pair of the **mammary glands** are integrated structurally and functionally to support the processes of ovulation, fertilisation, pregnancy, birth and child care.

c) Ovaries are the primary female sex organs that produce the female gamete (ovum) and several steroid hormones (ovarian hormones).

d) The ovaries are located one on each side of the lower abdomen.

Which of the above statement are/is correct?

1. a and c both

2. d only

3. a,b,c,d

4. b and d both

12. **Go through the following statements-**

ASSERTION(A). Each ovary is about 2 to 4 cm in length and is connected to the pelvic wall and uterus by ligaments.

REASON(R). Each ovary is covered by a thin epithelium which encloses the ovarian stroma.

1. A correct and R is correct explanation of A

2. A correct and R is also correct but R is not correct explanation of A

3. A correct but R incorrect

4. A and R both are incorrect

13. **Find out incorrect statement -**

1. The female reproductive system consists of a pair of **ovaries** alongwith a pair of **oviducts, uterus, cervix, vagina** and the **external genitalia** located in pelvic region.

2. These parts of the system alongwith a pair of the **mammary glands** are integrated structurally and functionally to support the processes of ovulation, fertilisation, pregnancy, birth and child care.

3. Ovaries are the primary female sex organs that produce the female gamete (ovum) and several steroid hormones (ovarian hormones).

4. The ovaries are located one on each side of the upper abdomen.

14. **Read the following statements and find out correct option-**

a) Each ovary is about 2 to 4 cm in length and is connected to the pelvic wall and uterus by ligaments.

b) Each ovary is covered by a thin epithelium which encloses the ovarian stroma.

c) The stroma is divided into two zones – a peripheral cortex and an inner medulla.

d) The oviducts (fallopian tubes), uterus and vagina constitute the female accessory ducts.

e) Each fallopian tube is about 10-12 cm long and extends from the periphery of each ovary to the uterus

How many of them are correct-

1. four

2. five

3. two

4. three

15. Consider the following statements and find out the correct option

STATEMENT 1. Immediately after implantation, the inner cell mass (embryo) differentiates into an outer layer called **ectoderm** and an inner layer called **endoderm**.

STATEMENT 2. A **mesoderm** soon appears between the ectoderm and the endoderm.

1. Both are wrong statements

2. Only statement 1 correct

3. Both are correct statements

4. Only statement 2 correct

16. Match the list 1 and 2 with respect to organogenesis-

List 1	List 2
a. 1st month	Heart
b. *2nd month*	limb
c. 3rd month	organ sytem
d. *5th month*	Movement

How many of them are correctly matched-

1. one

2. two

3. three

4. four

17. Consider the following -

a) The edges of the infundibulum possess finger-like projections called **fimbriae**, which help in collection of the ovum after ovulation.

b) The infundibulum leads to a wider part of the oviduct called **ampulla**.

c) The last part of the oviduct, **isthmus** has a narrow lumen and it joins the uterus.

d) The uterus is single and it is also called **womb**.

Which of the above statements are correct?

1. b and a only

2. c and b only

3. a,b,c only

4. a,b,c,d

18. Match the list 1 and 2-

List 1	List 2
a. After implantation, finger-like projections appear on	the trophoblast called **chorionic villi** which are surrounded by the uterine tissue and maternal blood.

b. The chorionic villi and uterine tissue become	interdigitated with each other and jointly form a structural and functional unit between developing embryo (foetus) and maternal body called placenta
c. The placenta facilitate	the supply of oxygen and nutrients to embryo and also removal of carbon dioxide and excretory/waste materials produced by the embryo.
d. Placenta also acts as an endocrine tissue and produces several hormones	like human chorionic gonadotropin (hCG), human placental lactogen (hPL), estrogens, progestogens, etc.

How many of them are/is correctly matched-

1. one

2. two

3. three

4. four

19. Consider the following statements -

a) The shape of the uterus is like an inverted pear.

b) It is supported by ligaments attached to the pelvic wall.

c) The uterus opens into vagina through a narrow cervix.

d) The cavity of the cervix is called **cervical canal** which along with vagina forms the birth canal.

How many of them are/is correct for human female-

1. one

2. two

3. three

4. four

20. Read the following statements-

I. The wall of the uterus has three layers of tissue.

II. The external thin membranous **perimetrium,** middle thick layer of smooth muscle, **myometrium** and inner glandular layer called **endometrium** that lines the uterine cavity.

III. The endometrium undergoes cyclical changes during menstrual cycle.

IV. The myometrium exhibits strong contraction during delivery of the baby.

How many of them are/is correct **statements-**

1. two

2. three

3. four

4. one

21. Consider the following statements and find out the correct option for humans-

STATEMENT 1. The female external genitalia include mons pubis, labia majora, labia minora, hymen and clitoris

STATEMENT 2. Mons pubis is a cushion of fatty tissue covered by skin and pubic hair.

1. Both are wrong statements

2. Only Statement 1 correct

3. Both are correct statements

4. Only statement 2 correct

22. Go through the following statements and find out the correct option-

ASSERTION(A). The **labia majora** are fleshy folds of tissue, which extend down from the mons pubis and surround the vaginal opening.

REASON(R). The **labia minora** are paired folds of tissue under the labia majora.

1. A correct and R is correct explanation of A

2. A correct and R is also correct but R is not correct explanation of A

3. A correct but R incorrect

4. A and R both are incorrect

23. Go through the following statements and find out the correct option-

A. The opening of the vagina is often covered partially by a membrane called **hymen**.

B. The **clitoris** is a tiny finger-like structure which lies at the upper junction of the two labia minora above the urethral opening.

C. The hymen is often torn during the first coitus (intercourse).

D. Hymen can also be broken by a sudden fall or jolt, insertion of a vaginal tampon, active participation in some sports like horseback riding, cycling, etc.

Which of the above statement are correct -

1. A, B, C only

2. C and D only

3. D and A only

4. All are correct

24. Read the statements given below-

A. A functional mammary gland is characteristic of few female mammals.

B. The mammary glands are paired structures (breasts) that contain glandular tissue and variable amount of fat.

C. The glandular tissue of each breast is divided into 30-40 **mammary lobes** containing clusters of cells called alveoli.

D. The cells of alveoli secrete milk, which is stored in the cavities (lumens) of alveoli.

E. The alveoli open into mammary tubules.

F.   The tubules of each lobe join to form a **mammary duct**.

Which of the above statement are incorrect?

1. A and C only

2. E only

3. D and E only

4. A,B,C,D,E,F

25. Read the statements given below-

A.   In some women the hymen persists even after coitus.

B.   The presence or absence of hymen is not a reliable indicator of virginity or sexual experience.

C.   The cells of alveoli of mammary gland secrete milk, which is stored in the cavities (lumens) of alveoli.

D.   The alveoli open into mammary tubules.

Which of the above statement are correct?

1. A and C only

2. A only

3. D and C only

4. A,B,C,D

26. Consider the following statements-

I.   The cells of alveoli secrete milk, which is stored in the cavities (lumens) of alveoli.

II.   The alveoli open into mammary tubules.

III.   The tubules of each lobe join to form a **mammary duct**.

IV.   Several mammary ducts join to form a wider mammary ampulla which is connected to **lactiferous duct** through which milk is sucked out.

How many of them are correct-

1. one

2. two

3. three

4. four

27. Match the list 1 and 2-

List 1   List 2 (life span)

a. Dog	100-150 year
b. Parrot	25-30 year
c. Tortoise	120 year
d. Crocodile	60 year

How many of them are correctly matched-

1. one

2. two

3. three

4. four

28. Read the following statements-

   a) The primary sex organs – the testis in the males and the ovaries in the females – produce gametes, i.e, sperms and ovum, respectively, by the process called gametogenesis.

   b) In testis, the immature spermatogonia produce sperms by **spermatogenesis** that begins at puberty.

   c) The **spermatogonia** present on the inside wall of seminiferous tubules multiply by mitotic division and increase in numbers.

   d) Each spermatogonium is diploid and contains 23 chromosomes.

Which of the above statements are/is correct-

1. a and c only

2. a,b,c only

3. d and c only

4. a,b,c,d

29. Consider the following statements and find out incorrect one-

   1. In testis, the immature male germ cells (spermatogonia) produce sperms by **spermatogenesis** that begins at puberty.

   2. The **spermatogonia** (sing. spermatogonium) present on the outside the wall of seminiferous tubules multiply by mitotic division and increase in numbers.

   3. Each spermatogonium is diploid and contains 46 chromosomes.

   4. Some of the spermatogonia called **primary spermatocytes** periodically undergo meiosis.

30. Read the following facts -

   A. The reproductive cycle in the female primates (e.g. monkeys, apes and human beings) is called Oestrus cycle.

   B. The first menstruation begins at puberty and is called **menarche**.

   C. In human females, menstruation is repeated at an average interval of about 28/29 days, and the cycle of events starting from one menstruation till the next one is called the **menstrual cycle**.

   D. One ovum is released (ovulation) during approx the end of each menstrual cycle.

   E. The cycle starts with the menstrual phase, when menstrual flow occurs and it lasts for 3-5 days.

How many of them are correct with respect to Menstrual cycle-

1. four

2. two

3. three

4. five

31.Read the following statements and find out the correct option

STATEMENT 1. The mitotic division starts as the zygote moves through the isthmus of the oviduct called **cleavage** towards the uterus and forms 2, 4, 8, 16 daughter cells called **blastomere.**

STATEMENT 2. The embryo with 80 to 160 blastomeres is called a morula which, continues to divide and transforms into blastocyst as it moves further into the uterus.

1. Both are wrong statements

2. Both are correct statements

3. Only statement 1 correct

4. Only statement 2 correct

32. Go through the following statement and find out the correct option-

ASSERTION(A). A primary spermatocyte completes the first meiotic division (reduction division) leading to formation of two equal, haploid cells called **secondary spermatocytes**, which have only 23 chromosomes each.

REASON(R). The secondary spermatocytes undergo the second meiotic division to produce four equal, haploid **spermatids**

1. A correct and R is correct explanation of A

2. A correct and R is also correct but R is not correct explanation of A

3. A correct but R incorrect

4. A and R both are incorrect

33. Go through the following statements and find out the correct option-

ASSERTION(A). The spermatids are transformed into **spermatozoa (sperms)** by the process called **spermiogenesis.**

REASON(R). Spermatogenesis starts at the age of puberty due to significant increase in the secretion of gonadotropin releasing hormone(GnRH).

1. A correct and R is correct explanation of A

2. A correct and R is also correct but R is not correct explanation of A

3. A. correct but R incorrect

4. A and R both are incorrect

34. Read the following statements-

a) The spermatids are transformed into **spermatozoa (sperms)** by the process called **spermiogenesis.**

b) After spermiogenesis,sperm heads become embedded in the **Sertoli cells,** and are finally released from the seminiferous tubules by the process called **spermiation.**

c) Spermatogenesis starts at the age of puberty due to significant increase in the secretion of gonadotropin releasing hormone(GnRH).

Which above statements is/are correct-

1. a only   2. b only

3. c, a only   4. a,b,c

35. Which of the following is/are correct -

    I. The increased levels of GnRH then acts at the anterior pituitary gland and stimulates secretion of two gonadotropins – luteinising hormone (LH) and follicle stimulating hormone (FSH).

    II. LH acts at the Leydig cells and stimulates synthesis and secretion of androgens.

    III. Androgens, in turn, stimulate the process of spermatogenesis.

    IV. FSH acts on the Leydig cells and stimulates secretion of some factors which help in the process of spermiogenesis.

How many of above are/is incorrect-

1. three

2. four

3. two

4. one

36. Consider the following statements -

    i. Sperm is a microscopic structure composed of a **head, neck,** a **middle piece** and a **tail**.

    ii. A plasma membrane envelops the whole body of sperm.

    iii. The sperm head contains an elongated haploid nucleus, the anterior portion of which is covered by a cap-like structure, **acrosome.**

    iv. The acrosome is filled with enzymes that help fertilisation of the ovum.

Which above statements are correct-

1. i,ii only

2. i, iii,iv only

3. i,ii,iii only

4 all are correct

37. Read the following statements-

    i. The middle piece possesses numerous mitochondria, which produce energy for the movement of tail that facilitate sperm motility essential for fertilisation.

    ii. The human male ejaculates about 200 to 300 million sperms during a coitus of which, for normal fertility, at least 06 per cent sperms must have normal shape and size and for at least 40 per cent of them must show vigorous motility.

    iii. Sperms released from the seminiferous tubules, are transported by the accessory ducts.

    iv. Secretions of epididymis, vas deferens, seminal vesicle and prostate are essential for maturation and motility of sperms.

Which above statements is/are incorrect-

1. v and ii only

2. ii only

3. i and ii only

4. All are correct

38. Consider the following statements-

A. The seminal plasma along with the sperms constitute the **semen**.

B. The functions of male sex accessory ducts and glands are maintained by the testicular hormones (androgens).

C. The process of formation of a mature female gamete is called **oogenesis** which is markedly different from spermatogenesis.

D. Oogenesis is initiated during the embryonic development stage when a couple of million gamete mother cells (**oogonia**) are formed within each fetal ovary; no more oogonia are formed and added after birth.

How many of above are/is correct-

1. three

2. four

3. two

4. one

39. Read the following statements and find out the correct option-

STATEMENT 1. The primary follicles get surrounded by more layers of granulosa cells and a new theca and called **secondary follicles**.

STATEMENT 2. The secondary follicle soon transforms into a tertiary follicle which is characterised by a fluid filled cavity called **antrum**.

1. Both are wrong statements

2. Both are correct statements

3. Only statement 1 correct

4. Only statement 2 correct

40. Read the following statements-

a) Each primary oocyte gets surrounded by a layer of granulosa cells and then called the **primary follicle**.

b) A large number of these follicles degenerate during the phase from birth to puberty.

c) Therefore, at puberty only 60,000-80,000 primary follicles are left in each ovary.

d) The primary follicles get surrounded by more layers of granulosa cells and a new theca and called **secondary follicles**.

e) The secondary follicle soon transforms into a tertiary follicle which is characterised by a fluid filled cavity called **antrum**.

Which of the above are correct?

1. a and b only

2. b and c only

3. c and d only

4. a,b,c,d,e

41. Go through the following statement and find out the correct option-

ASSERTION(A). The tertiary follicle further changes into the mature follicle or **Graafian follicle**

REASON(R). The Graafian follicle ruptures to release the primary oocyte from the ovary.

1. A correct and R is correct explanation of A

2. A correct and R is also correct but R is not correct explanation of A

3. A correct but R incorrect

4. A and R both are incorrect

42. Read the following statement -

A. Menstruation only occurs if the released ovum is not fertilised.

B. Lack of menstruation may be indicative of pregnancy.

C. Menstruation may also be caused due to some other underlying causes like stress, poor health etc.

D. The menstrual phase is followed by the follicular phase.

E. During this phase, the primary follicles in the ovary grow to become a fully mature Graafian follicle and simultaneously the endometrium of uterus regenerates through proliferation.

How many of above are correct-

1. three

2. four

3. two

4.five

43. Consider the following statements-

A. The secretion of gonadotropins (LH and FSH) increases gradually during the follicular phase, and stimulates follicular development as well as secretion of estrogens by the growing follicles.

B. Both LH and FSH attain a peak level in the middle of cycle (about 14th day).

C. Rapid secretion of LH leading to its maximum level during the mid-cycle called LH surge induces rupture of Graafian follicle and thereby the release of ovum (**ovulation**).

D. The ovulation (ovulatory phase) is followed by the luteal phase during which the remaining parts of the Graafian follicle transform as the **corpus luteum**

How many of them are correct-

1. one

2. three

3. four

4. two

44. Read the following statements and find out the correct option-

STATEMENT 1. The corpus luteum secretes large amounts of progesterone which is essential for maintenance of the endometrium.

STATEMENT 2. Such an endometrium is necessary for implantation of the fertilized ovum and other events of pregnancy.

1. Both are correct statements

2. Both are wrong statements

3. Only statement 1 correct

4. Only statement 2 correct

45. **Find out the incorrect statement -**

    1. During pregnancy all events of the menstrual cycle stop and there is no menstruation.

    2. In the absence of fertilisation, the corpus luteum degenerates.

    3. The absence of fertilisation causes disintegration of the endometrium leading to menstruation, marking a new menstrual cycle.

    4. In human beings, menstrual cycles ceases around 35 years of age; that is termed as **menopause.**

46. **Read the following statements and find out the correct option-**

    STATEMENT 1. During copulation (coitus) semen is released by the penis into the vagina (insemination).

    STATEMENT 2. The motile sperms swim rapidly, pass through the cervix, enter into the uterus and finally reach the ampulla of the fallopian tube.

    1. Both are correct statements

    2. Both are wrong statements.

    3. Only statement 1 correct

    4. Only statement 2 correct

47. **Go through the following statements and find out the correct option-**

    ASSERTION(A). The average duration of human pregnancy is about 9 months which is called the gestation period. Vigorous contraction of the uterus at the end of pregnancy causes expulsion/ delivery of the foetus. This process of delivery of the foetus (childbirth) is called **parturition.**

    REASON(R). Parturition is induced by a complex neuroendocrine mechanism.

    1. A correct and R is correct explanation of A

    2. A correct and R is also correct but R is not correct explanation of A

    3. A correct but R incorrect

    4. A and R both are incorrect

48. **Read the following statements -**

    a) The signals for parturition originate from the fully developed foetus and the placenta which induce mild uterine contractions called **foetal ejection reflex.**

    b) This triggers release of oxytocin from the maternal pituitary.

    c) Oxytocin acts on the uterine muscle and causes stronger uterine contractions, which in turn stimulates further secretion of oxytocin.

d) The stimulatory reflex between the uterine contraction and oxytocin secretion continues resulting in stronger and stronger contractions.

How many of them are/is correct-

1. one

2. two

3. three

4. four

49. Consider the following statements -

A. The mammary glands of the female undergo differentiation during pregnancy and starts producing milk towards the end of pregnancy by the process called **lactation**.

B. This helps the mother in feeding the newborn.

C. The milk produced during the initial few days of lactation is called **colostrum** which contains several antibodies absolutely essential to develop resistance for the new-born babies.

D. Breast-feeding during the initial period of infant growth is recommended by doctors for bringing up a healthy baby.

Which of the above statements are correct-

1. A and C only

2. A,B,C only

3. B and D only

4. All are correct

50. Read the following statements-

A. By the end of the second month of pregnancy, the foetus develops limbs and digits.

B. By the end of 12 weeks (first trimester), most of the major organ systems are formed, for example, the limbs and external genital organs are well-developed.

C. The first movements of the foetus and appearance of hair on the head are usually observed during the fifth month.

D. By the end of 24 weeks (second trimester), the body is covered with fine hair, eye-lids separate, and eyelashes are formed.

E. By the end of nine months of pregnancy, the foetus is fully developed and is ready for delivery.

Which of the above statements are correct-

1. A and C only

2. A,B,C only

3. B and D only

4. A,B,C,D,E

REPRODUCTIVE HEALTH

11.1 Reproductive Health –Problems and Strategies

11.2 Population Explosion and Birth Control

11.3 Medical Termination of Pregnancy

11.4 Sexually Transmitted Diseases

11.5 Infertility

- **According** to the **World Health Organisation** (WHO), reproductive health means a total well-being in all aspects of reproduction, i.e., physical, emotional, behavioural and social.

- A society with people having physically and functionally normal reproductive organs and normal **emotional** and **behavioural** interactions among them in all sex-related aspects might be called reproductively healthy.

11.1 REPRODUCTIVE HEALTH –PROBLEMS AND STRATEGIES

- Our **nation** was the first nation in the world to **initiate** various action plans at national level towards attaining a reproductively healthy society.

- **Family planning in India** started in**1951**.

- The **primary** step towards reproductive health are-

  - Awareness among people about reproductive organs

  - Adolescence and associated changes

  - Safe and hygienic sexual practices

  - Sexually transmitted diseases (STDs) including AIDS, etc.

- Reproduction-related areas are currently in operation under the popular name '**Reproductive and Child Health Care (RCH) programmes**'.

- **Reproductive and Child Health Care (RCH) programmes'** in India started in**1997**.

- The awareness among people about various reproduction related aspects and providing facilities and support for building up a reproductively healthy society are the major tasks under these programmes.

- The **governmental** and **non-governmental** agencies have taken various steps to create awareness among the people about reproduction-related aspects with the help of audio-visual and print-media.

- **Parents, relatives, teachers and friends,** can also play a major role in the dissemination of the above information.

- **The sex education** in schools should also be encouraged to provide right information to the young so as to discourage children from believing in myths and having misconceptions about sex-related aspects.

- **Educating people**, especially fertile couples and those in **marriageable** age group, about available birth control options, care of pregnant mothers, post-natal care of the **mother** and child, importance of breast feeding, equal **opportunities** for the male and the female child, etc., would address the **importance** of bringing up socially conscious healthy families of desired size.

- **The Awareness of problems** due to uncontrolled population growth, social evils like sex-abuse and sex-related crimes, etc., need to be created to enable people to think and take up **necessary** steps to prevent them and so can **build** up a socially responsible and healthy society.

- The successful implementation of various action plans to attain **reproductive** health requires strong **infrastructural** facilities, professional expertise and material support.

- These are essential to provide medical assistance and care to people in reproduction-related problems like **pregnancy, delivery, STDs, abortions, contraception, menstrual problems, infertility,** etc. Implementation of better techniques and new strategies from time to time are also required to provide more efficient care and **assistance** to people.

Amniocentesis

- In **aminocentesis** some of the amniotic fluid of the developing foetus is taken to analyse the fetal cells and dissolved substances.

- **Aminocentesis** is used to test for the presence of certain genetic disorders such as, down syndrome, haemoplilia, sickle-cell anemia, etc., determine the survivability of the foetus.

- **Statutory ban** on amniocentesis for sex-determination to legally check increasing menace of female foeticides, massive child immunisation, etc., are some programmes that merit mention in this connection.

Saheli

- 'Saheli'–a new oral contraceptive for the females–was developed by scientists at Central Drug Research Institute (CDRI) in Lucknow, India.

Points to remember-

- Improved reproductive health of the society indicated by-
  - Better awareness about sex related matters,
  - Increased number of medically assisted deliveries and better post-natal care leading to decreased maternal and infant mortality rates,
  - Increased number of couples with small families, better detection and cure of STDs and overall increased medical facilities for all sex-related problems, etc.

- **Research** on various reproduction-related areas are encouraged and supported by **governmental** and **non-governmental** agencies done to find out new methods and/or to improve upon the existing ones.

11.2 POPULATION EXPLOSION AND BIRTH CONTROL

- The world population which was around **2 billion (2000 million) in 1900.**
- The world population about 6 billions by **2000.**
- In **2011 world population was 7.2 Billion.**
- Indian population which was approximately **350 million** at the time of our independence reached close to the billion mark by 2000 and crossed **1 billion** in May 2000.
- In **2011 Indian population was 1.2 Billion.**
- That means, every sixth person in the world is an Indian.
- A rapid decline in death rate, **maternal mortality rate** (MMR) and **infant mortality rate** (IMR) as well as an increase in number of people in reproducible age are probable reasons for this.
- By RCH programmes, though we could bring down the population growth rate, it was only marginal.
- According to the **2001 census report**, the population growth rate was **around 1.7 percent, i.e., 17/1000/year.**
- According to the **2011** census report, the population growth rate was less than 2 per cent, i.e., 20/1000/year, a rate at which our population could increase rapidly.
- **At this rate** our population could double in **33 years.**
- Such an alarming growth rate could lead to an absolute scarcity of even the basic requirements, i.e., food, shelter and clothing, in spite of significant progress made in those areas.
- The government was forced to take up **serious measures** to check this population growth rate.
- The most important step to overcome this problem is to motivate smaller families by using various contraceptive methods.
- In advertisements in the media as well as posters/bills, etc., we can see a slogan *Hum Do Hamare Do* (we two, our two).
- Presently many couples, mostly the young, urban, working ones have even adopted **'one child norm'.**
- Statutory raising of marriageable age of the female to **18 years** and that of males to **21 years**, and incentives given to couples with small families are two of the other measures taken to tackle this problem.

Properties of an ideal contraceptive

- An ideal **contraceptive** should be-
    - ➢ user-friendly
    - ➢ easily available
    - ➢ effective
    - ➢ reversible with no or least side-effects
    - ➢ no way interfere with the sexual drive, desire and/or the sexual act of the user.

Contraceptive methods

- A wide range of **contraceptive** methods are presently available which could be broadly grouped into the following categories, namely Natural/Traditional, Barrier, IUDs, Oral contraceptives, Injectables, Implants and Surgical methods.

a.Natural methods

- **Natural methods** work on the principle of avoiding chances of ovum and sperms meeting.

i. Periodic abstinence

- **Periodic abstinence** is one such method in which the couples avoid or abstain from coitus from day 10 to 17 of the menstrual cycle when ovulation could be expected.
- As chances of fertilisation are very high during this period, it is called the fertile period.
- **Abstaining** from coitus during this period, conception could be prevented.

ii. Withdrawal or **coitus interruptus**

- **Withdrawal** or **coitus interruptus** is another method in which the male partner withdraws his penis from the vagina just before ejaculation so as to avoid insemination.

iii. Lactational amenorrhea

- **Lactational amenorrhea** (absence of menstruation) method is based on the fact that ovulation and therefore the cycle do not occur during the period of intense lactation following **parturition**.
- Therefore, as long as the mother breast-feeds the child fully, chances of conception are almost nil.
- **Lactational amenorrhea** method has been reported to be effective only upto a maximum period of six months following parturition.
- As no medicines or devices are used in these methods, side effects are almost nil.
- Chances of failure, **lactational amenorrhea** are also high.

b. Barrier methods

- In **barrier** methods, ovum and sperms are prevented from physically meeting with the help of barriers.
- Such methods are available for **both males and females.**

Condoms

- **Condoms** are barriers made of thin rubber/ latex sheath.
- **Condoms** are used to cover the penis in the male or vagina and cervix in the female, just before coitus so that the ejaculated semen would not enter into the female reproductive tract.
- **Condoms** can prevent conception.
- **'Nirodh'** is a popular brand of condom for the male.
- Use of condoms has increased in recent years they protect from STDs like AIDS.
- Both the male and the female condoms are disposable, can be self-inserted and thereby gives privacy to the user.

Diaphragms, cervical caps and **vaults**

- **Diaphragms, cervical caps** and **vaults** are also barriers made of rubber that are inserted into the female reproductive tract to cover the cervix during coitus.

- **Diaphragms, cervical caps** and **vaults** prevent conception by blocking the entry of sperms through the cervix.

- **Diaphragms, cervical caps** and **vaults** are reusable.

- Spermicidal creams, jellies and foams are usually used along with these barriers to increase their **contraceptive** efficiency.

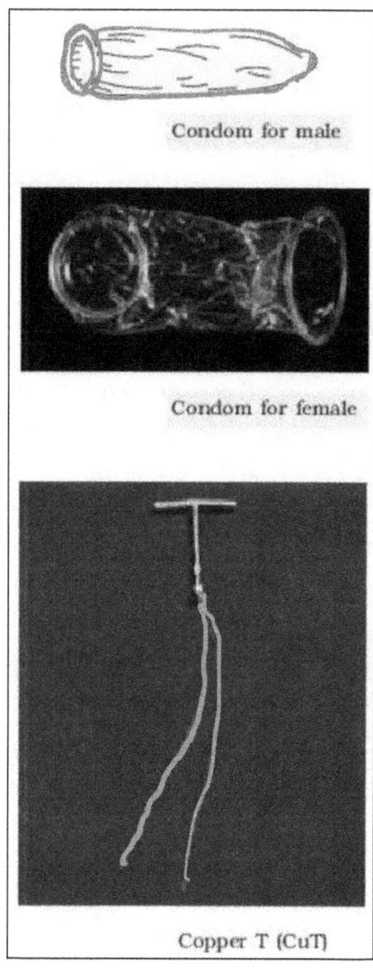

c.Intra Uterine Devices (IUDs).

- **Intra Uterine Devices (IUDs) is** effective and popular method of contraception.

- **Intra Uterine Devices (IUDs)** devices are inserted by doctors or expert nurses in the uterus through vagina.

- These Intra Uterine Devices are presently three types-

    ➢ the non-medicated IUDs e.g., **Lippes loop**

    ➢ copper releasing IUDs e.g. **CuT, Cu7, Multiload 375**

    ➢ the hormone releasing IUDs e.g. **Progestasert, LNG-20**

- IUDs increase **phagocytosis** of sperms within the uterus.

- The Cu ions released suppress sperm motility and the **fertilising** capacity of sperms.
- The hormone releasing IUDs, in addition, make the **uterus** unsuitable for implantation and the cervix **hostile** to the sperms.
- IUDs are ideal **contraceptives** for the females who want to delay pregnancy and/or space children.
- It is one of most widely accepted methods of **contraception** in India.

d.Oral pills

- Oral administration of small doses of **progestogens** or **progestogen**–estrogen combinations is another contraceptive method used by the females.
- They are used in the form of tablets and hence are popularly called the **pills**.
- **Pills** have to be taken daily for **a period of 21 days** starting preferably within the first five days of menstrual cycle.
- After a gap of **7 days** (during which menstruation occurs) it has to be repeated in the same pattern till the female desires to prevent conception.
- They inhibit **ovulation and implantation** as well as alter the quality of cervical mucus to prevent/retard entry of sperms.
- **Pills** are very effective with lesser side effects and are well accepted by the females.

Points to remember-

- *Saheli* –the new oral contraceptive for the females contains a non-steroidal preparation.
- It is a **'once a week'** pill with very few side effects and high contraceptive value.
- **Progestogens** alone or in combination with estrogen can also be used by females as **injections or implants** under the skin.

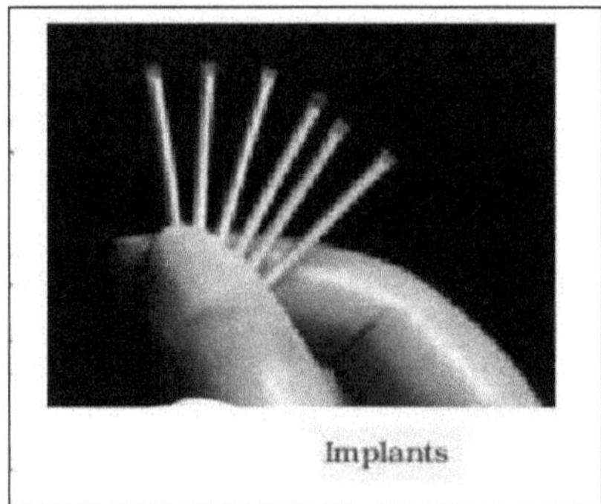

Implants

- The mode of action **injections or implants** is similar to that of pills but their effective periods are much longer.
- Administration of **progestogens or progestogen-estrogen combinations or IUDs** within **72 hours** of coitus have been found to be very effective as emergency contraceptives as they could be used to avoid possible pregnancy due to rape or casual **unprotected intercourse.**

e.Surgical methods

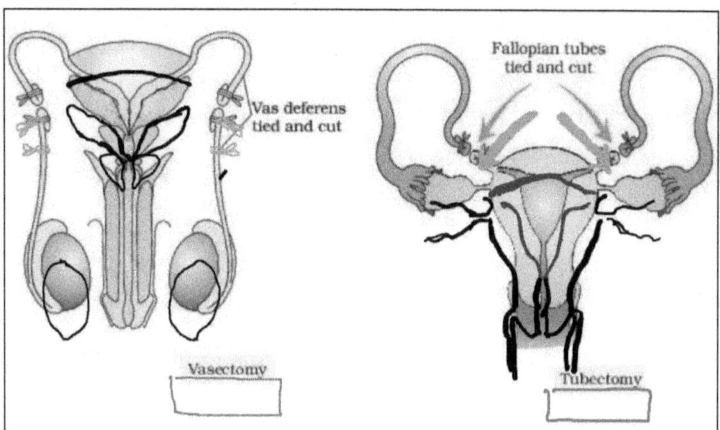

- Surgical methods, also called **sterilisation**, are generally advised for the male/female partner as a terminal method to prevent any more pregnancies.

- Surgical intervention blocks gamete transport and thereby prevent conception.

- Sterilisation procedure in the male is called '**vasectomy**'and that in the female, '**tubectomy**'.

Vasectomy and tubectomy

- In **vasectomy**, a small part of the vas deferens is removed or tied up through a small incision on the scrotum.

- In tubectomy, a small part of the **fallopian** tube is removed or tied up through a small incision in the abdomen or through vagina.

- These techniques are highly effective but their **reversibility** is very poor.

Points to remember-

- It needs to be **emphasised** that the selection of a suitable contraceptive method and its use should always be undertaken in **consultation** with **qualified** medical professionals.

- One must also remember that **contraceptives** are not regular requirements for the maintenance of reproductive health.

- In fact, they are **practiced** against a natural reproductive event, i.e., conception/pregnancy.

- One is forced to use these methods either to **prevent** pregnancy or to delay or space pregnancy due to **personal** reasons.

- No doubt, the **widespread** use of these methods have a significant role in checking uncontrolled growth of population.

Side effect of Contraceptive devices

- ➢ Nausea

- ➢ abdominal pain

- ➢ breakthrough bleeding

- ➢ irregular menstrual bleeding or even breast cancer etc.

11.3 MEDICAL TERMINATION OF PREGNANCY (MTP)

- Intentional or voluntary termination of pregnancy before full term is called **medical termination of pregnancy** (MTP) or induced abortion.

- **Nearly 45 to 50 million MTPs** are performed in a year all over the world which accounts to **1/5th of the** total number of conceived pregnancies in a year.

- **MTP** has a significant role in decreasing the population though it is not meant for that purpose.

- Whether to accept / legalise MTP or not is being debated upon in many countries due to emotional, ethical, religious and social issues involved in it.

- Government of India legalised **MTP in 1971** with some strict conditions to avoid its misuse.

- Such restrictions are all the more important to check indiscriminate and illegal female foeticides which are reported to be high in India.

- **MTP done to-**
  - ➢ get rid of unwanted pregnancies either due to casual unprotected intercourse or failure of the contraceptive used during coitus or rapes.

- **MTPs are also essential –**
  - ➢ in certain cases where continuation of the pregnancy could be harmful or even fatal either to the mother or to the foetus or both.

- **MTPs are considered relatively safe -**
  - ➢ during the first trimester, i.e., upto 12 weeks of pregnancy. Second trimester abortions are much more riskier.

- **The Medical Termination of Pregnancy (Amendment) Act, 2017** was enacted by the government of India with the intension of reducing the incidence of illegal abortion and consequent maternal mortality and morbidity.

- According to this Act, a pregnancy may be terminated on certain considered grounds within the first 12 **weeks** of pregnancy on the opinion of one registered medical practitioner.

- If the pregnancy has lasted more than **12 weeks**, but fewer than **24 weeks**, two registered medical **practitioners** must be of the opinion, formed in good faith, that the required ground exist.

- The grounds for such **termination** of pregnancies are:-

  (i) The **continuation** of the pregnancy would involve a risk to the life of the pregnant woman or of grave injury physical or mental health; or

  (ii)There is a **substantial** risk that of the child were born, it would suffer from such physical or mental abnormalities as to be **seriously** handicapped.

- Such **practices** should be avoided because these are dangerous both for the young mother and the foetus.

- Effective **counselling** on the need to avoid unprotected coitus and the risk factors involved in illegal abortions as well as providing more health care facilities could reverse the mentioned **unhealthy** trend.

- One **disturbing** trend observed is that a majority of the **MTPs** are performed illegally by unqualified

quacks which are not only **unsafe** but could be fatal too.

- Another **dangerous** trend is the misuse of **amniocentesis** to determine the sex of the unborn child.

- Frequently, if the **foetus** is found to be female, it is followed by MTP - this is totally against what is legal.

- Such practices should be **avoided** because these are dangerous both for the young mother and the foetus.

- Effective counselling on the need to avoid **unprotected coitus** and the risk factors involved in illegal abortions as well as providing more health care **facilities** could reverse the mentioned unhealthy trend.

11.4 SEXUALLY TRANSMITTED DISEASES (STDS)

- Diseases or infections which are transmitted through sexual intercourse are collectively called **sexually transmitted diseases (STD) or venereal diseases (VD) or reproductive tract infections (RTI).**

- **Gonorrhoea, syphilis, genital herpes, chlamydiasis, genital warts, trichomoniasis, hepatitis-B** and **HIV leading** to AIDS are some of the common STDs.

- Among these, **HIV infection is most dangerous.**

- Some of these infections like **hepatitis–B and HIV** can also be transmitted by sharing of injection needles, surgical instruments, etc., with infected persons, transfusion of blood, or from an infected mother to the foetus too.

- Except for **hepatitis-B, genital herpes and HIV** infections, other diseases are completely curable if detected early and treated properly.

- **Early symptoms** of most of **STDs** are-
    - ➢ minor and include itching
    - ➢ fluid discharge
    - ➢ slight pain
    - ➢ swellings, etc., in the genital region.

- **The complications of STDs** are-
    - ➢ pelvic inflammatory diseases (PID)
    - ➢ abortions
    - ➢ still births
    - ➢ ectopic pregnancies
    - ➢ infertility
    - ➢ even cancer of the reproductive tract.

- **STDs** are a major threat to a healthy society.

- Infected females with STDs may often be **asymptomatic** and hence, may remain undetected for long.

- Absence or less **significant** symptoms in the early stages of infection and the social stigma attached to the STDs, deter the infected persons from **going** for timely detection and proper treatment.

- Therefore, **prevention** or early detection and cure of these diseases are given prime consideration **under** the **reproductive health-care programmes.**

- STDs commonly seen in the age group of **15-24 years.**

- **Don't panic with STDs.**

- Prevention is in our hands.

- To free from these infections if we follow the simple principles given below:

  - Avoid sex with **unknown** partners/multiple partners.

  - Always use **condoms** during coitus.

  - In case of doubt, go to a qualified doctor for early **detection** and get complete treatment if **diagnosed** with disease.

11.5 INFERTILITY

- A large number of couples all over the world including India are infertile, i.e., they are unable to produce children after unprotected sexual co-habitation.

- The reasons for this could be many–**physical, congenital, diseases, drugs, immunological or even psychological.**

- In India, mostly the female is blamed for the couple being childless, but the problem may also lies in the male partner.

- Specialised health care units (infertility clinics, etc.) could help in diagnosis and corrective treatment of some of these disorders and enable these couples to have children.

- When such corrections are not possible, the couples could be assisted to have children through certain special techniques commonly known as **assisted reproductive technologies** (ART).

- *In vitro* fertilisation (IVF–fertilisation outside the body in almost similar conditions as that in the body) followed by **embryo transfer** (ET) is one of such methods.

- In **test tube baby** programme, ova from the wife/donor (female) and sperms from the husband/donor (male) are collected and are induced to form zygote under simulated conditions in the laboratory.

- Embryos formed by **in-vivo fertilisation** (fusion of gametes within the female) also could be used for such transfer to assist those females who cannot conceive.

a. ZIFT

- The zygote or early embryos (with upto 8 blastomeres) could then be transferred into the fallopian tube (ZIFT–**zygote intra fallopian transfer**).

b. IUT

- The embryos with more than 8 blastomeres, into the uterus (IUT – **intra uterine transfer**), to complete its further development.

c. GIFT

- Transfer of an ovum collected from a donor into the fallopian tube (GIFT – **gamete intra fallopian transfer**) of another female who cannot produce one, but can provide suitable environment for fertilisation and further development is another method attempted.

d. ICSI

- **Intra cytoplasmic sperm injection** (ICSI) is another specialised procedure to form an embryo in the laboratory in which a sperm is directly injected into the ovum.

e. AI

- Infertility cases either due to inability of the male partner to inseminate the female or due to very low sperm counts in the ejaculates, could be corrected by **artificial insemination** (AI) technique.

- In this technique, the semen collected either from the husband or a healthy donor is artificially introduced into the vagina.

f. IUI

- In this technique, the semen collected either from the husband or a healthy donor is artificially introduced into the uterus (IUI – **intra-uterine insemination**) of the female.

Points to remember-

- Though options are many, all these techniques require extremely high precision handling by specialised professionals and expensive instrumentation.

- Therefore, these facilities are presently available only in very few centres in the country.

- Obviously their benefits is affordable to only a limited number of people.

- Emotional, religious and social factors are also deterrents in the adoption of these methods.

- Since the ultimate aim of all these procedures is to have children, in India we have so many orphaned and destitute children, who would probably not survive till maturity, unless taken care of.

- Our laws permit legal adoption and it is as yet, one of the best methods for couples looking for parenthood.

1. Consider the following statements and find out the correct option for humans-

STATEMENT 1. Natural methods work on the principle of avoiding chances of ovum and sperms meeting.

STATEMENT 2. Periodic abstinence is one such method in which the couples avoid or abstain from coitus from day 10 to 17 of the menstrual cycle when ovulation could be expected.

1. Both are wrong statements

2. Only statement 1 correct

3. Both are correct statements

4. Only statement 2 correct

2. Go through the following statements and find out the correct option-

ASSERTION(A). Withdrawal or **coitus interruptus** is another method in which the male partner withdraws his penis from the vagina just before ejaculation so as to avoid insemination.

REASON(R). Lactational amenorrhea is based on the fact that ovulation and therefore the cycle do not occur during the period of intense lactation following parturition.

1. A correct and R is correct explanation of A

2. A correct and R is also correct but R is not correct explanation of A

3. A correct but R incorrect

4. A and R both are incorrect

3. Go through the following statements and find out the correct option-

A. Reproduction-related areas are currently in operation under the popular name 'Reproductive and Child Health Care (RCH) programmes'.

B. Creating awareness among people about various reproduction related aspects and providing facilities and support for building up a reproductively healthy society are the major tasks under these programmes.

C. With the help of audio-visual and the print-media governmental and non-governmental agencies have taken various steps to create awareness among the people about reproduction-related aspects.

D. Parents, other close relatives, teachers and friends, also have a major role in the dissemination of the above information.

E. Introduction of sex education in schools should also be encouraged to provide right information to the young so as to discourage children from believing in myths and having misconceptions about sex-related aspects.

Which of the above statements are correct -

1. A and C only

2. C and E only

3. A,B,C,D only

4. A,B,C,D,E,

4. Read the statements given below-

A. **Diaphragms, cervical caps** and **vaults** are also barriers made of rubber that are inserted into the female reproductive tract to cover the cervix during coitus.

B. They prevent conception by blocking the entry of sperms through the cervix.

C. They are reusable. Spermicidal creams, jellies and foams are usually used alongwith these barriers to increase their contraceptive efficiency.

D. IUDs are inserted by doctors or expert nurses in the uterus through fallopian tube.

E. These Intra Uterine Devices are presently available as the non-medicated IUDs (e.g., Lippes loop), copper releasing IUDs (CuT, Cu7, Multiload 375) and the hormone releasing IUDs (Progestasert, LNG-20).

Which of the above statement is/are incorrect?

1. A and C only

2. B only

3.D and A only

4. D only

5. Which statement is incorrect w.r.t. contraceptive device-

1. Saheli are very effective with lesser side effects and are well accepted by the females.

2. *Saheli* –the new oral contraceptive for the females contains a non-steroidal preparation.

3. Progestogens alone or in combination with estrogen can also be used by females as injections or implants under the skin.

4. IUDs within 172 hours of coitus have been found to be very effective as emergency contraceptives as they could be used to avoid possible pregnancy due to rape or casual unprotected intercourse.

6. Consider the following statements-

A. The zygote or early embryos (with upto 8 blastomeres) could then be transferred into the fallopian tube (ZIFT–**zygote intra fallopian transfer**) and embryos with more than 8 blastomeres, into the uterus (IUT – **intra uterine transfer**), to complete its further development.

B. Embryos formed by **in-vivo fertilisation** (fusion of gametes within the female) also could be used for such transfer to assist those females who cannot conceive.

C. Transfer of an ovum collected from a donor into the fallopian tube (GIFT – **gamete intra fallopian transfer**) of another female who cannot produce one, but can provide suitable environment for fertilisation and further development is another method attempted.

D. **Intra cytoplasmic sperm injection** (ICSI) is another specialised procedure to form an embryo in the laboratory in which a sperm is directly injected into the ovum.

How many of them are/is correct-

1. one

2. two

3. three

4. four

7. Read the following statements w.r.t. STDs/RTIs-

a) Except for hepatitis-B, genital herpes and HIV infections, other diseases are completely curable if detected early and treated properly.

b) Early symptoms of most of these are minor and include itching, fluid discharge, slight pain, swellings, etc., in the genital region.

c) Infected females may often be asymptomatic and hence, may remain undetected for long.

d) Absence or less significant symptoms in the early stages of infection and the social stigma attached to the STDs, deter the infected persons from going for timely detection and proper treatment.

e) STDs could lead to complications later, which include pelvic inflammatory diseases (PID), abortions, still births, ectopic pregnancies, infertility or even cancer of the reproductive tract. STDs are a major threat to a healthy society.

Which of the above statements is/are correct-

1. a, b,c

2. a,b,c,d

3. b,c

4. all are correct

8. Find out the incorrect option-

1. Spermicidal creams, jellies and foams are usually used alongwith these barriers to increase their contraceptive efficiency.

2. Another effective and popular method is the use of **Intra Uterine Devices (IUDs)**.These devices are inserted by doctors or expert nurses in the uterus through vagina.

3. Sterilisation procedure in the male is called 'vasectomy' and that in the female, 'tubectomy'.

4. Sterilisation procedure techniques are highly effective with high reversibility.

9. Consider the following statements-

I. Government of India legalised MTP in 1971 with some strict conditions to avoid its misuse.

II. MTPs are considered relatively safe during the first trimester, i.e., upto 12 weeks of pregnancy. Second trimester abortions are much more riskier.

III. One disturbing trend observed is that a majority of the MTPs are performed illegally by unqualified quacks which are not only unsafe but could be fatal too.

IV. MTPs are also essential in certain cases where continuation of the pregnancy could be harmful or even fatal either to the mother or to the foetus or both.

How many of above are correct-

1. three

2. four

3. one

4. two

10. Amniocentesis is mainly for:-

(1) analysis of chemical composition of fluids of pregnant woman

(2) withdrawal of allantoic fluid from pregnant women

(3) withdrawal of chorionic fluid from pregnant women

(4) study of metaphase chromosomes from amniotic fluid to identify chromosomal abnormality

11. What is correct about test tube baby?

(1) Fertilisation inside female genital tract and growth in test tube

(2) Rearing of prematurely born baby in incubator

(3) Fertilisation outside and gestation inside womb of mother

(4) Both fertilisation and development outside the female genital tract

12. Study of chromosomal abnormalities by taken out the amniotic fluid of embryo is called:-

(1) endoscopy

(2) amniocentesis

(3) laproscopy

(4) natal endoscopy

13. Which one of the following is not legitimate for reducing birth rate?

(1) Ban on marriages

(2) Medical termination of pregnancy

(3) Use of contraceptives

(4) Late marriages

14. Purpose of tubectomy is to prevent:-

(1) egg formation

(2) embryonic development

(3) fertilisation

(4) coitus

15. Vasectomy is:-

(1) Cutting of fallopian tube

(2) Cutting of vas deferens

(3) A factor of population growth

(4) Cutting of vasa efferentia

16. An example of IUD is:-

(1) vasectomy

(2) copper T

(3) condom

(4) All of the above

17. Example(s) of contraceptive is/are:-

(1) condom, cervical cap and diaphragm

(2) intrauterine device

(3) pill

(4) All of the above

18. A contraceptive pill contains:-

(1) progesterone and estrogen

(2) spermicidal agents

(3) chemicals that cause abortion

(4) chemicals that prevent fertilization of ovum

19. The partner(s) responsible for sex of the child is/are:-

(1) male

(2) female

(3) both male and female

(4) at times male & at times female

20. Full form of MTP with respect to reproductive health is:-

(1) Magnetic tape processor

(2) Mid-term plan

(3) Motion to proceed

(4) Medical termination of pregnancy

21. A contraceptive pill prevents ovulation by:-

(1) blocking fallopian tube

(2) inhibiting release of FSH and LH

(3) stimulating release of FSH and LH

(4) causing immediate degeneration of released ovum

22. Amniocentesis is commonly used for determining:-

(1) heart disease

(2) brain disease

(3) hereditary disease of embryo

(4) All of the above

23. Family planning programmes were initiated in:-

(1) 1947

(2) 1951

(3) 1977

(4) 1955

24. Given below are four methods (A–D) and their modes of action (a–d) in achieving contraception. Select their correct matching from the four options that follow: Method Mode of Action

A. Mala D	(a) Prevents sperms reaching cervix
B. Condom	(b) Prevents implantation
C. Vasectomy	(c) Prevents ovulation
D. LNG-20	(d) Semen contains no sperms

Match the above:

(1) A – (c), B – (d), C – (a), D – (b)

(2) A – (b), B – (c), C – (a), D – (d)

(3) A – (c), B– (a), C – (d), D – (b)

(4) A – (d), B– (a), C – (b), D – (c)

25. Consider the statements given below regarding contraception and answer as directed there after:

(A) Medical Termination of Pregnancy (MTP) during first trimester is generally safe

(B) Generally, chances of conception are nil until mother breast-feeds the infant upto two years

(C) Intrauterine devices like copper T are effective contraceptives

(D)Contraception pills may be taken up to one week after coitus to prevent conception

Which two of the above statements are correct?

(1) A, C   (2) A, B

(3) B, C   (4) C, D

26. In vitro fertilisation is a technique that involves transfer of which one of the following into the fallopian tube?

(1) Zygote only

(2) Embryo only, up to 80 cell stage

(3) Either zygote or early embryo up to 8 cell stage

(4) Embryo of 32 cell stage only

27. The permissible use of the technique amniocentesis is for:

(1) Detecting any genetic abnormality

(2) Detecting sex of the unborn foetus

(3) Artificial insemination

(4) Transfer of embryo into the uterus of a surrogate mother

28. Which one of the following is the most widely accepted method of contraception in India, as at present?

(1) Cervical caps

(2) Tubectomy

(3) Diaphragms

(4) IUDs' (Intra uterine devices)

29. Medical Termination of Pregnancy (MTP) is considered safe up to have many weeks of pregnancy?
(1) Eight weeks

(2) Twelve weeks

(3) Eighteen weeks

(4) Six weeks

30. One of the legal methods of birth control is:

(1) by a premature ejaculation during coitus

(2) abortion by taking an appropriate medicine

(3) by abstaining from coitus from day 10 to 17 of menstrual cycle

(4) by having coitus at the time of day break

31. Which of the following approaches does not give the defined action of contraceptive?

(1) Barrier Methods - Prevent fertilization

(2) Intrauterine Devices - Increase phagocytosis of sperm, Suppress sperm motility and fertilising Capacity of sperms

(3) Hormonal contraceptives - Prevent/retard entry of sperms, prevents ovulation and Fertilization

(4) Vasectomy - Prevents spermatogenesis

32. The main function of copper ions in copper releasing IUD's is:

(1) They inhibit gametogenesis

(2) They make uterus unsuitable for implantation

(3) They inhibit ovulation

(4) The suppress sperm motility and fertilising capacity of sperms

33. The contraceptive 'SAHELI':

(1) blocks estrogen receptors in the uterus, preventing eggs from getting implanted

(2) increases the concentration of estrogen and prevents ovulation in females

(3) is an IUD

(4) is a post-coital contraceptive

34. Match List - I with List - II with respect to methods of Contraception and their respective actions.

List-I

(a) Diaphragms

(b) Contraceptive Pills

(c) Intra uterine Devices

(d) Lactational Amenorrhea

List-II

(i) Inhibit ovulation and Implantation

(ii) Increase phagocytosis of sperm within Uterus

(iii) Absence of Menstrual cycle and ovulation following parturition

(iv) They cover the cervix blocking the entry of sperms

Choose the correct answer from the options given below:

(1) (a)–(iv), (b)–(i), (c)–(ii), (d)–(iii)

(2) (a)–(ii), (b)–(iv), (c)–(i), (d)–(iii)

(3) (a)–(iii), (b)–(ii), (c)–(i), (d)–(iv)

(4) (a)–(iv), (b)–(i), (c)–(iii), (d)–(ii)

35. Consider the following and find out correct option-

Assertion(A): Reproductive health encompasses physical, emotional, and social aspects related to reproduction.

Reason(R): It includes the well-being of reproductive organs along with emotional and social factors.

1. A correct and R is correct explanation of A

2. A correct and R is also correct but R is not correct explanation of A

3. A correct but R incorrect

4. A and R both are incorrect

36. Consider the following and find out correct option-

Assertion(A): Sex education in schools can dispel myths and misconceptions about reproduction.

Reason(R): Providing accurate information can improve responsible sexual behavior.

1. A correct and R is correct explanation of A

2. A correct and R is also correct but R is not correct explanation of A

3. A correct but R incorrect

4. A and R both are incorrect

37. Consider the following and find out correct option-

Assertion(A): Condoms are used to cover the penis in males.

Reason(R): They prevent the entry of ejaculated semen into the female reproductive tract.

1. A correct and R is correct explanation of A

2. A correct and R is also correct but R is not correct explanation of A

3. A correct but R incorrect

4. A and R both are incorrect

38. Consider the following and find out correct option-

Assertion(A): Saheli is an oral contraceptive developed for females.

Reason(R): It provides a weekly contraceptive option with minimal side effects.

1. A correct and R is correct explanation of A

2. A correct and R is also correct but R is not correct explanation of A

3. A correct but R incorrect

4. A and R both are incorrect

39 Consider the following and find out correct option-

Assertion(A): In Lactational amenorrhea menstruation not occur during intense lactation so prevent conception.

Reason(R): It is effective as long as the mother fully breastfeeds the child for up to sixteen months after the child birth.

1. A correct and R is correct explanation of A

2. A correct and R is also correct but R is not correct explanation of A

3. A correct but R incorrect

4. A and R both are incorrect

40. Consider the following and find out correct option-

Assertion(A): Intra Uterine Devices (IUDs) are not suitable for females who want to delay pregnancy or space children.

Reason(R): IUDs are effective contraceptives inserted into the uterus to prevent fertilization only.

1. A correct and R is correct explanation of A

2. A correct and R is also correct but R is not correct explanation of A

3. A correct but R incorrect

4. A and R both are incorrect

41. Consider the following and find out correct option-

Assertion(A): Oral contraceptives inhibit ovulation and alter the quality of cervical mucus to prevent conception.

Reason(R): They are always taken daily for a specified period and are highly effective with no side effects.

1.A correct and R is correct explanation of A

2. A correct and R is also correct but R is not correct explanation of A

3. A correct but R incorrect

4. A and R both are incorrect

42. Consider the following and find out correct option-

Assertion(A): Progestogens alone or in combination with estrogen can be administered as injections or implants for contraception.

Reason(R): They have a similar mode of action to oral contraceptives but offer longer effective periods.

1.A correct and R is correct explanation of A

2. A correct and R is also correct but R is not correct explanation of A

3. A correct but R incorrect

4. A and R both are incorrect

43. Consider the following and find out correct option-

Assertion(A): Surgical methods, such as vasectomy and tubectomy, are reversible methods of contraception.

Reason(R): They permanently prevent further pregnancies by blocking the cervix or vas deferens.

1.A correct and R is correct explanation of A

2. A correct and R is also correct but R is not correct explanation of A

3. A correct but R incorrect

4. A and R both are incorrect

44. Consider the following and find out correct option-

Assertion(A): Sex education in schools can lead to increased awareness among adolescent.

Reason(R): Providing information about reproduction and safe sexual practices promotes responsible behavior and reduces risky sexual activity.

1.A correct and R is correct explanation of A

2. A correct and R is also correct but R is not correct explanation of A

3. A correct but R incorrect

4. A and R both are incorrect

45. Consider the following and find out correct option-

Assertion(A): Second-trimester abortions are riskier compared to those performed during the first trimester.

Reason(R): Majority of the MTPs are performed illegally by unqualified quacks, leading to unsafe practices.

1.A correct and R is correct explanation of A

2. A correct and R is also correct but R is not correct explanation of A

3. A correct but R incorrect

4. A and R both are incorrect

46. Consider the following and find out correct option-

Assertion(A): Sexually Transmitted Infections (STIs) are a major threat to a healthy society.

Reason(R): Prevention or early detection and cure of STIs are given prime consideration under reproductive health-care programmes.

1.A correct and R is correct explanation of A

2. A correct and R is also correct but R is not correct explanation of A

3. A correct but R incorrect

4. A and R both are incorrect

47. Consider the following and find out correct option-

Assertion(A): Infertility affects a large number of couples worldwide, and various factors contribute to it.

Reason(R): Specialized healthcare units and assisted reproductive technologies (ART) help diagnose and treat infertility.

1.A correct and R is correct explanation of A

2. A correct and R is also correct but R is not correct explanation of A

3. A correct but R incorrect

4. A and R both are incorrect

48. Consider the following and find out correct option-

Assertion(A): In vitro fertilization (IVF) involves, fertilization outside the body and is commonly known as the test tube baby program.

Reason(R): It allows the formation of zygotes under simulated conditions in the laboratory before transferring them into the fallopian tube or uterus.

1. A correct and R is correct explanation of A

2. A correct and R is also correct but R is not correct explanation of A

3. A correct but R incorrect

4. A and R both are incorrect

49. Consider the following and find out correct option-

Assertion(A): Adoption is one of the best methods for couples seeking parenthood, considering the challenges and limitations of assisted reproductive technologies.

Reason(R): Legal adoption provides an opportunity for couples to become parents while also addressing the issue of orphaned and destitute children.

1.A correct and R is correct explanation of A

2. A correct and R is also correct but R is not correct explanation of A

3. A correct but R incorrect

4. A and R both are incorrect

50. Consider the following and find out correct option-

Assertion(A): Prevention of sexually transmitted infections (STIs) involves following simple principles such as avoiding sex with unknown or multiple partners and using condoms during intercourse.

Reason(R): These practices reduce the risk of contracting STIs and promote sexual health.

1.A correct and R is correct explanation of A

2. A correct and R is also correct but R is not correct explanation of A

3. A correct but R incorrect

4. A and R both are incorrect

EVOLUTION

12.1 ORIGIN OF LIFE

- The earth itself is almost only a speck.
- The universe is very old – almost 20 billion years old.
- Huge clusters of galaxies comprise the universe.
- Galaxies contain stars and clouds of gas and dust.
- Considering the size of universe, earth is indeed a speck.

i. Big Bang theory

- The **Big Bang** theory attempts to explain to us the origin of universe.
- Study of Universe Called as Cosmology.
- **Big Bang** theory given by Abbe Laimatrie.
- Big Bang was thermos-nuclear explosion.
- It talks of a singular huge explosion unimaginable in physical terms.
- The universe expanded and hence, the temperature came down. Hydrogen and Helium formed sometime later.
- The gases condensed under gravitation and formed the galaxies of the present day universe.

- In the solar system of the milky way galaxy, earth was supposed to have been formed about 4.5 billion years back.

ii. Early earth

- There was no atmosphere on early earth.

- Water vapour, methane, carbondioxide and ammonia released from molten mass covered the surface.

- The UV rays from the sun brokeup water into Hydrogen and Oxygen and the lighter H2 escaped. Oxygen combined with ammonia and methane to form water, CO2 and others.

- The ozone layer was formed.

- As it cooled, the water vapor fell as rain, to fill all the depressions and form oceans.

iii. Life appeared

- Life appeared 500 million years after the formation of earth, i.e., almost four billion years back.

iv. Did life come from outerspace?

- Some scientists believe that it came from outside.

- Early Greek thinkers thought units of life called **spores** were transferred to different planets including earth.

- 'Panspermia' is still a favourite idea for some astronomers.

v. Theory of spontaneous generation

- For a long time it was also believed that life came out of decaying and rotting matter like straw, mud, etc.

- This was the theory of spontaneous generation.

- Louis Pasteur by careful experimentation demonstrated that life comes only from pre-existing life.

- He showed that in pre-sterilised flasks, life did not come from killed yeast while in another flask open to air, new living organisms arose from 'killed yeast'.

- Spontaneous generation theory was dismissed once and for all.

- However, this did not answer how the first life form came on earth.

vi. Oparin theory and S.L. Miller experiment

- Also called Oparin Haldane theory/ Naturalistic Theory/Biochemical Theory.

- Oparin of Russia and Haldane was British born Indian scientist.

- They proposed that the first form of life could have come from pre-existing non-living organic molecules (e.g. RNA, protein, etc.) and that formation of life was preceded by chemical evolution, i.e., formation of diverse organic molecules from inorganic constituents.

- The conditions on primitive earth were – high temperature, volcanic storms, reducing atmosphere containing CH_4, NH_3, etc.

- In 1953, **S.L. Miller,** an American scientist created similar conditions in a laboratory scale.

- He created electric discharge in a closed flask containing CH_4, H_2, NH_3 and water vapor at 800^0C.

- Ratio of CH_4, H_2, NH_3 was 2:2:1

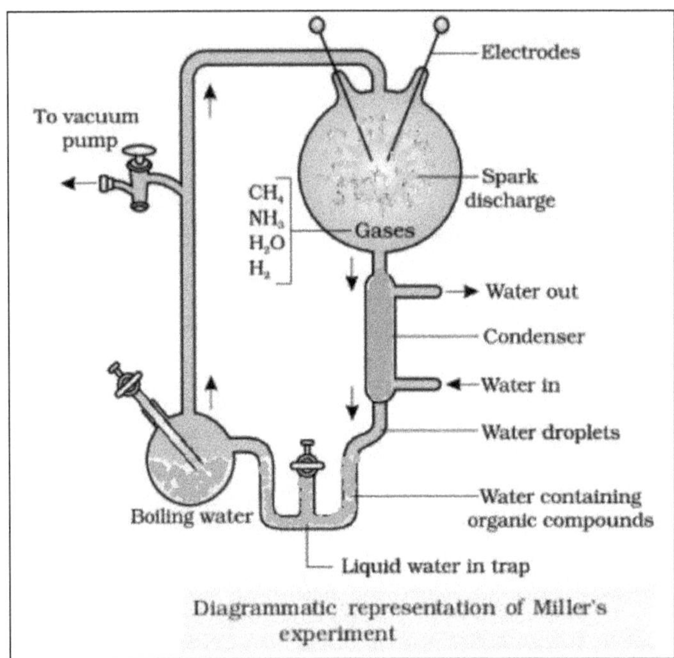

Diagrammatic representation of Miller's experiment

- He observed formation of amino acids.

- First molecular compound was water/NH_3.

- First organic compound was methane.

- In similar experiments others observed, formation of sugars, nitrogen bases, pigment and fats. Analysis of meteorite content also revealed similar compounds indicating that similar processes are occurring elsewhere in space.

- With this limited evidence, the first part of the conjectured story, i.e., chemical evolution was more or less accepted.

- We have no idea about how the first self replicating metabolic capsule of life arose.

- Carbohydrate and large protein combine together and form Coacervates.

- Lipid bilayer and protein forms Microsphere.

- Coacervates and Microsphere are protobiont.

vii. The first non-cellular forms of life

- The first non-cellular forms of life could have originated 3 billion years back.

- Nucleoprotein was first sign of life.

- They would have been giant molecules (RNA, Protein, Polysaccharides, etc.).

- These capsules reproduced their molecules perhaps.

viii. The first cellular form of life

- The first cellular form of life did not possibly originate till about 2000million years ago.

- These were probably single-cells.

- All life forms were in water environment only.

- The first form of life arose slowly through evolutionary forces from non-living molecules is accepted by majority.

- The first cellular forms of life could have evolved into the complex biodiversity of today is the fascinating story that will be discussed below.

12.2 EVOLUTION OF LIFE FORMS – A THEORY

- Conventional religious literature tells us about the theory of special creation.

i. The theory of special creation

- This theory has three connotations.
- **One,** that all living organisms (species or types) that we see, today were created as such.
- **Two,** that the diversity was always the same since creation and will be the same in future also.
- **Three,** that earth is about 4000 years old.
- All these ideas were strongly challenged during the nineteenth century.
- These are supported by Mythology.

ii. H.M.S. Beagle and Darwin

- Based on observations made during a **sea voyage** in a sail ship called **H.M.S. Beagle** round the world, **Charles Darwin** concluded that existing living forms share similarities to varying degrees not only among themselves but also with life forms that existed millions of years ago.
- Many such life forms do not exist any more.
- There had been extinctions of different life forms in the years gone by just as new forms of life arose at different periods of history of earth.
- There has been gradual evolution of life forms.
- Any population has built in variation in characteristics.
- Those characteristics which enable some to survive better in natural conditions (climate, food, physical factors, etc.) would outbreed others that are less-endowed to survive under such natural conditions.
- Another word used is fitness of the individual or population.

iii. The fitness

- **The fitness**, according to Darwin, refers ultimately and only to reproductive fitness.
- Those who are better fit in an environment, leave more progeny than others.
- These, therefore, will survive more and hence are selected by nature.

iv. Alfred Wallace

- He called it natural selection and implied it as a mechanism of evolution.
- **The Alfred Wallace**, a naturalist who worked in **Malay Archepelago** had also come to similar conclusions around the same time.

Points to remember-

- In due course of time, **apparently new types** of organisms are recognisable.
- **All the existing life forms** share similarities and share common ancestors.

- However, these ancestors were present at different periods in the history of earth (epochs, periods and eras).
- **The geological history of earth** closely correlates with the biological history of earth.
- **A common permissible conclusion** is that earth is very old, not thousand of years as was thought earlier but billions of years old.

12.3 What are the Evidences for Evolution?

i. Paleontological evidences/ Fossil evidences

- Evidence that evolution of life forms has indeed taken place on earth has come from many quarters. **Fossils are remained of hard parts** of life-forms found in rocks.
- **Rocks form sediments** and a cross-section of earth's crust indicates the arrangement of sediments one over the other during the long history of earth.
- Different-**aged rock sediments contain fossils** of different life-forms who probably died during the formation of the particular sediment.
- Some of them appear similar to **modern organisms**.
- They represent **extinct organisms** (e.g., Dinosaurs).
- A study of fossils in different **sedimentary layers indicates the geological period** in which they existed.
- **The study showed** that life-forms varied over time and certain life forms are restricted to certain geological time-spans.
- Hence, new forms of life have arisen at different times in the history of earth.
- **All this is** called **paleontological evidence.**

ii. Evidences from comparative anatomy and morphology

- Comparative anatomy and morphology shows similarities and differences among organisms of today and those that existed years ago.
- Homolous and Analogous organs comes under these evidences.
- Homolous and Analogous organs can help to understand whether common ancestors were shared or not.

iii. Homology

- The **whales, bats, Cheetah and human** (all mammals) share similarities in the pattern of bones of forelimbs.
- Though these forelimbs perform different functions in these animals, they have similar anatomical structure – all of them have **humerus, radius, ulna, carpals, metacarpals and phalanges** in their forelimbs.
- In these animals, the same structure developed along different directions due to adaptions to different needs. This is **divergent evolution** and these structures are **homologous**.
- Homology indicates common ancestry.

- Other examples are vertebrate hearts or brains. In plants also, the thorn and tendrils of *Bougainvillea* and *Cucurbita* represent homology.

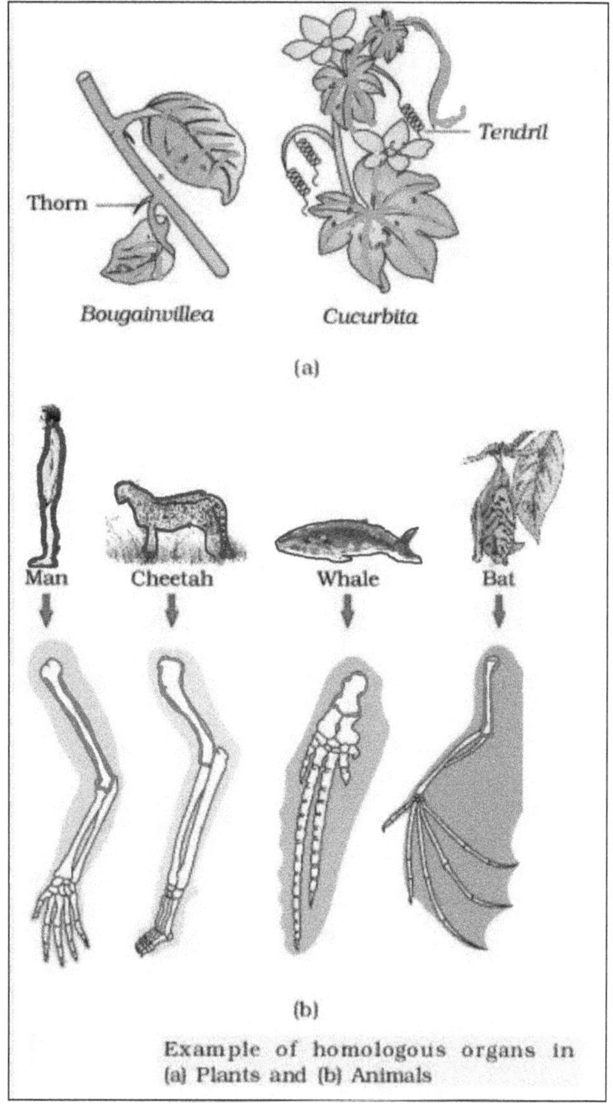

Example of homologous organs in (a) Plants and (b) Animals

- Homology is based on divergent evolution whereas analogy refers to a situation exactly opposite.

iv. Analogy

- The wings of butterfly and of birds look alike.
- They are not anatomically similar structures though they perform similar functions and called as analogous organs.
- Analogous structures are a result of **convergent evolution** - different structures evolving for the same function and hence having similarity.
- Other examples of analogy are the eye of the octopus and of mammals or the flippers of Penguins and Dolphins.
- One can say that it is the similar habitat that has resulted in selection of similar adaptive features in different groups of organisms but toward the same function.
- Sweet potato (root modification) and potato (stem modification) is another example for analogy.

Points to remember-

- In the same line of argument, similarities in proteins and genes performing a given function among diverse organisms give clues to common ancestry.
- These biochemical similarities point to the same shared ancestry as structural similarities among diverse organisms.

iv. Breeding programme can help in evolution

- Man has bred selected plants and animals for agriculture, horticulture, sport or security.
- Man has domesticated many wild animals and crops.
- This intensive breeding programme has created breeds that differ from other breeds (e.g., dogs) but still are of the same group.
- It is argued that if within hundred of years, man could create new breeds, could not nature have done the same over millions of years?

v. Observation supporting evolution by natural selection comes from England

- In a collection of moths made in **1850s**, i.e., before **industrialisation** set in, it was observed that there were more **white-winged moths** on trees than dark-winged or melanised moths.
- It was observed by **Ford, Fisher and Kettlewell.**
- However, in the collection carried out from the same area, but after **industrialisation,** i.e., in **1920,** there were more dark-winged moths in the same area, i.e., the proportion was reversed.
- The explanation put forth for this observation was that 'predators will spot a moth against a contrasting background'.

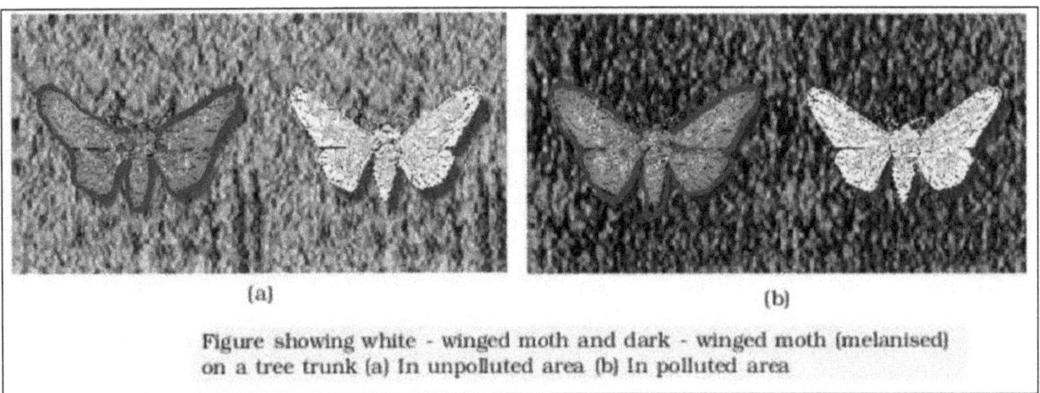

Figure showing white - winged moth and dark - winged moth (melanised) on a tree trunk (a) In unpolluted area (b) In polluted area

- During post **industrialisation period,** the tree trunks became dark due to industrial smoke and soots. Under this condition the white-winged moth did not survive due to predators, dark-winged or melanised moth survived.
- Before **industrialisation** set in, thick growth of almost white-coloured lichen covered the trees - in that background the white winged moth survived but the dark-coloured moth were picked out by predators.
- The *lichens can be used as **industrial pollution indicators.***
- They will not grow in areas that are polluted.
- These moths that were able to camouflage themselves, i.e., hide in the background, survived.

- This understanding is supported by the fact that in areas where industrialisation did not occur e.g., in rural areas, the count of **melanic moths** was low.

- This showed that in a mixed population, those that can better-adapt, survive and increase in population size.

- No variant is completely wiped out.

Points to remember-

- Similarly, excess use of **herbicides, pesticides,** etc., has only resulted in selection of resistant varieties in a much lesser time scale.

- This is also true **for microbes against** which we employ antibiotics or drugs against eukaryotic organisms/cell.

- The resistant organisms/cells are appearing in a time scale of months or years and not centuries. These are examples of evolution by **anthropogenic action.**

- This also tells us that evolution is not a direct process in the sense of **determinism.**

- It is a **stochastic process** based on chance events in nature and chance mutation in the organisms.

12.4 What Is Adaptive Radiation?

a. Darwin's Finches

- During his journey **Darwin went to Galapagos Islands.**

- There he observed an amazing diversity of creatures.

- Of particular the **small black birds** later called **Darwin's Finches** amazed him.

- He realised that there were many varieties of finches in the same island.

- All the varieties, he conjectured, evolved on the island itself.

- From the **original seed-eating features**, many other forms with altered beaks arose, enabling them to become insectivorous and vegetarian finches.

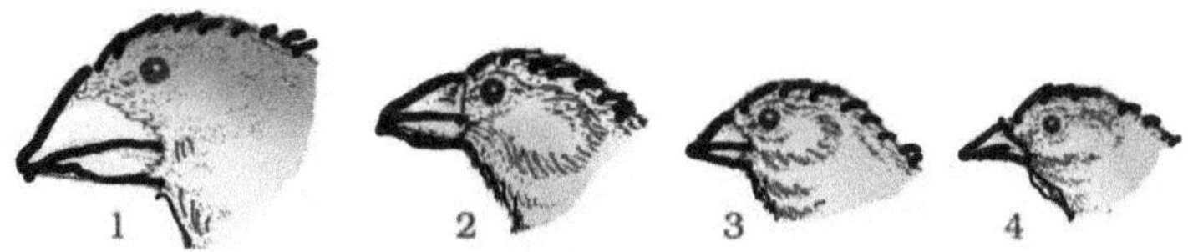

Variety of beaks of finches that Darwin found in Galapagos Island

b. Adaptive radiation.

- This process of evolution of different species in a given geographical area starting from a point and literally radiating to other areas of geography (habitats) is called **adaptive radiation.**

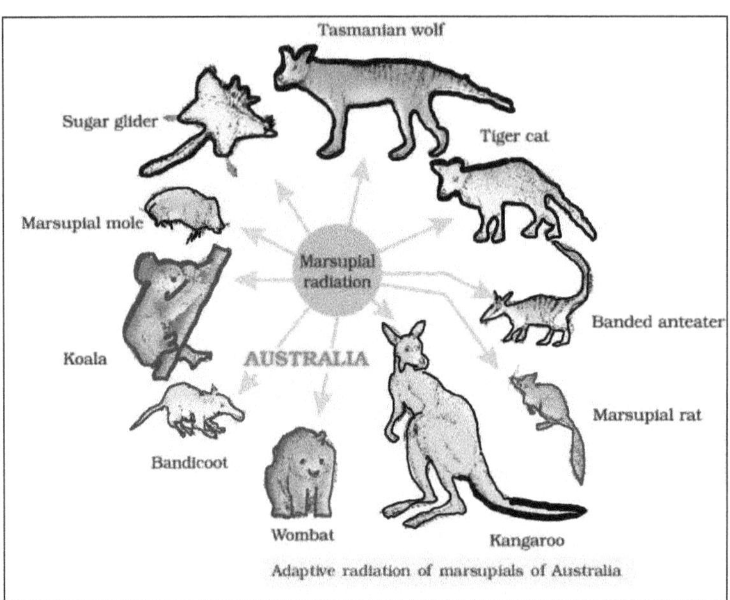

Adaptive radiation of marsupials of Australia

c. Examples of Adaptive radiation.

- Darwin's finches represent one of the best examples of this phenomenon.

- The Australian marsupials is another example **adaptive radiation.**

- A number of marsupials, each different from the other evolved from an ancestral stock, but all within the Australian island continent.

d. Convergent evolution.

- When more than one adaptive radiation appeared to have occurred in an isolated geographical area (representing different habitats), it is called as convergent evolution.

- Placental mammals in Australia also exhibit adaptive radiation in evolving into varieties of such placental mammals each of which appears to be 'similar' to a corresponding marsupial

(e.g., Placental wolf and Tasmanian wolfmarsupial).

12.5 BIOLOGICAL EVOLUTION

- Evolution by **natural selection**, in a true sense would have started when cellular forms of life with differences in metabolic capability originated on earth.

- The essence of **Darwinian theory** about evolution is natural selection.

- Book of **Darwin origin of species** by Natural Selection **(1859)**

- The rate of appearance of new forms is linked to the life cycle or the life span.

- **Natural selection** can also be explained with the help of Microbes.

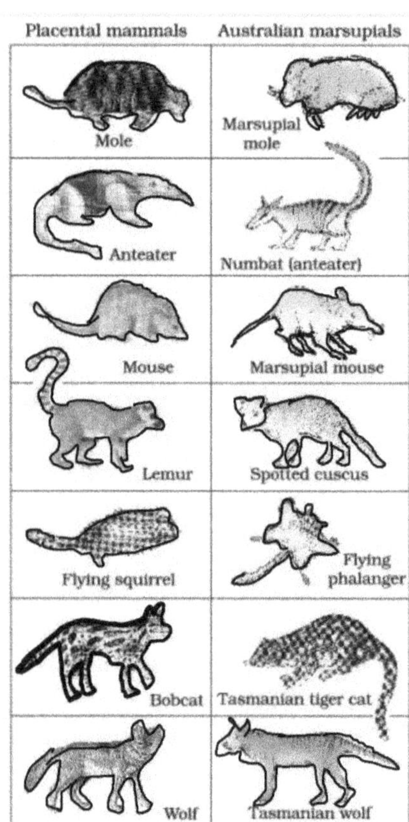

Picture showing convergent evolution of Australian Marsupials and placental mammals

- Microbes that divide fast have the ability to multiply and become millions of individuals within hours.

- A colony of bacteria **(say A)** growing on a given medium has builtin variation in terms of ability to utilise a feed component.

- **A change in the medium composition** would bring out only that part of the population (say B) that can survive under the new conditions.

- In due course of time this **variant population** outgrows the others and appears as new species.

- This would happen within days.

- For the same thing to happen in a fish or fowl would take **million of years** as life spans of these animals are in years.

- We say that **fitness of B is better than that of A** under the new conditions.

- Nature selects for fitness.

- One must remember that the so-called fitness is based on characteristics which are inherited. Hence, there must be a genetic basis for getting selected and to evolve.

- Another way of saying the same thing is that some organisms are better adapted to survive in an otherwise hostile environment.

- **Adaptive ability** is inherited.

- It has a genetic basis. Fitness is the end result of the ability to adapt and get selected by nature.

- **Branching descent** and **natural selection** are the two key concepts of Darwinian Theory of Evolution.

- Even before Darwin, **a French naturalist Lamarck had said that evolution of life forms had occurred but driven by use and disuse of organs.**

- He gave the examples of Giraffes who in an attempt to forage leaves on tall trees had to adapt by elongation of their necks.

- As they passed on this acquired character of elongated neck to succeeding generations, Giraffes, slowly, over the years, came to acquire long necks.

- Nobody believes this conjecture any more.

a. Is evolution a process or the result of a process?

- The world we see, inanimate and animate, is only the success stories of evolution.

- When we describe the story of this world we describe evolution as a process.

- On the other hand when we describe the story of life on earth, we treat evolution as a consequence of a process called natural selection.

- We are still not very clear whether to regard evolution and natural selection as processes or end result of unknown processes.

b. Thomas Malthus

- It is possible that the work of Thomas Malthus on populations influenced Darwin.

- Natural selection is based on certain observations which are factual.

- For example, natural resources are limited, populations are stable in size except for seasonal fluctuation, members of a population vary in characteristics (infact no two individuals are alike) even though they look superficially similar, most of variations are inherited etc.

- The fact that theoretically population size will grow exponentially if everybody reproduced maximally (this fact can be seen in a growing bacterial population) and the fact that population sizes in reality are limited, means that there had been competition for resources.

- Only some survived and grew at the cost of others that could not flourish.

c. The novelty and brilliant insight of Darwin

- The novelty and brilliant insight of Darwin was this: he asserted that variations, which are heritable and which make resource utilisation better for few (adapted to habitat better) will enable only those to reproduce and leave more progeny.

- Hence for a period of time, over many generations, survivors will leave more progeny and there would be a change in population characteristic and hence new forms appear to arise.

12.6 Mechanism Of Evolution

- Darwin either ignored these observations or kept silence.

- In **the first decade of twentieeth century, Hugo deVries(1901)** based on his work on evening primrose (***Oenothera lamarkiana***) brought forth the idea of mutations – large difference arising suddenly in a population.

- He believed that it is mutation which causes **evolution** and not the minor variations (heritable) that Darwin talked about.

- Mutations are random and directionless while **Darwinian variations** are small and directional.

- Evolution for Darwin was gradual while **De Vries** believed mutation caused speciation and hence called it **saltation** (single step large mutation).

12.7 Hardy-Weinberg Principle

- **By this principle** one can find out the frequency of occurrence of alleles of a gene or a locus.

- This frequency is supposed to **remain fixed** and even remain the same through generations if no evolutionary force works.

- Hardy-Weinberg principle stated it using algebraic equations.

a. Genetic equilibrium

- This principle says that allele frequencies in a population are stable and is constant from generation to generation.

- The gene pool (total genes and their alleles in a population) remains a constant called as genetic equilibrium.

- **Sum total of all the allelic frequencies is 1**. Individual frequencies, for example, can be named p, q, etc. In a diploid, p and q represent the frequency of allele A and allele a.

- The frequency of AA individuals in a population is simply p^2.

- This is simply stated in another ways, i.e., the probability that an allele A with a frequency of p appear on both the chromosomes of a diploid individual is simply the product of the probabilities, i.e., p^2. Similarly of aa is q^2, of Aa is 2pq.

- Hence, $\mathbf{p^2+2pq+q^2=1}$.

- This is a binomial expansion of $\mathbf{(p+q)^2}$.

- When frequency measured, differs from expected values, the difference (direction) indicates the extent of evolutionary change.

- Disturbance in genetic equilibrium, or Hardy - Weinberg equilibrium, i.e., change of frequency of alleles in a population would then be interpreted as resulting in evolution.

b. Five factors are known to affect Hardy-Weinberg equilibrium.

- These are gene migration or **gene flow, genetic drift, mutation, genetic recombination and natural selection.**

- **When migration** of a section of population to another place and population occurs, gene frequencies change in the original as well as in the new population.

- **New genes/alleles** are added to the new population and these are lost from the old population.

- There would be a gene flow if this **gene migration, happens multiple times.**

- If the same change occurs by chance, **it is called genetic drift.**

- Sometimes the change in allele frequency is so different in the new sample of population that they become a different species.

c. Founder effect

- The original drifted population becomes founders and the effect is called **founder effect.**

- The phenomenon which occurs when a small group of population isolated from a large population.

d. Bottle neck effect

- It is an extreme example of genetic drift that happens when the size of a population is highly reduced.

- It occur due to natural disaster.

Points to remember-

- **Microbial experiments show** that pre-existing advantageous mutations when selected will result in observation of new phenotypes.

- **Over few generations**, this would result in Speciation.

- **Natural selection** is a process in which heritable variations enabling better survival are enabled to reproduce and leave greater number of progeny.

- **A critical analysis** makes us believe that variation due to mutation or variation due to recombination during gametogenesis, or due to gene flow or genetic drift results in changed frequency of genes and alleles in future generation.

- Coupled to **enhance reproductive success**, natural selection makes it look like different population.

d. Types of Natural selection

- Natural selection can be three types-

    - ➤ stabilisation (in which more individuals acquire mean character value),

    - ➤ directional change (more individuals acquire value other than the mean character value)

    - ➤ disruption (more individuals acquire peripheral character value at both ends of the distribution curve).

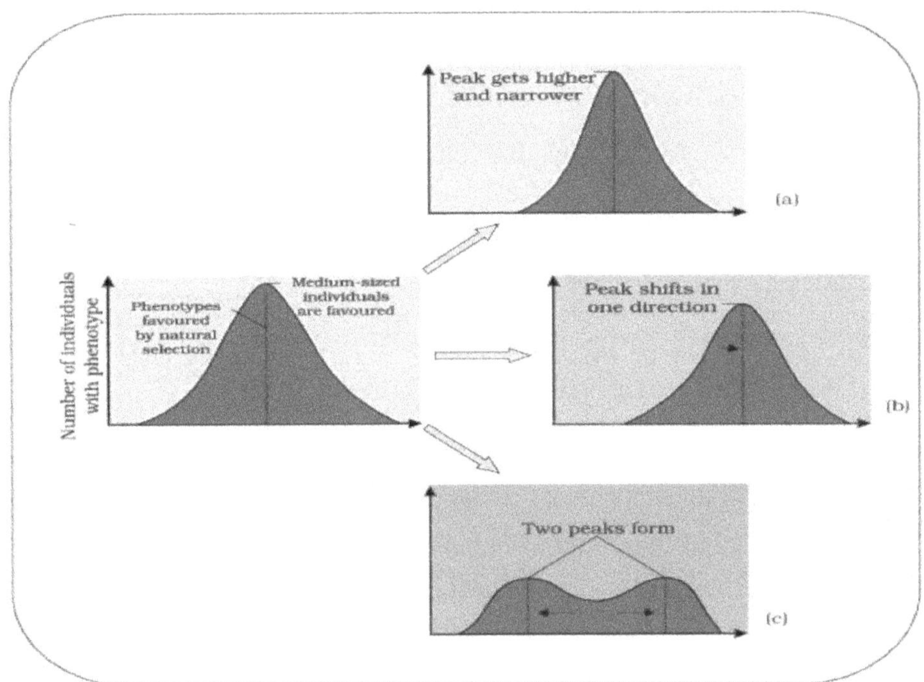

Diagrammatic representation of the operation of natural selection on different traits : (a) Stabilising (b) Directional and (c) Disruptive

7.8 A BRIEF ACCOUNT OF EVOLUTION

- About 2000 million years ago (mya) the first cellular forms of life appeared on earth.

- The mechanism of how non-cellular aggregates of giant macromolecules could evolve into cells with membranous envelop is not known.

- Some of these cells had the ability to release O2.

- The reaction could have been similar to the light reaction in photosynthesis in which water is split with the help of solar energy captured and channelised by appropriate light harvesting pigments.

- Slowly single-celled organisms evolved multi-cellular life forms.

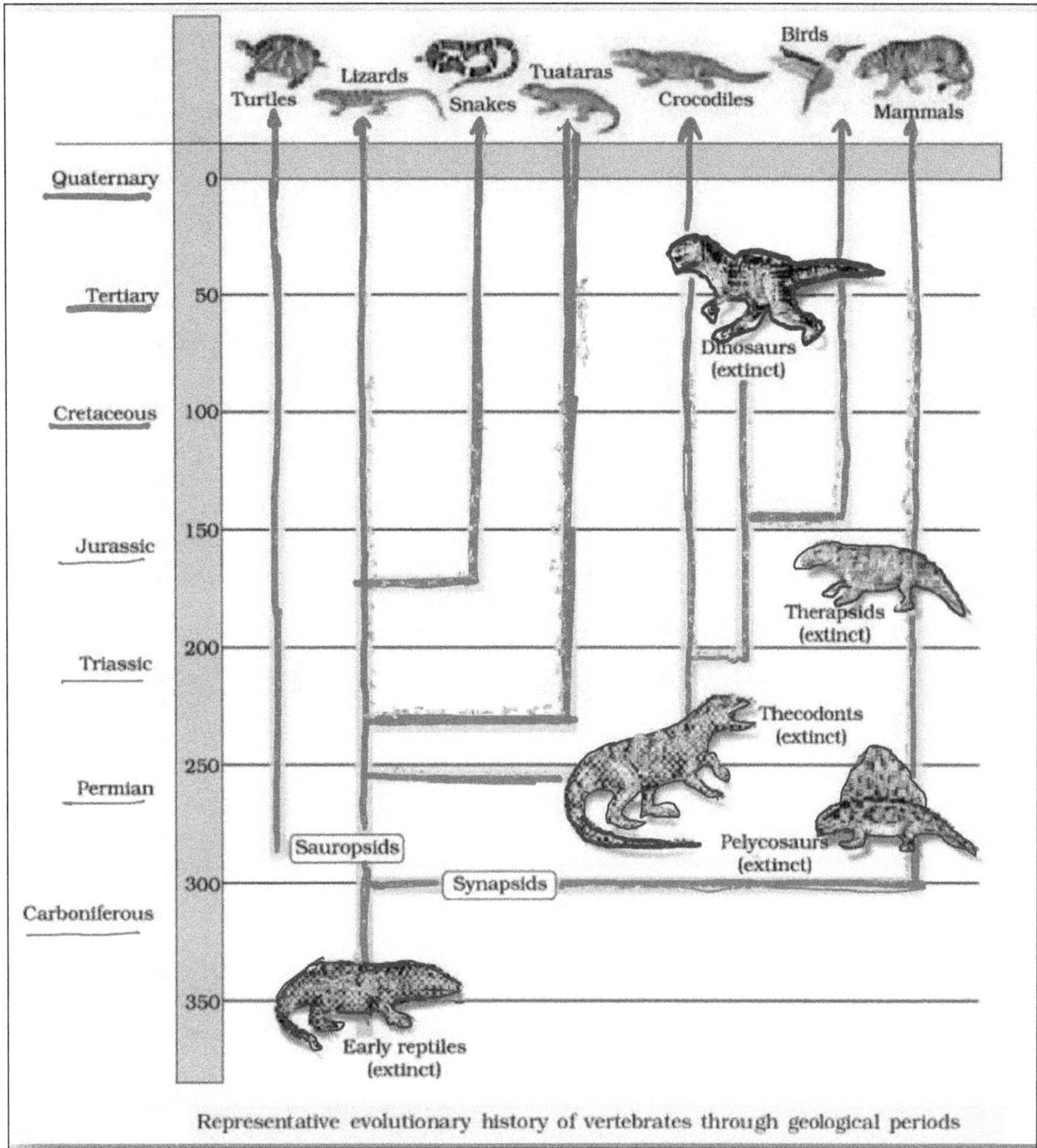

Representative evolutionary history of vertebrates through geological periods

- By the time of **500 mya**, invertebrates were formed and active.
- Jawless fish probably evolved around **350 mya**.
- Sea weeds and few plants existed probably around **320 mya**.
- The first organisms that invaded land were plants.
- They were widespread on land when animals invaded land.
- Fish with stout and strong fins could move on land and go back to water. This was about **350 mya.**
- In **1938**, a fish caught in South Africa happened to be a **Coelacanth** which was thought to be extinct.
- Coelacanth called lobefins fishes evolved into the first amphibians that lived on both land and water.
- There are no specimens of these left with us.
- Coelacanth were ancestors of modern day **frogs and salamanders.**
- The **amphibians** evolved into reptiles.

- Reptiles lay thick shelled eggs which do not dry up in sun unlike those of amphibians.

- The descendents of reptiles the turtles, tortoises and crocodiles.

- In the next **200 millions years** or so, reptiles of different shapes and sizes dominated on earth.

- Giant ferns (pteridophytes) were present but they all fell to form coal deposits slowly.

- Some of these land reptiles went back into water to evolve into fish like reptiles probably **200 mya** (**e.g. *Ichthyosaurs*).**

- The land reptiles were, of course, the dinosaurs.

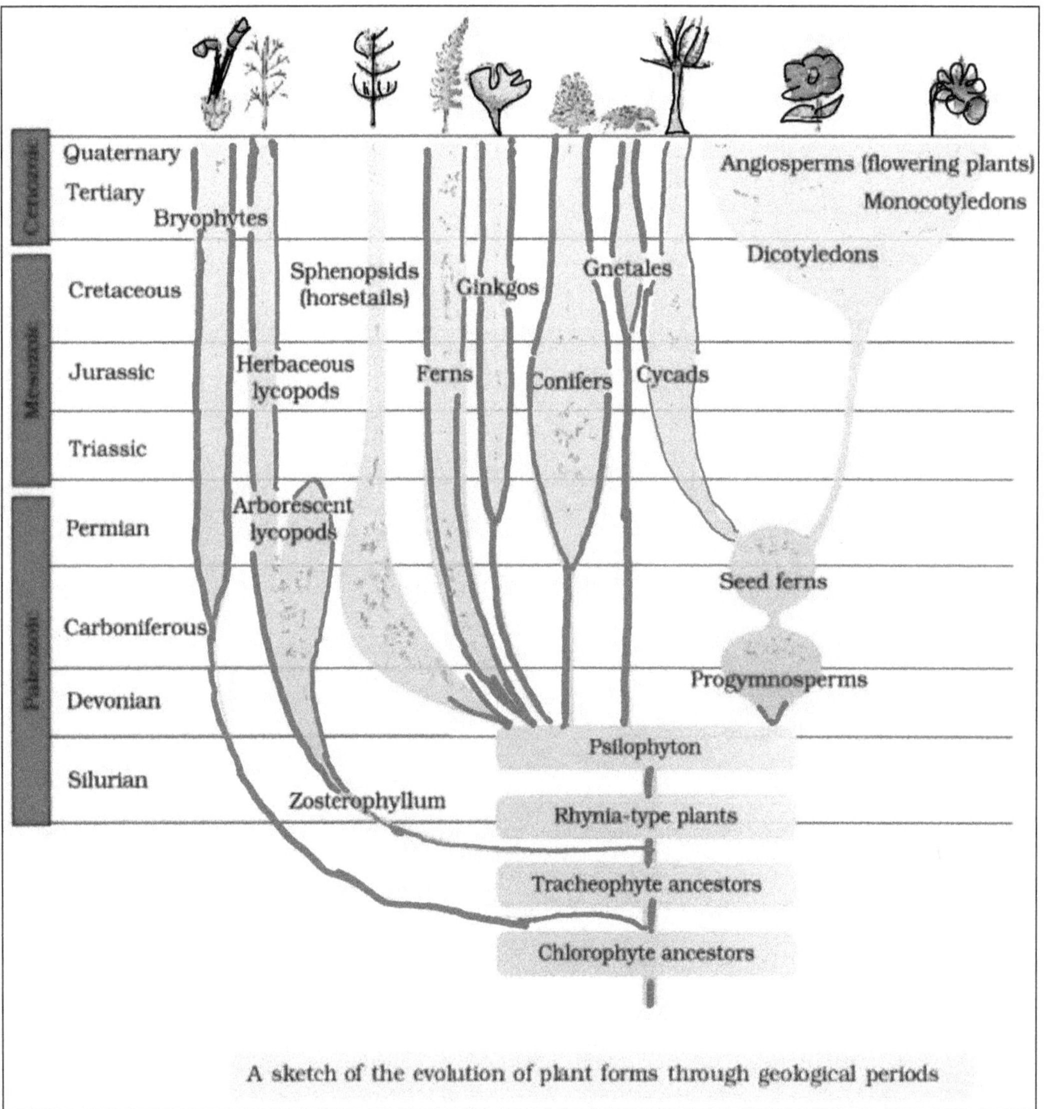

A sketch of the evolution of plant forms through geological periods

- The biggest of them, i.e., ***Tyrannosaurus rex*** was about 20 feet in height and had huge fearsome dagger like teeth.

- About **65 mya,** the dinosaurs suddenly disappeared from the earth.

- We do not know the exact reason.

- Some say climatic changes killed them. Some say most of them evolved into birds.

- The truth may live in between. Small sized reptiles of that era still exist today.

- **The first mammals were like shrews.**
- The fossils of these mammals are small sized.
- Mammals were **viviparous** and protected their unborn young inside the mother's body.
- Mammals were **more intelligent** in sensing and avoiding danger at least.
- When reptiles came down mammals took over this earth.
- There were in **South America** mammals resembling horse, hippopotamus, bear, rabbit, etc.
- Due to continental drift, when South America joined North America, these animals were overridden by **North American fauna.**
- Due to the same **continental drift pouched mammals of Australia** survived because of lack of competition from any other mammal.
- Some mammals live totally in water. Whales, dolphins, seals and sea cows are some examples.
- Evolution of horse, elephant, dog, etc., are also represents evolution.
- The most successful story is the evolution of man with language skills and self-consciousness.
- A rough sketch of the evolution of life forms, their times on a geological scale are indicated in figure-

12.9 ORIGIN AND EVOLUTION OF MAN

a. *Dryopithecus* and *Ramapithecus*

- About 15 mya, primates called *Dryopithecus* and *Ramapithecus* were existing.
- They were hairy and walked like gorillas and chimpanzees.
- *Ramapithecus* was more man-like while *Dryopithecus* was more ape-like.

b. *Australopithecus*

- Few fossils of man-like bones have been discovered in Ethiopia and Tanzania.
- These revealed hominid features leading to the belief that about 3-4 mya, man-like primates walked in eastern Africa.
- They were probably not taller than 4 feet but walked up right.
- Two mya, *Australopithecines* probably lived in East African grasslands.
- Evidence shows they hunted with stone weapons but essentially ate fruit.
- Also known as first ape Man.
- Connecting link between ape and man.

c. *Homo habilis/Able man/Skillful man*

- Some of the bones among the bones discovered were different.
- This creature was called the first human-like being the hominid and was called *Homo habilis*.
- The brain capacities were between **650-800cc.**
- They probably did **not eat meat.**

d. *Homo erectus/Java man*

- Fossils discovered in **Java in 1891** revealed the next stage, i.e., *Homo erectus* about 1.5 mya.

- *Homo erectus* had a large brain around **900cc.**

- *Homo erectus* probably **ate meat**.

- Firstly use fire by java man.

e. Neanderthal man/*Homo sapiens neanderthalensis*

- The Neanderthal man with a brain size of 1400cc.

- They lived in near east and central Asia between 1,00,000-40,000 years back.

- Heavy eyebrows.

- They used hides to protect their body and buried their dead.

f. Homo sapiens

- *Homo sapiens* arose in Africa and moved across continents and developed into distinct races.

- During ice age between 75,000-10,000 years ago modern *Homo sapiens* arose.

- Pre-historic cave art developed about 18,000 years ago.

- Agriculture came around 10,000 years back and human settlements started.

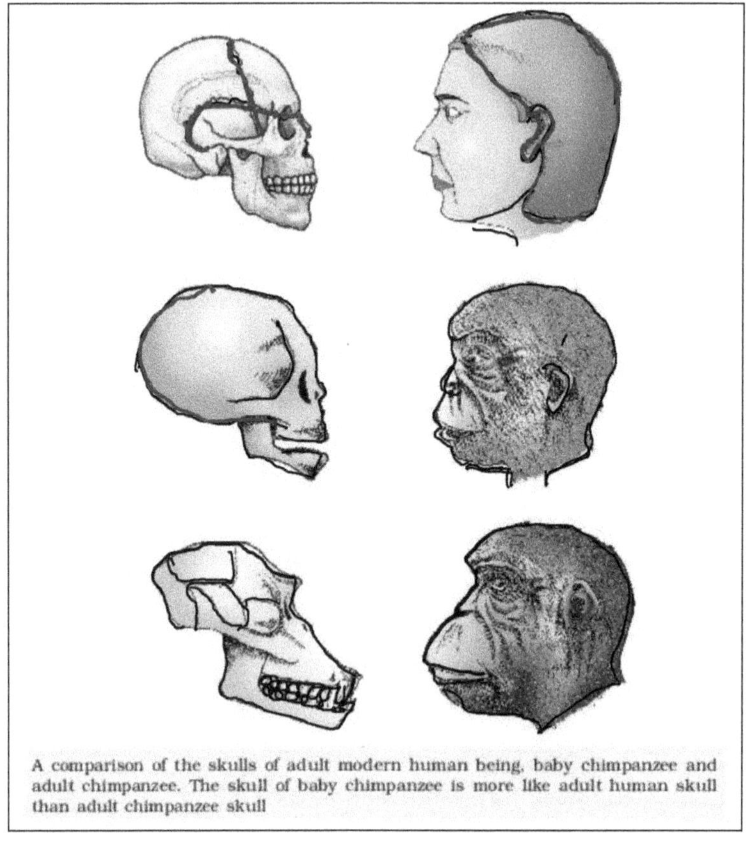

A comparison of the skulls of adult modern human being, baby chimpanzee and adult chimpanzee. The skull of baby chimpanzee is more like adult human skull than adult chimpanzee skull

- The skull of baby chimpanzee is more like adult human skull than adult chimpanzee skull

1. Consider the following statements and find out the correct option-

   A. The earth itself is almost only a speck.

   B. The universe is very old – almost 20 billion years old.

   C. Huge clusters of galaxies comprise the universe.

   D. Galaxies contain stars and clouds of gas and dust.

   E. Considering the size of universe, earth is indeed a speck.

   Which of the above are correct -

   1. A,E,C

   2. B,C

   3. D,E,A

   4. A,B,C,D,E

2. Match the list 1 and 2-

   List 1   List 2

a. Life appeared on earth	j. 1953
b. S.L. Miller experiment	k. 3 billion years back.
c. First non-cellular forms	l. 4 billion years back.
d. Jawless fish evolved	m. 350 mya

   Find out the correct option –

   1. a.k, b.j, c.l, d.m

   2. a.k,b.l,c.j,d.m

   3. a.l,b.j,c.k,d.m

   4. a.l,b.j,c.m,d.k

3. Consider the following statements-

   a) The **Big Bang** theory attempts to explain to us the origin of universe.

   b) The **Big Bang** theory talks of a singular huge explosion unimaginable in physical terms.

c) The universe expanded and hence, the temperature came down.

d) Hydrogen and Helium formed sometime later.

e) The gases condensed under gravitation and formed the galaxies of the present day universe.

Which of the above are/is correct -

1. only a and d

2. a,b,c,d,e

3. only c and d

4. a,e,c

4. Consider the following statements-

a) There was oxidizing atmosphere on early earth.

b) Water vapour, methane, carbondioxide and ammonia released from molten mass covered the surface.

c) The UV rays from the sun brokeup water into Hydrogen and Oxygen and the lighter H2 escaped.

d) Oxygen combined with ammonia and methane to form water, CO2 and others.

e) The ozone layer was formed. As it cooled, the water vapor fell as rain, to fill all the depressions and form oceans.

Which of the above are/is incorrect -

1. a

2. a,b

3. b,d

4. e

5. Consider the following statements and find out the correct option

STATEMENT 1. Early Greek thinkers thought units of life called **spores** were transferred to different planets including earth.

STATEMENT 2. The geological history of earth closely correlates with the biological history of earth.

1. Both are correct statements

2. Only statement 1 correct

3. Both are wrong statements

4. Only statement 2 correct

6. Go through the following statement w.r.t. first non-cellular forms-

ASSERTION(A). The first non-cellular forms of life could have originated 3 billion years back.

REASON(R). They would have been giant molecules (RNA, Protein, Polysaccharides, etc.).

1. A correct and R is correct explanation of A

2. A correct and R is also correct but R is not correct explanation of A

3. A correct but R incorrect

4. A and R both are incorrect

7. Which statement is incorrect w.r.t. theory of special creation-

1. Conventional religious literature tells us about the theory of special creation.

2. This theory has three connotations. One, that all living organisms (species or types) that we see, today were created as such.

3. Two, that the diversity was always the same since creation and will be the same in future also.

4. Three, that earth is about 4000 billion years old, All these ideas were strongly challenged during the nineteenth century.

8. Go through the following statements-

I. Based on observations made during a sea voyage in a sail ship called H.M.S. Beagle round the world, Charles Darwin concluded that existing living forms share similarities to varying degrees not only among themselves but also with life forms that existed millions of years ago.

II. Many such life forms do not exist any more.

III. There had been extinctions of different life forms in the years gone by just as new forms of life arose at different periods of history of earth.

IV. There has been gradual evolution of life forms. Any population has built in variation in characteristics.

How many of them are correct-

1. two

2. three

3. four

4. One

9. Match the list 1 and 2-

List 1   List 2

a. invertebrates were formed and active.	j. 350 mya.
b. Jawless fish probably evolved around	k. 320 mya.
c. Sea weeds and few plants existed probably around	l. 500 mya,
d. fish like reptiles probably	m. 200 mya

Find out the correct option –

1. a.k, b.j, c.l, d.m

2. a.k,b.l,c.j,d.m

3. a.l,b.j,c.k,d.m

4. a.l,b.j,c.m,d.k

10. Consider the following statements and find out the correct option-

STATEMENT 1. The fitness, according to Darwin, refers ultimately and only to reproductive fitness.

STATEMENT 2. Those who are better fit in an environment, leave more progeny than others.

1. Both are wrong statements

2. Only statement 1 correct

3. Both are correct statements

4. Only statement 2 correct

11. Read the following statements very carefully and find out the correct-

a) Alfred Wallace, a naturalist who worked in Malay Archepelago had also come to similar conclusions like Darwin.

b) In due course of time, apparently new types of organisms are originated.

c) Many life forms share similarities and share common ancestors.

d) However, these ancestors were present at different periods in the history of earth (epochs, periods and eras).

Which of the above statement is/are correct?

1. a and c both

2. d only

3. a,b,c,d

4. b and d both

12. Go through the following statements-

ASSERTION(A). Sweet potato (root modification) and potato (stem modification) is an example for analogy.

REASON(R). In proteins and genes performing a same function among diverse organisms give clues to common ancestry.

1. A correct and R is correct explanation of A

2. A correct and R is also correct but R is not correct explanation of A

3. A correct but R incorrect

4. A and R both are incorrect

13. Find out the incorrect statement -

1. Homology indicates common ancestry.

2. The thorn and tendrils of *Bougainvillea* and *Cucurbita* represent analogy.

3. Homology is based on divergent evolution whereas analogy refers to a situation exactly opposite.

4. Wings of butterfly and of birds look alike.

14. Read the following statements and find out correct option-

I. The biochemical similarities point to the same shared ancestry as structural similarities among diverse organisms.

II. Man has bred selected plants and animals for agriculture, horticulture, sport or security.

III. Man has domesticated many wild animals and crops.

IV. This intensive breeding programme has created breeds that differ from other breeds (e.g., dogs) but still are of the same group.

V. It is argued that if within hundred of years, man could create new breeds.

How many of them are correct-

1. four

2. five

3. two

4. three

15. Consider the following statements and find out the correct option-

STATEMENT 1. The original drifted population becomes founders and the effect is called **founder effect**.

STATEMENT 2. Microbial experiments show that pre-existing advantageous mutations when selected will result in observation of new phenotypes.

1. Both are wrong statements

2. Only statement 1 correct

3. Both are correct statements

4. Only statement 2 correct

16. Match the list 1 and 2 -

List 1	List 2
a. Dryopithecus found	15 mya
b. Neanderthal man	1,00,000-40,000 years back
c. Modern *Homo sapiens*	75,000-10,000 years ago
d. Agriculture came around	10,000 years back

How many of them are correctly matched-

1. one	2. two
3. three	4. four

17. Consider the following -

a) During his journey Darwin went to Galapagos Islands.

b) There he observed an amazing diversity of creatures.

c) Of particular interest, small black birds found on Galapagos island later called Darwin's Finches amazed him.

d) He realised that there were many varieties of finches in the same island.

e) All the varieties, he conjectured, evolved on the island itself.

Which of the above statements are/is correct?

1. b and a only	2. a,b,c only
3. d and e only	4. a,b,c,d,e

18. Match the list 1 and 2-

List 1   List 2

List 1	List 2
a. A fish caught in South Africa happened to be a Coelacanth which was thought to be extinct.	In 1938
b. Sea weeds and few plants existed probably around	320 mya.
c. was about 20 feet in height and had huge fearsome dagger like teeth.	*Tyrannosaurus rex*
d. The amphibians evolved into	reptiles.

How many of them are correctly matched-

1. one

2. two

3. three

4. four

19. Consider the following statements -

I. Disturbance in genetic equilibrium, or Hardy - Weinberg equilibrium, i.e., change of frequency of alleles in a population would then be interpreted as resulting in evolution.

II. Five factors are known to affect Hardy-Weinberg equilibrium.

III. These factors are gene migration or gene flow, genetic drift, mutation, genetic recombination and natural selection.

IV. When migration of a section of population to another place and population occurs, gene frequencies change in the original as well as in the new population.

How many of them are/is correct-

1. one

2. two

3. three

4. four

20. Read the following statements-

I. New genes/alleles are added to the new population and these are lost from the old population.

II. There would be a gene flow if this gene migration, happens multiple times.

III. If the same change occurs by chance, it is called genetic drift.

IV. Sometimes the change in allele frequency is so different in the new sample of population that they become a different species.

How many of them are/is correct **statements-**

1. two

2. three

3. four

4. one

21. Consider the following statements and find out the correct option -

STATEMENT 1. Natural selection is a process in which heritable variations enabling better survival are enabled to reproduce and leave greater number of progeny.

STATEMENT 2. A critical analysis makes us believe that variation due to mutation or variation due to recombination during gametogenesis, or due to gene flow or genetic drift results in changed frequency of genes and alleles in future generation.

1. Both are wrong statements

2. Only statement 1 correct

3. Both are correct statements

4. Only statement 2 correct

22. Go through the following statements and find out the correct option-

ASSERTION(A). The mechanism of how non-cellular aggregates of giant macromolecules could evolve into cells with membranous envelop is not known.

REASON(R). Some of these cells had the ability to release O_2.

1. A correct and R is correct explanation of A

2. A correct and R is also correct but R is not correct explanation of A

3. A correct but R incorrect

4. A and R both are incorrect

23. Go through the following statements and find out the correct option-

A. Fish with stout and strong fins could move on land and go back to water. This was about 350 mya.

B. In 1938, a fish caught in South Africa happened to be a Coelacanth which was thought to be extinct.

C. These animals called lobefins evolved into the first amphibians that lived on both land and water.

D. There are no specimens of lobed fin left with us.

Which above statements are correct -

1. A and C only

2. C and D only

3. D and A only

4. All are correct

24. Read the statements given below-

A. By the time of 500 mya, invertebrates were formed and active.

B. Jawless fish probably evolved around 50 mya.

C. Sea weeds and few plants existed probably around 320 mya.

D. The first organisms that invaded land were plants.

E. They were widespread on land when animals invaded land.

Which of the above statements are/is incorrect?

1. A and C only

2. B only

3. D and E only

4. A,C,D,E

25. **Read the statements given below -**

A. In 1978, a fish caught in South Africa happened to be a Coelacanth which was thought to be extinct.

B. These animals called lobefins evolved into the first amphibians that lived on both land and water.

C. There are no specimens of coelacanth left with us.

D. Coelacanth were ancestors of modern day frogs and salamanders.

E. The amphibians evolved into reptiles.

Which of the above statements is/are incorrect?

1. A and C only

2. A only

3. D and C only

4. A,B,C,D,E

26. **Consider the following statements-**

I. Giant ferns (pteridophytes) were present but they all fell to form coal deposits slowly.

II. Some land reptiles went back into water to evolve into fish like reptiles probably 200 mya (e.g. *Ichthyosaurs*).

III. The most of land reptiles were, dinosaurs.

IV. The biggest of them, i.e., *Tyrannosaurus rex* was about 200 feet in height and had huge fearsome dagger like teeth.

How many of them are/is incorrect-

1. one

2. two

3. three

4. four

27. **Match the list 1 and 2-**

<table>
<tr><td></td><td>List1</td><td>List2</td></tr>
<tr><td>A. Stabilising selection</td><td colspan="2">in which more individuals acquire mean character value</td></tr>
<tr><td>B. directional selection</td><td colspan="2">more individuals acquire value other than the mean character value</td></tr>
<tr><td>C. disruptive selection</td><td colspan="2">more individuals acquire peripheral character value at both ends of the distribution curve</td></tr>
</table>

Which of them are correctly matched-

1. A

2. A and B

3. A and C

4. A, B, C

28. Read the following statements-

a) Evolution by natural selection, in a true sense would have started when cellular forms of life with differences in metabolic capability originated on earth.

b) The essence of Darwinian theory about evolution is natural selection.

c) The rate of appearance of new forms is linked to the life cycle or the life span.

d) Microbes that divide fast have the ability to multiply and become millions of individuals within hours.

Which of the above statements are/is correct-

1. a and c only

2.a only

3.d and c only

4. a,b,c,d

29. Consider the following statements-

1. A colony of bacteria (say A) growing on a given medium has built in variation in terms of ability to utilise a feed component.

2. A change in the medium composition would bring out only that part of the population (say B) that can survive under the new conditions.

3. In due course of time this variant population outgrows the others and appears as new species.

4. This would happen within days. For the same thing to happen in a fish or fowl would take million of years as life spans of these animals are in years.

Which of the above statements are/is correct-

1. a and c only

2. a only

3. d and c only

4. a,b,c,d

30. Read the following facts -

I. Mammals were viviparous and protected their unborn young inside the mother's body.

II. Mammals were more intelligent in sensing and avoiding danger at least.

III. There were in South America mammals resembling horse, hippopotamus, bear, rabbit, etc.

IV. Due to continental drift, when South America joined North America, these animals were overridden by North American fauna.

V. Due to the same continental drift pouched mammals of Australia survived because of lack of competition from any other mammal.

How many of them are correct –

1. four

2. two

3. three

4. five

31. Read the following statements and find out the correct option

STATEMENT 1. The most successful story is the evolution of man with language skills and self-consciousness.

STATEMENT 2. The mechanism of how non-cellular aggregates of giant macromolecules could evolve into cells with membranous envelop is not known.

1. Both are wrong statements

2. Both are correct statements

3. Only statement 1 correct

4. Only statement 2 correct

32. Go through the following statement and find out the correct option-

ASSERTION(A). The origin of life on earth can be understood only against the background of origin of universe especially earth.

REASON(R). Most scientists believe chemical evolution, i.e., formation of biomolecules preceded the appearance of the first cellular forms of life.

1. A correct and R is correct explanation of A

2. A correct and R is also correct but R is not correct explanation of A

3. A correct but R incorrect

4. A and R both are incorrect

33. Find out the incorrect option-

1. Diversity of life forms on earth has been changing over millions of years.

2. It is generally believed that variations in a population result in variable fitness.

3. Other phenomena like habitat fragmentation and genetic drift may accentuate these variations leading to appearance of new species and hence evolution.

4. Homology is not accounted for by the idea of branching descent.

34. Read the following statements-

a) During ice age between 75,000-10,000 years ago modern *Homo sapiens* arose.

b) Pre-historic cave art developed about 58,000 years ago.

c) Agriculture came around 10,000 years back and human settlements started.

Which of the above statements is/are correct-

1. a only

2. b only

3. c, a only

4. a,b,c

35. Which of the following is/are correct -

I. The first human-like being the hominid and was called *Homo habilis*.

II. The brain capacities *Homo habilis* were between 650-800cc.

III. *Homo habilis* probably did not eat meat.

IV. The skull of baby chimpanzee is more like adult human skull than adult chimpanzee skull

How many of above are/is correct-

1. three

2. four

3. two

4. one

36. Read the statements given below-

i. About 65 mya, the dinosaurs suddenly disappeared from the earth.

ii. We do not know the true reason for disappearance of dinosaurs.

iii. Some say climatic changes killed dinosaurs some say most of them evolved into birds.

iv. Small sized reptiles of that era still exist today.

Which of the above statements are correct-

1. i,ii only

2. i, iii,iv only

3. i,ii,iii only

4. all are correct

37. Read the following statements-

i. When we describe the story of this world we describe evolution as a process.

ii. On the other hand when we describe the story of life on earth, we treat evolution as a consequence of a process called natural selection.

iii. We are still not very clear whether to regard evolution and natural selection as processes or end result of unknown processes.

iv. It is possible that the work of Thomas Malthus on populations influenced Darwin.

Which of the above statements is/are correct-

1. i and ii only

2. ii only

3. i and iii only

4. All are correct

38. Consider the following statements-

I. During his journey Darwin went to Galapagos Islands.

II. There he observed an amazing diversity of creatures.

III. The small black birds later called Darwin's Finches amazed him.

IV. Darwin realised that there were many varieties of finches in the same island.

V. All the varieties, he conjectured, evolved on the island itself.

VI. From the original seed-eating features, many other forms with altered beaks arose, enabling them to become insectivorous and vegetarian finches

How many of above are/is correct-

1. three

2.four

3.two

4. six

39. Read the following statements and find out the correct option-

STATEMENT 1. The novelty and brilliant insight of Darwin was this: he asserted that variations, which are heritable and which make resource utilisation better for few (adapted to habitat better) will enable only those to reproduce and leave more progeny.

STATEMENT 2. Hence for a period of time, over many generations, survivors will leave more progeny and there would be a change in population characteristic and hence new forms appear to arise.

1.Both are wrong statements

2.Both are correct statements

3. Only statement 1 correct

4.Only statement 2 correct

40. Read the following statements-

a) The process of evolution of different species in a given geographical area starting from a point and literally radiating to other areas of geography (habitats) is called **adaptive radiation**.

b) Darwin's finches represent one of the best examples of above phenomenon.

c) Another example is Australian marsupials, A number of marsupials, each different from the other evolved from an ancestral stock, but all within the Australian island continent.

d) When more than one adaptive radiation appeared to have occurred in an isolated geographical area (representing different habitats), one can call this convergent evolution.

Which of the above is/are correct?

1. a and b only

2. a,b,c only

3. c and d only

4. a,b,c,d

41. Go through the following statements and find out the correct option-

ASSERTION(A). Placental mammals in Australia also exhibit adaptive radiation in evolving into varieties of such placental mammals each of which appears to be 'similar' to a corresponding marsupial.

REASON(R). When more than one adaptive radiation appeared to have occurred in an isolated geographical area (representing different habitats), one can call this convergent evolution.

1.A correct and R is correct explanation of A

2. A correct and R is also correct but R is not correct explanation of A

3. A correct but R incorrect

4. A and R both are incorrect

42. Read the following statement -

I. Early Greek thinkers thought units of life called **spores** were transferred to different planets including earth.

II. 'Panspermia' is still a favourite idea for some astronomers.

III. For a long time it was also believed that life came out of decaying and rotting matter like straw, mud, etc, was the theory of spontaneous generation.

IV. Louis Pasteur by careful experimentation demonstrated that life comes only from pre-existing life.

V. Louis Pasteur showed that in pre-sterilised flasks, life did not come from killed yeast while in another flask open to air, new living organisms arose from 'killed yeast'.

How many of above are correct-

1. three

2. four

3. two

4. five

43.Consider the following statements-

a) Oparin of Russia and Haldane of England proposed that the first form of life could have come from pre-existing non-living organic molecules (e.g. RNA, protein, etc.) and that formation of life was preceded by chemical evolution, i.e., formation of diverse organic molecules from inorganic constituents.

b) The conditions on primitive earth were – high temperature, volcanic storms, reducing atmosphere containing CH_4, NH_3, etc.

c) In 1953, S.L. Miller, an American scientist created similar conditions in a laboratory scale.

d) S.L. Miller created electric discharge in a closed flask containing CH_4, H_2, NH_3 and water vapour at 800^0C.

e) S.L. Miller observed formation of amino acids.

How many of them are correct-

1. five

2. three

3. four

4. two

44. Read the following statements and find out the correct option with respect to sewage treatment-

STATEMENT 1. Due to continental drift, when South America joined North America, these animals were overridden by North American fauna.

STATEMENT 2. Due to the same continental drift pouched mammals of Australia survived because of lack of competition from any other mammal.

1. Both are correct statements

2. Both are wrong statements

3. Only statement 1 correct

4. Only statement 2 correct

45. Which statements is incorrect -

1. About 2000 billion years ago (bya) the first cellular forms of life appeared on earth.

2. The mechanism of how non-cellular aggregates of giant macromolecules could evolve into cells with membranous envelop is not known.

3. Some of above cells had the ability to release O_2.

4. The reaction could have been similar to the light reaction in photosynthesis where water is split with the help of solar energy captured and channelised by appropriate light harvesting pigments.

46. Read the following statements and find out the correct option

STATEMENT 1. The first mammals were like shrews and their fossils are small sized.

STATEMENT 2. Mammals were viviparous and protected their unborn young inside the mother's body.

1. Both are correct statements

2. Both are wrong statements.

3. Only statement 1 correct

4. Only statement 2 correct

47. Go through the following statement and find out the correct option-

ASSERTION(A). The skull of baby chimpanzee is more like adult human skull than adult chimpanzee skull

REASON(R). The Neanderthal man with a brain size of 1400cc lived in near east and central Asia between 1,00,000-40,000 years back.

1. A correct and R is correct explanation of A

2. A correct and R is also correct but R is not correct explanation of A

3. A correct but R incorrect

4. A and R both are incorrect

48. Read the following statements -

a) *Homo erectus* had a large brain around 1900cc.

b) *Homo erectus* probably ate meat.

c) The Neanderthal man with a brain size of 400cc lived in near east and central Asia between 1,00,000-40,000 years back.

d) Neanderthal man used hides to protect their body and buried their dead.

e) *Homo sapiens* arose in Africa and moved across continents and developed into distinct races.

How many of them are correct-

1.one

2.two

3.three

4.four

49.Consider the following statements -

A. Two mya, *Australopithecines* probably lived in East African grasslands.

B. Evidence shows they hunted with stone weapons but essentially ate fruit.

C. Some of the bones among the bones discovered were different.

D. This creature was called the first human-like being the hominid and was called *Homo habilis*.

Which above statements are correct-

1. A and C only

2.D and A only

3. B and D only

4. All are correct

50. Read the following facts-

A. About 15 mya, primates called *Dryopithecus* and *Ramapithecus* were existing.

B. They were hairy and walked like gorillas and chimpanzees.

C. *Ramapithecus* was more ape-like while *Dryopithecus* was more man-like.

D. Few fossils of man-like bones have been discovered in Ethiopia and Tanzania

Which of the above statements are/is incorrect-

1. A and C only

2.D and A only

3. C only

4. A,C,D

HUMAN HEALTH AND DISEASE

Health

- The term **health** is very frequently used by everybody.
- It is a state of complete **physical, mental, social and psychological well-being**.
- Diseases like **typhoid, cholera, pneumonia, fungal infections of skin, malaria** and many others are a major cause of distress to human beings.
- Health does not simply mean 'absence of disease' or 'physical fitness'.

Black bile concept/ black bile concept.

- **Good humor hypothesis** given by Greeks - Hippocrates.
- **Good humor hypothesis** supported by Indian Ayurveda.
- Humor are fluid of the body which if become darker than person feel sick. This concept was known as **black bile concept.**
- According to black bile concept the person with blackbile belonged to hot personality and would have fevers. This concept **Supported by Indian Ayurveda.**
- This concept disproved by **William Harvey.**

Point to remember

- When people are healthy, they are more efficient at work.
- **Physical fitness increases** productivity and brings economic prosperity.
- Good Health also increases **longevity** of people and reduces infant and **maternal** mortality.
- Balanced diet, personal hygiene and regular exercise are very important to maintain good health.
- **Yoga** has been practised to achieve **physical** and **mental** health.

- Awareness about diseases and their effect on different bodily functions, vaccination (immunisation) against infectious diseases, proper disposal of wastes, control of vectors and maintenance of hygienic food and water resources are necessary for achieving good health.

Infectious and non-infectious diseases

- When the functioning of one or more organs or systems of the body is adversely affected, characterised by various signs and symptoms, we say that we are not healthy, i.e., we have a **disease**.

- Diseases can be broadly grouped into **infectious** and **non-infectious**.

- Diseases which are easily transmitted from one person to another, are called **infectious diseases**.

- **Infectious** diseases are very common and every one of us suffers from these at sometime or other.

- Some of the infectious diseases like **AIDS**, **Pneumonia**, **Plague** are fatal.

- Among non-infectious diseases, **cancer** is the major cause of death.

- **Drug** and **alcohol** abuse also affect our health adversely.

13.1 COMMON DISEASES IN HUMANS

a. Pathogens.

- A wide range of **organisms** belonging to bacteria, viruses, fungi, protozoans, helminths, etc., could cause diseases in man.

- The disease causing organisms are called **pathogens**.

- The **parasites** are pathogens because they cause harm to the host by living in (or on) them.

- The pathogens can enter our body by various means, multiply and interfere with normal vital activities, resulting in morphological and functional damage.

- **Pathogens** have to adapt to life within the environment of the host.

- The **pathogens** that enter the gut must know a way of surviving in the stomach at low pH and resisting the various digestive enzymes.

b. Typhoid

- *Salmonella typhi* is a pathogenic bacterium.

- *Salmonella typhi* causes **typhoid** fever in human beings.

- *Salmonella typhi* generally enter the small intestine through food and water contaminated with them and migrate to other organs through blood.

- Sustained high fever (39° to 40°C), weakness, stomach pain, constipation, headache and loss of appetite are some of the common symptoms of this disease.

- Intestinal perforation and death may occur in severe cases.

- Typhoid fever could be confirmed by **Widal test**.

- A classic case in medicine, that of **Mary Mallon** nicknamed *Typhoid Mary*.

- Mary Mallon was a cook by profession and was a typhoid carrier who continued to spread typhoid for several years through the food she prepared.

c. Pneumonia

- Bacteria like *Streptococcus pneumoniae* and *Haemophilus influenza* are responsible for the disease **pneumonia** in humans which infects the alveoli (air filled sacs) of the lungs.
- The alveoli get filled with leading to severe problems in respiration.
- The symptoms of **pneumonia** include **fever, chills, cough and headache.**
- In **severe cases**, the lips and finger nails may turn gray to bluish in colour.
- A healthy person can infected by inhaling the droplets/aerosols released by an infected person or even by sharing glasses and utensils with an infected person.

Points to remember

- **Dysentery, plague, diphtheria,** etc., are some of the other bacterial diseases in man.
- **Many viruses** also cause diseases in human beings.

d. Common cold

- **Rhino viruses** represent one such group of viruses which cause one of the **most infectious** human disease – the **common cold.**
- **Rhino viruses** infect the nose and respiratory passage but not the lungs.
- The common cold is characterised by nasal congestion and discharge, sore throat, hoarseness, cough, headache, tiredness, etc., which usually last for **3-7 days.**
- **Droplets spreads** by cough or sneezes of an infected person are either inhaled directly or transmitted through contaminated objects such as pens, books, cups, doorknobs, computer keyboard or mouse, etc., and cause infection in a healthy person.

e. Malaria

- Malaria, a protozoan disease of man.
- *Plasmodium,* a tiny protozoan is responsible for this disease.
- Different species of *Plasmodium* (**P. vivax, P. malaria** and **P. falciparum**) are responsible for different types of malaria.
- The **malignant malaria** caused by *Plasmodium falciparum* is the most serious one and can even be fatal.
- *Plasmodium* enters the human body as **sporozoites (infectious form)** through the bite of infected female *Anopheles* mosquito.
- The **parasites firstly multiply within the liver cells** and then attack the **red blood cells** (RBCs) resulting in their rupture.
- The rupture of RBCs is associated with release of a toxic substance, **haemozoin,** which is responsible for the chill and high fever recurring every three to four days.
- When a female *Anopheles* mosquito bites an infected person, these parasites enter the mosquito's body and undergo further development.
- The parasites multiply within them to form **sporozoites** that are stored in their salivary glands.

- When these mosquitoes bite a human, the **sporozoites** are introduced into his/ her body, thereby initiating the events mentioned above.

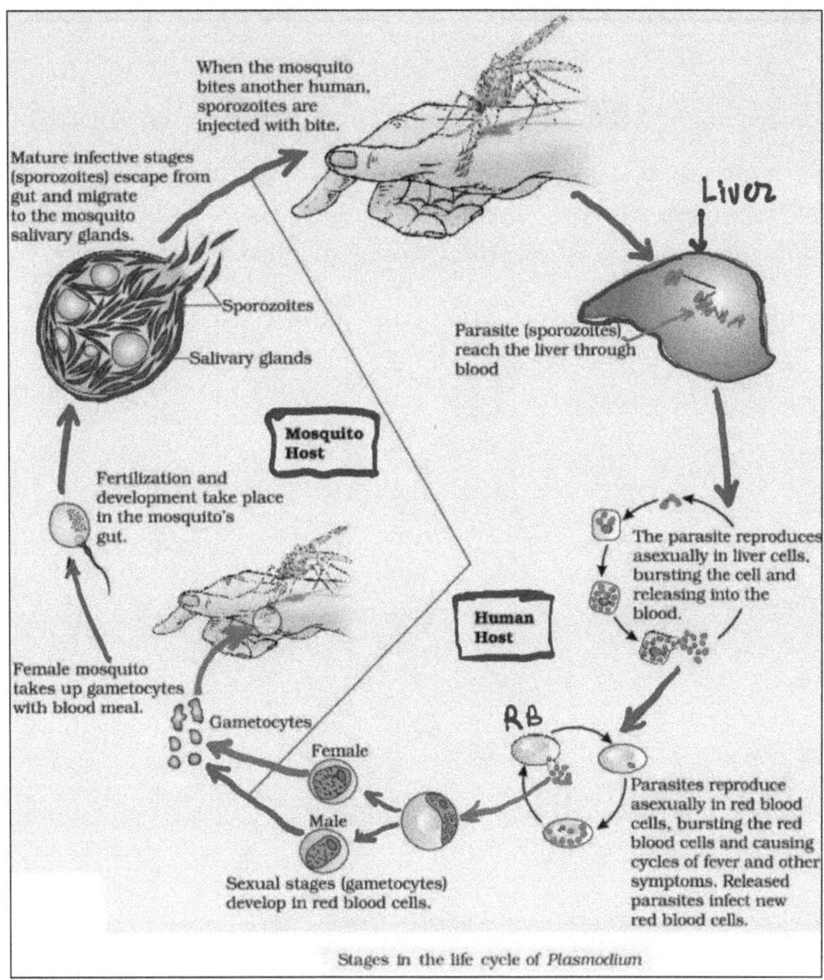

Stages in the life cycle of *Plasmodium*

- The malarial parasite requires two hosts to complete its life cycle – human and mosquitoes the female *Anopheles* mosquito is also act as the vector.

f. Amoebiasis

- *Entamoeba histolytica* is a protozoan parasite in the large intestine of human which causes **amoebiasis (amoebic dysentery)**.

- Symptoms of this disease include **constipation, abdominal pain and cramps, stools with excess mucous and blood clots.**

- **Houseflies act as mechanical carriers** and serve to transmit the parasite from faeces of infected person to food and food products, thereby contaminating them.

- Drinking water and food contaminated by the faecal matter are the main source of infection.

g. Ascariasis

- *Ascaris*, the common round worm and *Wuchereria*, the filarial worm, are some of the helminths which are known to be pathogenic to man. *Ascaris*, an intestinal parasite causes **ascariasis**.

- Symptoms of **ascariasis** include **internal bleeding, muscular pain, fever, anemia and blockage of the intestinal passage.**

- The eggs of the parasite are excreted along with the faeces of infected persons which contaminate soil, water, plants, etc.
- Oil of chenopodium use treat **ascariasis.**

h. Filariasis

- A healthy person acquires this infection through contaminated water, vegetables, fruits, etc.
- *Wuchereria (W. bancrofti* **and** *W. malayi),* the filarial worms cause a slowly developing chronic inflammation of the organs in which they live for many years, usually the lymphatic vessels of the lower limbs and the disease is called **elephantiasis** or **filariasis.**

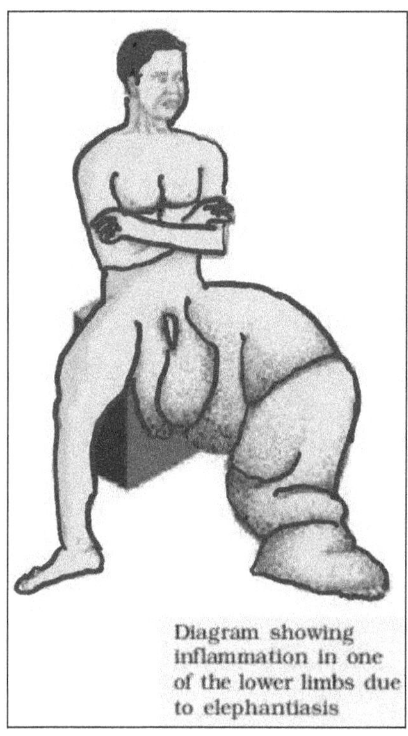

Diagram showing inflammation in one of the lower limbs due to elephantiasis

- The genital organs are may also be affected, resulting in gross deformities.
- The pathogens are transmitted to a healthy person through the bite by the female mosquito vectors.

i. Ringworms

- Many fungi belonging to the genera *Microsporum, Trichophyton* and *Epidermophyton* are responsible for **ringworms** which is one of the most common infectious diseases in man.

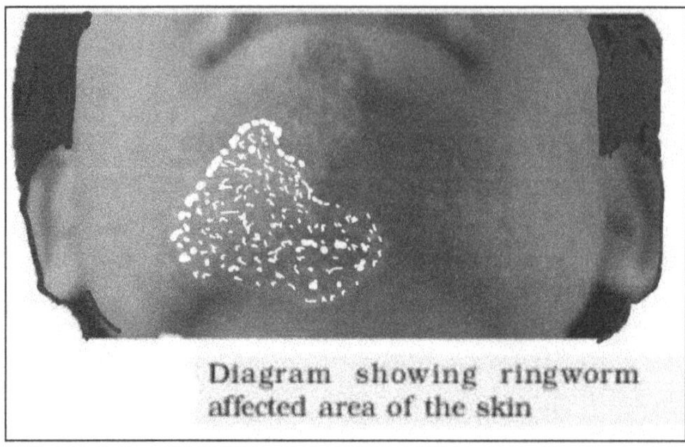

Diagram showing ringworm affected area of the skin

- **Appearance of dry, scaly lesions** on various parts of the body such as skin, nails and scalp are the main symptoms of the disease.

- **These lesions** are accompanied by **intense itching.**

- **Heat and moisture** help these fungi to grow, which makes them thrive in skin folds such as those in the groin or between the toes.

- **Ringworms** are generally acquired from soil or by using towels, clothes or even the comb of infected individuals.

Points to remember

- **Maintenance** of personal and public hygiene is very important for prevention and control of many infectious diseases.

- Measures for personal **hygiene** include keeping the body clean; consumption of clean drinking water, food, vegetables, fruits, etc.

- Public hygiene includes proper disposal of waste and excreta; **periodic** cleaning and disinfection of water **reservoirs**, pools, cesspools and tanks and observing standard practices of **hygiene** in public catering.

- These **measures** are particularly essential where the **infectious** agents are transmitted through food and water such as typhoid, amoebiasis and ascariasis.

- In cases of air-borne diseases such as **pneumonia** and common cold, in addition to the above **measures**, close contact with the infected persons or their belongings should be avoided.

- For **diseases** such as malaria and filariasis that are transmitted through insect vectors, the most important measure is to control or eliminate the **vectors** and their breeding places.

- This can be achieved by avoiding **stagnation** of water in and around **residential** areas, regular cleaning of household coolers, use of mosquito nets, introducing fishes like *Gambusia* in ponds that feed on mosquito larvae, **spraying** of insecticides in ditches, drainage areas and swamps, etc. In addition, doors and windows should be provided with wire mesh to prevent the entry of **mosquitoes.**

- Such precautions have become all the more important especially in the light of recent widespread incidences of the vector-borne (*Aedes* mosquitoes) diseases like dengue and **chikungunya** in many parts of India.

- The advancements made in **biological** science have armed us to effectively deal with many infectious diseases.

- The use of vaccines and **immunisation** programmes have enabled us to completely eradicate a deadly disease like smallpox.

- A large number of other infectious diseases like polio, diphtheria, pneumonia and tetanus have been controlled to a large extent by the use of **vaccines.**

- **Biotechnology** helps to make newer and safer vaccines.

- Discovery of **antibiotics** and various other drugs has also helps us to effectively treat infectious diseases.

13.2 IMMUNITY

- We are exposed to large number of **infectious** agents. But, only a few of these exposures result in disease. This is due to the fact that the body is able to defend itself from most of these foreign agents.
- The ability of the host to fight the disease-causing organisms, by the immune system is called **immunity**.

Type of Immunity

- Immunity is of two types: (i) Innate immunity and (ii) Acquired immunity.

13.2.1 Innate Immunity

- **Innate immunity** is non-specific type of defence.
- **Innate immunity** is present at the time of birth.
- This is accomplished by providing different types of barriers to the entry of the foreign agents into our body.
- **Innate immunity** consist of four types of barriers. These are —
    (i) *Physical barriers:*
    - ➤ Skin and Mucus coating included under these barriers.
    - ➤ Skin on our body is the main barrier which prevents entry of the micro-organisms.
    - ➤ Mucus coating of the epithelium lining the respiratory, gastrointestinal and urogenital tracts also help in trapping microbes entering our body.
    (ii) *Physiological barriers:*
    - ➤ Acid in the stomach, saliva in the mouth, tears from eyes–all prevent microbial growth.
    (iii) *Cellular barriers:*
    - ➤ Certain types of leukocytes (WBC) of our body like polymorpho-nuclear leukocytes (PMNL-neutrophils) and monocytes and natural killer (type of lymphocytes) in the blood as well as macrophages in tissues can phagocytose and destroy microbes.
    (iv) *Cytokine barriers:*
    - ➤ Virus-infected cells secrete proteins called **interferons** which protect non-infected cells from further viral infection.

13.2.2 Acquired Immunity

- Acquired immunity is pathogen specific.
- Acquired immunity is characterised by memory.

a. Primary immune response

- When our body when it encounters a pathogen for the first time produces a response called **primary response** which is of low intensity.

b. Secondary or anamnestic immune response.

- Subsequent encounter with the same pathogen elicits a highly intensified **secondary or anamnestic response.**
- This is ascribed to the fact that our body appears to have memory of the first encounter.

c. Lymphocytes

- The primary and secondary immune responses are carried out with the help of two special types of lymphocytes present in our blood, i.e., **B**-lymphocytes and **T** lymphocytes.
- The B-lymphocytes produce an army of proteins in response to pathogens into our blood to fight with them.
- These proteins are called antibodies.
- The T-cells themselves do not secrete antibodies but help B cells to produce them.

d. Antibody molecule

- Each antibody molecule has four peptide chains, two small called **light chains** and two longer called **heavy chains**.

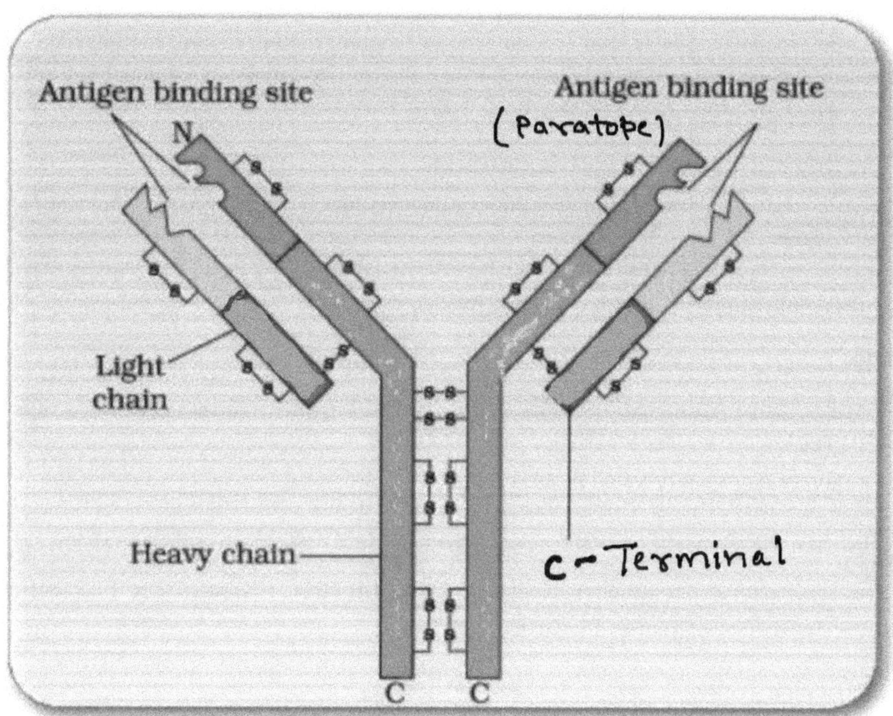

Structure of an antibody molecule

- Hence, an antibody is represented as **H2L2**.
- Different types of antibodies are produced in our body. **IgA, IgM, IgE, IgG** are some of them.

e. Humoral immune response/ Antibody mediated immune response

- The antibodies are found in the blood helps to fight against antigen this response called as **humoral immune response**.
- This is one of the two types of our acquired immune response – antibody mediated.

f. Cell-mediated immunity (CMI)

- The second type is called cell-mediated immune response or **cell-mediated immunity** (CMI).
- The T-lymphocytes mediate CMI.

g. Grafting/ Transplantation

> When some human organs like heart, eye, liver, kidney fail to function satisfactorily, transplatation is the only remedy to enable the patient to live a normal life. Then a search starts – to find a suitable donor.

> Grafts from just any source – an animal, another primate, or any human beings cannot be made since the grafts would be rejected sooner or later.

> Tissue matching, blood group matching are essential before undertaking any graft/transplant and even after this the patient has to take immuno–suppresants all his/her life.

> The body is able to differentiate 'self' and 'nonself' and the cell-mediated immune response is responsible for the graft rejection.

13.2.3 Active and Passive Immunity

a. Active immunity.

- When a host is exposed to antigens, which may be in the form of living or dead microbes or other proteins, antibodies are produced in the host body.
- This type of immunity is called **active immunity.**
- Active immunity is slow and takes time to give its full effective response.
- Injecting the microbes deliberately during immunisation or infectious organisms gaining access into body during natural infection induce active immunity.

b. Passive immunity.

- When ready-made antibodies are directly given to protect the body against foreign agents, it is called **passive immunity**.
- The yellowish fluid **colostrum** secreted by mother during the initial days of lactation has abundant antibodies (IgA) to protect the infant.
- The foetus also receives some antibodies from their mother, through the placenta during pregnancy. These are some examples of passive immunity.

13.2.4 Vaccination and Immunisation

- The principle of **immunisation or vaccination** is based on the property of 'memory' of the immune system.
- **In vaccination**, a preparation of antigenic proteins of pathogen or inactivated/weakened pathogen (vaccine) are introduced into the body.
- The antibodies produced in the body against these **antigens would neutralise the pathogenic agents** during actual infection.

Role of B and T-cells

- **The vaccines also generate memory – B and T-cells** that recognize the pathogen quickly on subsequent exposure and overwhelm the invaders with a massive production of antibodies.
- If a person is infected with some deadly microbes to which quick immune response is required as in tetanus, we need to directly inject the preformed **antibodies, or antitoxin** (a preparation containing antibodies to the toxin).

- Even in cases of snakebites, the injection which is given to the patients, contain **preformed antibodies against the snake venom.**

- The above type of immunisation is called **passive immunisation.**

- Recombinant DNA technology has allowed the production of antigenic polypeptides of pathogen in bacteria or yeast.

- Vaccines produced by recombinant DNA technology allow large scale production and **hence greater availability for immunisation,** e.g., hepatitis B vaccine produced from yeast.

8.2.5 Allergies

- The exaggerated response of the immune system to certain antigens present in the environment is called **allergy.**

- In a new place, suddenly you started sneezing, wheezing for no explained reason, and when you came away, your symptoms disappeared.

- The above-mentioned reaction could be because of allergy to pollen, mites, etc., which are different in different places.

- Some of us are sensitive to some particles in the environment.

- The substances to which such an immune response is produced are called allergens.

- Common examples of allergens are mites in dust, pollens, animal dander, etc.

- The antibodies produced to these are of **IgE** type.

a. Symptoms of allergic reactions

- Symptoms of allergic reactions include **sneezing, watery eyes, running nose and difficulty** in breathing.

b. Modern-day life style has resulted in lowering of immunity and more sensitivity

- Somehow, modern-day life style has resulted in lowering of immunity and more sensitivity to allergens – more and more children in metro cities of India suffer from allergies and asthma due to sensitivity to the environment.

- This could be because of the protected environment provided early in life.

c. Allergy Caused due to

- Allergy is due to the release of chemicals like histamine and serotonin from the mast cells. For determining the cause of allergy, the patient is exposed to or injected with very small doses of possible allergens, and the reactions studied.

d. Quickly relief from the symptoms of allergy

- The use of drugs like anti-histamine, adrenalin and steroids quickly reduce the symptoms of allergy.

8.2.6 Auto Immunity

- **Memory-based acquired immunity** evolved in higher vertebrates based on the ability to differentiate foreign organisms (e.g., pathogens) from self cells.

- The higher vertebrates can distinguish foreign molecules as well as foreign organisms.

- Most of the **experimental immunology deals** with this aspect.
- Sometimes, due to genetic and other unknown reasons, the body attacks self-cells.
- This results in damage to the body and is called **auto-immune** disease.
- Rheumatoid arthritis affects many people in our society is an example of auto-immune disease.

8.2.7 Immune System in the Body

- The human immune system consists of **lymphoid organs, tissues, cells and soluble molecules like antibodies.**
- **The immune system is unique in the sense that it recognises foreign antigens**, responds to these and remembers them.
- The immune system also plays an important role in allergic reactions, auto-immune diseases and organ transplantation.
- **Lymphoid organs:** These are the organs where origin and/or maturation and proliferation of lymphocytes occur.

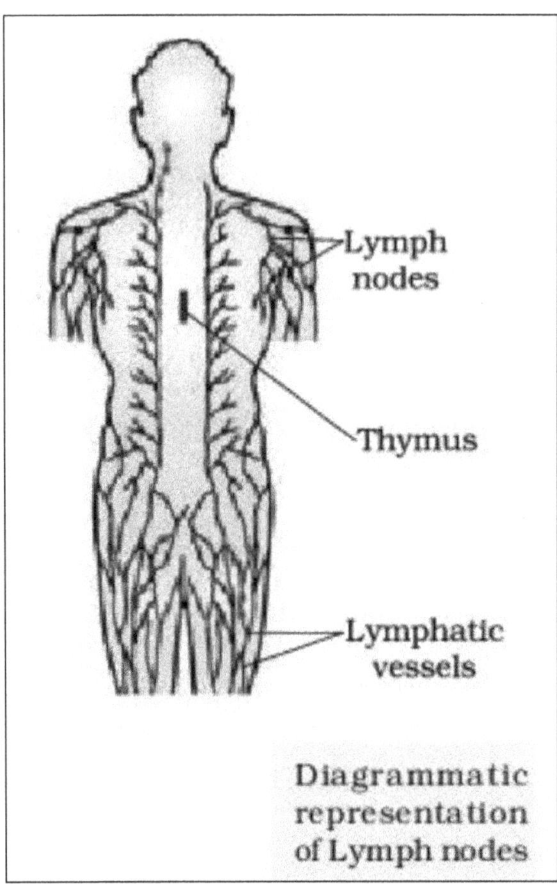

i. The primary lymphoid organs

- The primary lymphoid organs are **bone marrow** and **thymus** where immature lymphocytes differentiate into antigen-sensitive lymphocytes.
- The **bone marrow** is the main **lymphoid organ** where all blood cells including lymphocytes are produced.

- The **thymus is a lobed organ located** near the heart and beneath the breastbone.
- The thymus is quite large at the time of birth but keeps reducing in size with age and by the time puberty is attained it reduces to a very small size.
- Both bone-marrow and thymus provide micro-environments for the development and maturation of T-lymphocytes.

ii. The secondary lymphoid organs

- After maturation the lymphocytes migrate to secondary lymphoid organs like **spleen, lymph nodes, tonsils, Peyer's patches of small intestine and appendix.**
- The secondary lymphoid organs provide the sites for interaction of lymphocytes with the antigen, which then proliferate to become effector cells.

a. Spleen

- The spleen is a large bean shaped organ.
- Spleen mainly contains lymphocytes and phagocytes.
- Spleen acts as a filter of the blood by trapping blood-borne microorganisms.
- Spleen also has a large reservoir of erythrocytes.

b. Lymph Node

- The lymph nodes are small solid structures located at different points along the lymphatic system.
- Lymph nodes serve to trap the micro-organisms or other antigens, which happen to get into the lymph and tissue fluid.
- Antigens trapped in the lymph nodes are responsible for the activation of lymphocytes present there and cause the immune response.
- The lymphoid tissue also located within the lining of the major tracts (respiratory, digestive and urogenital tracts) called **mucosal associated lymphoid tissue** (MALT).
- MALT constitutes about 50 per cent of the lymphoid tissue in human body.

8.3 AIDS

- The word AIDS means **Acquired Immuno Deficiency Syndrome.**
- This means deficiency of immune system, acquired during the lifetime of an individual indicating that **it is not a congenital disease.**
- **'Syndrome' means a group of symptoms.**

a. History

- AIDS was first reported in **1981** and in the **last twenty-five years** or so, it has spread all over the world killing more than 25 million persons.

b. Caused By

- AIDS is caused by the Human Immuno deficiency Virus (HIV), a member of a group of viruses called **retrovirus**, which have an envelope enclosing the RNA genome.

c. Transmission By

- Transmission of HIV-infection generally occurs by

  (a) sexual contact with infected person,

  (b) by transfusion of contaminated blood and blood products,

  (c) by sharing infected needles as in the case of intravenous drug abusers and

  (d) from infected mother to her child through placenta.

d. High risk In People

- So, People who are at high risk of getting this infection includes - individuals who have multiple sexual partners, drug addicts who take drugs intravenously, individuals

- Who require repeated blood transfusions and children born to an HIV infected mother.

e. HIV/AIDS is not spread by mere touch or physical contact

- It is important to note that **HIV/AIDS** is not spread by mere touch or physical contact; it spreads only through body fluids.

- It is, hence, imperative, for the physical and psychological well-being, that the **HIV/AIDS** infected persons are not isolated from family and society.

f. Latent period

- There is always a time-lag between the infection and appearance of AIDS symptoms.

- **This period may vary from a few months to many years (usually 5-10 years).**

g. The virus enters into macro-phages

- After getting into the body of the person, the virus enters into macrophages

- Where RNA genome of the virus replicates to form viral DNA with the help of the enzyme reverse transcriptase.

- This viral DNA gets incorporated into host cell's DNA and directs the infected cells to produce virus particles.

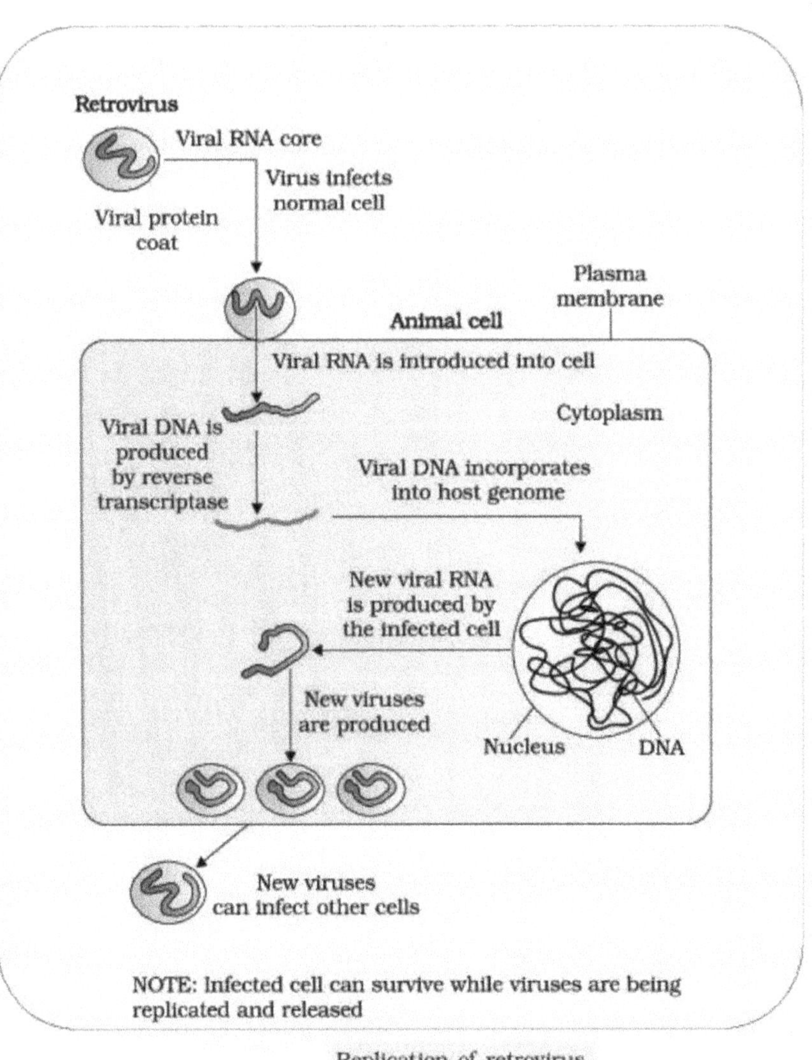

Replication of retrovirus

- The macrophages continue to produce virus and in this way acts like a **HIV factory.**

h. Progressive decrease in the number of helper T-lymphocytes

- **Simultaneously, HIV enters into helper T-lymphocytes (TH), replicates and produce progeny viruses. The progeny viruses released in the blood attack other helper T-lymphocytes.**

- This is repeated leading to a progressive decrease in the number of helper T-lymphocytes in the body of the infected person.

- During this period, the person suffers from bouts of fever, diarrhoea and weight loss.

- Due to decrease in the number of helper T lymphocytes, the person starts suffering from infections that could have been otherwise overcome such as those due to bacteria especially *Mycobacterium*, viruses, fungi and even parasites like *Toxoplasma*.

- The patient becomes so immuno-deficient that he/she is unable to protect himself/herself against these infections.

i. Enzyme linked immuno-sorbent assay (ELISA)

- A widely used diagnostic test for AIDS is **enzyme linked immuno-sorbent assay** (ELISA). Treatment of AIDS with anti-retroviral drugs is only partially effective.

- They can only prolong the life of the patient but cannot prevent death, which is inevitable.

j. Prevention of AIDS

- As AIDS has no cure, prevention is the best option.

- Moreover, HIV infection, more often, spreads due to conscious behavior patterns and is not something that happens inadvertently, like pneumonia or typhoid.

- Of course, infection in blood transfusion patients, new-borns (from mother) etc., may take place due to poor monitoring.

- The only excuse may be ignorance and it has been rightly said – "don't die of ignorance".

k. National AIDS Control Organisation (NACO) and other non-governmental organisation (NGOs)

- In our country the National AIDS Control Organisation (NACO) and other non-governmental organisation (NGOs) are doing a lot to educate people about AIDS.

- WHO has started a number of programmes to prevent the spreading of HIV infection.

Points to remember

- Making blood (from blood banks) safe from HIV, ensuring the use of only disposable needles and syringes in public and private hospitals and clinics, free distribution of condoms, controlling drug abuse, advocating safe sex and promoting regular check-ups for HIV in susceptible populations, are some such steps taken up.

- Infection with HIV or having AIDS is something that should not be hidden – since then, the infection may spread to many more people.

- HIV/AIDS-infected people need help and sympathy instead of being shunned by society.

- Unless society recognises it as a problem to be dealt with in a collective manner – the chances of wider spread of the disease increase manifold. It is a malady that can only be tackled, by the society and medical fraternity acting together, to prevent the spread of the disease.

8.4 CANCER

- **Cancer** is one of the most dreaded diseases of human beings and is a major cause of death all over the globe.
- More than a million Indians suffer from cancer and a large number of them die from it annually.
- The mechanisms that underlie development of cancer or oncogenic transformation of cells, its treatment and control have been some of the most intense areas of research in biology and medicine.
- In our body, cell growth and differentiation is highly controlled and regulated.
- In cancer cells, there is breakdown of these regulatory mechanisms.

a. Contact inhibition lost

- Normal cells show a property called **contact inhibition** by virtue of which contact with other cells inhibits their uncontrolled growth.
- Cancer cells appears to have lost contact inhibition property.

b. Tumors and its type

- As a result of this, cancerous cells just continue to divide giving rise to masses of cells called **tumors**.
- Tumors are of two types: benign and malignant.
- **Benign tumors** normally remain confined to their original location and do not spread to other parts of the body and cause little damage.
- The **malignant tumors**, on the other hand are a mass of proliferating cells called neoplastic or tumor cells.
- These cells grow very rapidly, invading and damaging the surrounding normal tissues.

c. Metastasis

- As these cells actively divide and grow they also starve the normal cells by competing for vital nutrients.
- Cells sloughed from such tumors reach distant sites through blood, and wherever they get lodged in the body, they start a new tumor there.
- This property called **metastasis** is the most feared property of malignant tumors.

d. Causes of cancer

- Transformation of normal cells into cancerous neoplastic cells may be induced by physical, chemical or biological agents.
- Cancer causing agents are called **carcinogens**.
- Ionizing radiations like X-rays and gamma rays.
- Non-ionizing radiations like UV cause DNA damage leading to neoplastic transformation.
- The chemical carcinogens present in tobacco smoke have been identified as a major cause of lung cancer.
- Cancer causing viruses called **oncogenic viruses** have genes called **viral oncogenes**.
- Several genes called **cellular oncogenes** (*c-onc*) or **proto oncogenes** have been identified in normal cells which, when activated under certain conditions, could lead to oncogenic transformation of the cells.

e. Cancer detection and diagnosis

- Early detection of cancers is essential as it allows the disease to be treated successfully in many cases.
- Cancer detection is based on **biopsy and histopathological studies** of the tissue and blood and bone marrow tests for increased cell counts in the case of leukemias.
- In biopsy, a piece of the suspected tissue cut into thin sections is stained and examined under microscope (histopathological studies) by a pathologist.
- Techniques like radiography (use of X-rays), CT (computed tomography) and MRI (magnetic resonance imaging) are very useful to detect cancers of the internal organs.
- **Computed tomography** uses X-rays to generate a three-dimensional image of the internals of an object.
- **MRI** uses strong magnetic fields and non-ionising radiations to accurately detect pathological and physiological changes in the living tissue.
- **Antibodies against cancer-specific antigens** are also used for detection of certain cancers.

Points to remember

- Techniques of molecular biology can be applied to detect genes in individuals with inherited susceptibility to certain cancers.
- Identification of such genes, which predispose an individual to certain cancers, may be very helpful in prevention of cancers.
- Such individuals may be advised to avoid exposure to particular carcinogens to which they are susceptible (e.g., tobacco smoke in case of lung cancer).

f. Treatment of cancer

- The common approaches for treatment of cancer are **surgery, radiation therapy and immunotherapy**.
- In radiotherapy, tumor cells are irradiated lethally, taking proper care of the normal tissues surrounding the tumor mass.
- Several **chemotherapeutic drugs** are used to kill cancerous cells.
- Some of these are specific for particular tumors.
- **Majority of drugs shows side effects like hair loss, anemia, etc.**
- Most cancers are treated by combination of surgery, radiotherapy and chemotherapy.

Points to remember

- Tumor cells have been shown to avoid detection and destruction by immune system.
- Therefore, the patients are given substances called biological response modifiers such as alpha-**interferon** which activate their immune system and help in destroying the tumor.

8.5 DRUGS AND ALCOHOL ABUSE

- The use of drugs and alcohol has been on the rise especially among the youth.
- This is a cause of concern as it could result in many harmful effects.

- Proper education and guidance would enable youth to safeguard themselves against these dangerous behaviour patterns and follow healthy lifestyles.
- The drugs, which are commonly abused are opioids, cannabinoids and coca alkaloids.
- Majority of these drugs are obtained from flowering plants.
- Some are obtained from fungi.

a. Opioids

- **Opioids** are the drugs, which bind to specific opioid receptors present in our central nervous system and gastrointestinal tract.
- Morphine is a very effective sedative and painkiller, and given after surgery.
- Heroin commonly called *smack* is chemically diacetylmorphine which is a white, odourless, bitter crystalline compound.
- This is obtained by acetylation of morphine, which is extracted from the latex of poppy plant **Papaver somniferum.**

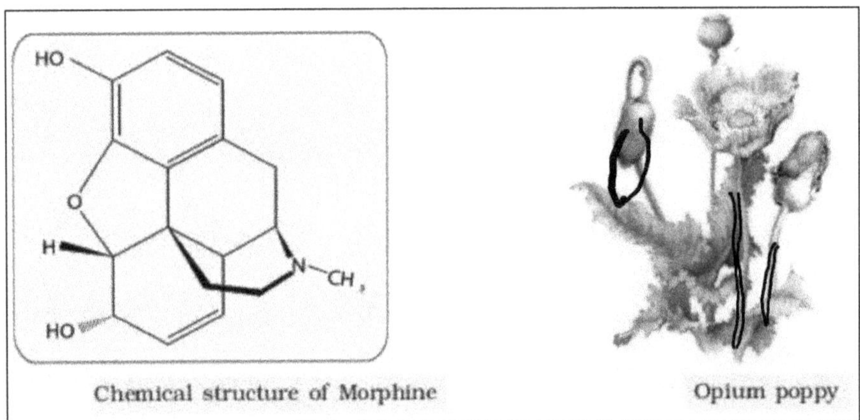

Chemical structure of Morphine   Opium poppy

- Generally taken by snorting and injection, heroin is a depressant and slows down body functions.

b. Cannabinoids

- **Cannabinoids** are a group of chemicals, which interact with cannabinoid receptors present principally in the brain.

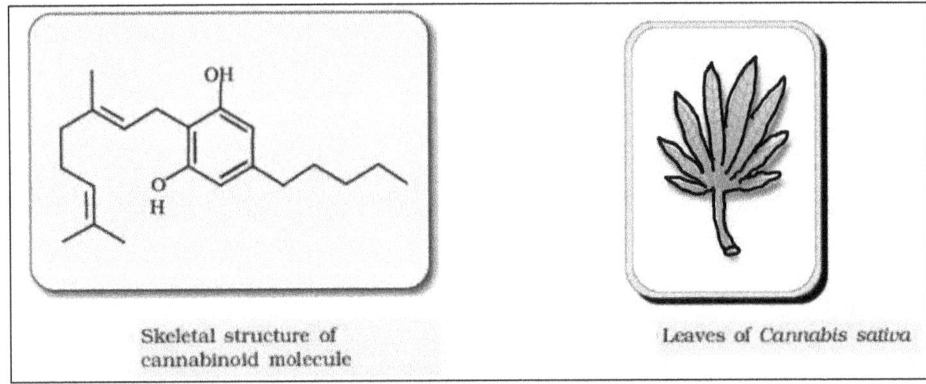

Skeletal structure of
cannabinoid molecule   Leaves of *Cannabis sativa*

- Natural cannabinoids are obtained from the inflorescences of the plant **Cannabis sativa.**

- The flower tops, leaves and the resin of cannabis plant are used in various combinations to produce marijuana, hashish, charas and ganja.
- It is taken by inhalation and oral ingestion, these are known for their effects on cardiovascular system of the body.

c. Coca alkaloid

- Coca alkaloid or **cocaine** is obtained from coca plant *Erythroxylum coca*, native to South America.
- It interferes with the transport of the neuro-transmitter dopamine.
- Cocaine, commonly called **coke** or **crack** is usually snorted.
- **cocaine** has a potent stimulating action on **central nervous system**, producing a sense of euphoria and increased energy.

Points to remember

- Excessive dosage of cocaine causes hallucinations. Other well-known plants with hallucinogenic properties are *Atropa belladona* and *Datura*.

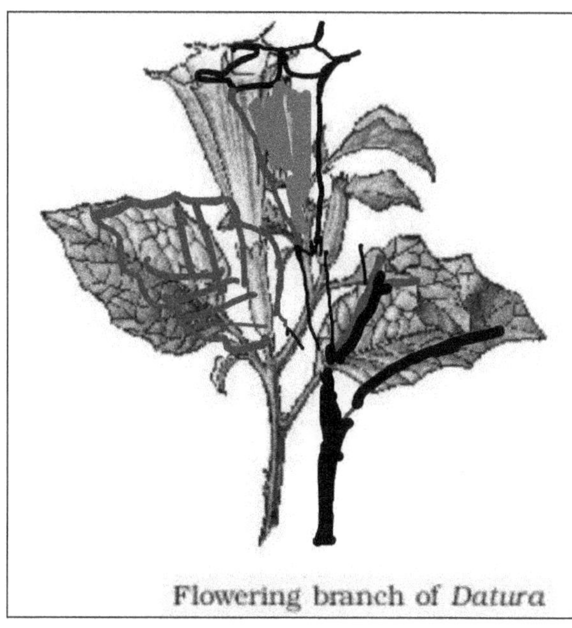

Flowering branch of *Datura*

- Presently cannabinoids are also being abused by some sportspersons.
- Drugs like **barbiturates, amphetamines, benzodiazepines, lysergic acid diethyl amides (LSD)**, and other similar drugs, that are normally used as medicines to help patients cope with mental illnesses like **depression and insomnia**, are often abused.
- Several plants, fruits and seeds having hallucinogenic properties have been used for hundreds of years in folk-medicine, religious ceremonies and rituals all over the globe.
- When these are taken for a purpose other than medicinal use or in amounts/frequency that impairs one's physical, physiological or psychological functions, it constitutes drug abuse.

Tobacco

- Smoking also paves the way to hard drugs.
- Tobacco has been used by human beings for more than 400 years.

- It is smoked, chewed or used as a snuff.

- Tobacco contains a large number of chemical substances including nicotine, an alkaloid.

- Nicotine stimulates adrenal gland to release adrenaline and nor-adrenaline into blood circulation, both of which raise blood pressure and increase heart rate.

- Nicotine stimulates sympathetic nervous system.

- Smoking is associated with increased incidence of cancers of lung, urinary bladder and throat, bronchitis, emphysema, coronary heart disease, gastric ulcer, etc.

- Tobacco chewing is associated with increased risk of cancer of the oral cavity.

- Smoking increases carbon monoxide (CO) content in blood and reduces the concentration of haem bound oxygen so causes oxygen deficiency in the body.

- At the time take packets of cigarettes one cannot miss the statutory warning that is present on the packing which warns against smoking and says how it is injurious to health.

- Smoking is very prevalent in society, both among young and old.

- Knowing the dangers of smoking and chewing tobacco, and its addictive nature, the youth and old need to avoid these habits.

- To get rid of addiction counselling and medical help require.

8.5.1 Adolescence and Drug/Alcohol Abuse

- **Adolescence** means both 'a period' and 'a process' during which a child becomes mature in terms of his/her attitudes and beliefs for effective participation in society.

- The period between **12-18 years** of age may be thought of as adolescence period.

- In other words, adolescence is a bridge linking childhood and adulthood.

- Adolescence is accompanied by **several biological and behavioural** changes. Adolescence, thus is a very vulnerable phase of mental and psychological development of an individual.

- **Curiosity, need for adventure and excitement, and experimentation**, constitute common causes, which motivate youngsters towards drug and alcohol use.

- A child's natural **curiosity** motivates him/her to experiment.

- This is complicated further by effects that might be perceived as benefits, of alcohol or drug use.

- Thus, the first use of drugs or **alcohol** may be out of curiosity or experimentation, but later the child starts using these to escape facing problems.

- Of late, stress, from pressures to excel in academics or **examinations**, has played a significant role in persuading the youngsters to try alcohol and drugs.

- The perception among youth that it is 'cool' or **progressive** to smoke, use drugs or alcohol, is also in a way a major cause for youth to start these habits.

- **Television**, movies, newspapers, internet also help to promote this perception.

- Other factors that have been seen to be associated with drug and alcohol abuse among **adolescents** are unstable or unsupportive family structures and peer pressure.

8.5.2 Addiction and Dependence

- Because of the perceived benefits, drugs are frequently used repeatedly.
- The most important thing, which one fails to realise, is the inherent addictive nature of alcohol and drugs.

Addiction

- **Addiction is a psychological attachment** to certain effects –such as euphoria and a temporary feeling of well-being – associated with drugs and alcohol.
- These drive people to take them even when these are not needed, or even when their use becomes **self-destructive**.
- With repeated use of drugs, the **tolerance** level of the receptors present in our body increases.
- Consequently the receptors respond only to higher doses of drugs or alcohol leading to greater intake and addiction.
- However, it should be **clearly** borne in mind that use of these drugs even once, can be a fore-runner to addiction.
- Thus, **the addictive potential of drugs and alcohol,** pull the user into a vicious circle leading to their regular use (abuse) from which he/she may not be able to get out.
- In the absence of any guidance or **counselling**, the person gets addicted and becomes dependent on their use.

Withdrawal syndrome

- Dependence is the tendency of the body to manifest a characteristic and unpleasant **withdrawal syndrome** if regular dose of drugs/alcohol is abruptly discontinued.
- This is characterised by **anxiety, shakiness, nausea and sweating**, which may be relieved when use is resumed again.
- In some cases, **withdrawal** symptoms can be severe and even life threatening and the person may need medical supervision.
- **Dependence** leads the patient to ignore all social norms in order to get sufficient funds to satiate his/her needs.
- These result in many social adjustment problems.

8.5.3 Effects of Drug/Alcohol Abuse

- The **immediate** adverse effects of drugs and alcohol abuse are manifested in the form of reckless behaviour, vandalism and violence.
- **Excessive** doses of drugs may lead to coma and death due to respiratory failure, heart failure or cerebral hemorrhage.
- A **combination** of drugs or their intake along with alcohol generally results in overdosing and even deaths.

The most common warning signs of drug and alcohol abuse among youth

The most common warning signs of drug and alcohol abuse among youth include –

- ➤ drop in academic performance
- ➤ unexplained absence from school/college
- ➤ lack of interest in personal hygiene
- ➤ withdrawal
- ➤ isolation
- ➤ depression
- ➤ fatigue
- ➤ aggressive and rebellious behaviour
- ➤ deteriorating relationships with family and friends
- ➤ loss of interest in hobbies
- ➤ change in sleeping and eating habits
- ➤ fluctuations in weight and appetite, etc.

Drug/alcohol abuse-Results

- There may even be some far-reaching implications of drug/alcohol abuse.
- If a abuser is unable to get money to buy drugs/alcohol he/she may turn to stealing.
- At times, a drug/alcohol addict becomes the cause of mental and financial distress to his/her entire family and friends.
- Those who take drugs intravenously (direct injection into the vein using a needle and syringe), are much more likely to acquire serious infections like **AIDS** and **hepatitis B**.
- The viruses, which are responsible for these diseases, are transferred from one person to another by sharing of infected needles and syringes. Both AIDS and Hepatitis B infections are chronic infections and ultimately fatal.
- AIDS can be transmitted to one's life partner through sexual contact while Hepatitis B is transmitted through infected blood.
- The use of alcohol during adolescence may also have long-term effects.
- The chronic use of **drugs and alcohol damages nervous system and liver (cirrhosis)**.
- The use of drugs and alcohol during pregnancy is also known to adversely affect the foetus.
- Another misuse of drugs is what certain sportspersons do to enhance their performance.
- They (mis)use **narcotic analgesics, anabolic steroids, diuretics and certain hormones** in sports to increase muscle strength and bulk and to promote aggressiveness and as a result increase athletic performance.

The side-effects of the use of anabolic steroids in females

- The side-effects of the use of anabolic steroids in females include-
  - ➤ masculinisation (features like males)
  - ➤ increased aggressiveness
  - ➤ mood swings

- ➤ depression
- ➤ abnormal menstrual cycles
- ➤ excessive hair growth on the face and body
- ➤ enlargement of clitoris
- ➤ deepening of voice.

The side-effects of the use of anabolic steroids in females

- In males it includes –
  - ✓ Acne
  - ✓ increased aggressiveness
  - ✓ mood swings
  - ✓ depression
  - ✓ reduction of size of the testicles
  - ✓ decreased sperm production
  - ✓ potential for kidney and liver dysfunction
  - ✓ breast enlargement
  - ✓ premature baldness
  - ✓ enlargement of the prostate gland.

Points to remember-

- These effects may be permanent with prolonged use.
- In the adolescent male or female, severe facial and body acne, and premature closure of the growth centres of the long bones may result in stunted growth.

8.5.4 Prevention and Control

- The prevention is better than cure holds true here also.
- It is also true that habits such as smoking, taking drug or alcohol are more likely to be taken up at a young age, more during adolescence.
- It is best to identify the situations that may push an adolescent towards use of drugs or alcohol, and to take remedial measures well in time.
- In this regard, the parents and the teachers have a special responsibility.
- Parenting that combines with high levels of nurturance and consistent discipline, has been associated with lowered risk of substance (alcohol/drugs/tobacco) abuse.
- Some of the measures mentioned here for prevention and control of alcohol and drugs abuse among adolescents

  - *(i) Avoid undue peer pressure –*
    - ✓ Every child has his/her own choice and personality, which should be respected and nurtured.
    - ✓ A child should not be pushed unduly to perform beyond his/her threshold limits; be it studies, sports or other activities.

(ii) *Education and counselling –*

✓ Educating and counselling him/ her to face problems and stresses, and to accept disappointments and failures as a part of life.

✓ It would also be worthwhile to channelize the child's energy into healthy pursuits like sports, reading, music, yoga and other extracurricular activities.

(iii) *Seeking help from parents and peers –*

✓ Help from parents and peers should be sought immediately so that they can guide appropriately.

✓ Help may even be sought from close and trusted friends.

✓ Besides getting proper advise to sort out their problems, this would help young to vent their feelings of anxiety and guilt.

(iv) *Looking for danger signs –*

✓ Parents and teachers need to look for and identify the danger signs.

✓ Even friends, if they find someone using drugs or alcohol, should not hesitate to bring this to the notice of parents or teacher in the best interests of the person concerned.

✓ Appropriate measures would then be required to diagnose the malady and the underlying causes.

✓ This would help in initiating proper remedial steps or treatment.

(v) *Seeking professional and medical help –*

✓ A lot of help is available in the form of highly qualified psychologists, psychiatrists, and deaddiction and rehabilitation programmes to help individuals who have unfortunately got in the quagmire of drug/alcohol abuse.

✓ With such help, the affected individual with sufficient efforts and will power, can get rid of the problem completely and lead a perfectly normal and healthy life.

1. Consider the following statements and find out the correct option-

A. Health does not simply mean 'absence of disease' or 'physical fitness'.

B. When people are healthy, they are more efficient at work.

C. Physical fitness increases productivity and brings economic prosperity.

D. Health also increases longevity of people and reduces infant and maternal mortality.

Which of the above are correct -

1. A,C

2. B,C

3. D,A

4. A,B,C,D

2. Match the Column 1 and Column 2-

Column 1   Column 2

a. *Salmonella typhi*	j. ELISA
b. AIDS	k. RT-PCR
c. *Corona*	l. Widal test
d. *Cancer*	m. Biopsy

Find out the correct option –

1. a.k, b.j, c.l, d.m

2. a.k,b.l,c.j,d.m

3. a.l,b.j,c.k,d.m

4. a.l,b.j,c.m,d.k

3. Consider the following statements-

a) Yoga has been practised since time immemorial to achieve physical and mental health.

b) Awareness about diseases and their effect on different bodily functions, vaccination (immunisation) against infectious diseases, proper disposal of wastes, control of vectors and maintenance of hygienic food and water resources are necessary for achieving good health.

c)   When the functioning of one or more organs or systems of the body is adversely affected, characterised by various signs and symptoms, we say that we are not healthy, i.e., we have a **disease**.

d)   Diseases can be broadly grouped into **infectious** and **non-infectious**.

e)   Diseases which are easily transmitted from one person to another, are called **infectious diseases**.

Which of the above statements are correct -

1. only a and d

2. a,b,c,e

3. a,b,c,d

4. all are correct

4. Consider the following statements-

a)   A wide range of organisms belonging to bacteria, viruses, fungi, protozoans, helminths, etc., could cause diseases in man.

b)   The disease causing organisms are called **pathogens**.

c)   The parasites are pathogens as they cause harm to the host by living in (or on) them.

d)   The pathogens can enter our body by various means, multiply and interfere with normal vital activities, resulting in morphological and functional damage.

e)   Pathogens do not to adapt to life within the environment of the host.

Which of the above statements are incorrect -

1. a

2. a,b

3. b,d

4. e

5. Consider the following statements and find out the correct option-

STATEMENT 1. The parasites are pathogens as they cause harm to the host by living in (or on) them.

STATEMENT 2. The pathogens can enter our body by various means, multiply and interfere with normal vital activities, resulting in morphological and functional damage.

1. Both are correct statements

2. Only Statement 1 correct

3. Both are wrong Statements

4. Only Statement 2 correct

6. Go through the following statement-

ASSERTION(A). *Salmonella typhi* is a pathogenic bacterium which causes **typhoid** fever in human beings.

REASON(R). These pathogens generally enter the small intestine through food and water contaminated with them and migrate to other organs through blood.

1. A correct and R is correct explanation of A

2. A correct and R is also correct but R is not correct explanation of A

3. A correct but R incorrect

4. A and R both are incorrect

7. Which statement is incorrect w.r.t. Typhoid-

1. Typhoid fever could be confirmed by **Schick test**.

2. Mary Mallon nicknamed as *Typhoid Mary*.

3. Mary Mallon was a cook by profession and was a typhoid carrier who continued to spread typhoid for several years through the food she prepared.

4. Intestinal perforation and death may occur in severe cases.

8. Go through the following statements-

A. Bacteria like *Streptococcus pneumoniae* and *Haemophilus influenza* are responsible

B. *Streptococcus pneumoniae* and *Haemophilus influenza* infects the alveoli (air filled sacs) of the lungs.

C. The alveoli get filled with fluid leading to severe problems in respiration.

D. The symptoms of pneumonia include fever, chills, cough and headache. In severe cases, the lips and finger nails may turn gray to bluish in colour.

E. A healthy person acquires the infection by inhaling the droplets/aerosols released by an infected person or even by sharing glasses and utensils with an infected person.

How many of them are correct for pneumonia in humans-

1. two

2. three

3. four

4. five

9. Consider the following statements and find out the correct option

STATEMENT 1. Cancer detection is based on widal test of the tissue and bone marrow tests for increased cell counts in the case of leukemias.

STATEMENT 2. In biopsy, a piece of the suspected tissue cut into thin sections is stained and examined under microscope (histopathological studies) by a pathologist.

1. Both are wrong statements

2. Only Statement 1 correct

3. Both are correct statements

4. Only statement 2 correct

10. Consider the following statements and find out the correct option

STATEMENT 1. Dysentery, plague, diphtheria, mumps are bacterial diseases in man.

STATEMENT 2. Rhino viruses causes common cold.

1. Both are wrong statements

2. Only Statement 1 correct

3. Both are correct statements

4. Only Statement 2 correct

11. Read the following statements very carefully and find out the correct-

a) The common cold is characterised by nasal congestion and discharge, sore throat, hoarseness, cough, headache and tiredness.

b) The common cold usually last for 3-7 days.

c) Droplets resulting from cough or sneezes of an infected person are either inhaled directly or transmitted through contaminated objects such as pens, books, cups, doorknobs, computer keyboard or mouse, etc., and cause infection in a healthy person.

Which of the above statements is/are correct?

1. a and c both

2. b only

3. a,b,c

4. b and c only

12. Go through the following statements-

ASSERTION(A). When a female *Anopheles* mosquito bites an infected person, malarial parasites enter the mosquito's body and undergo further development.

REASON(R). The parasites multiply within them to form sporozoites that are stored in their gastric glands.

1. A correct and R is correct explanation of A

2. A correct and R is also correct but R is not correct explanation of A

3. A correct but R incorrect

4. A and R both are incorrect

13. Find out the incorrect statement -

1. *Plasmodium*, a tiny bacteria is responsible for malaria.

2. Different species of *Plasmodium* (*P. vivax*, *P. malaria* and *P. falciparum*) are responsible for different types of malaria.

3. Of these, malignant malaria caused by *Plasmodium falciparum* is the most serious one and can even be fatal.

4. *Plasmodium* enters the human body as sporozoite (infectious form) through the bite of infected female *Anopheles* mosquito.

14. Find out incorrect statements –

1. The malarial parasite requires two hosts – human and mosquitoes – to complete its life cycle.

2. *Entamoeba histolytica* is a bacterial parasite in the small intestine of human which causes amoebiasis (amoebic dysentery).

3. Symptoms of amoebic dysentery disease include constipation, abdominal pain and cramps, stools with excess mucous and blood clots.

4. Houseflies act as mechanical carriers and serve to transmit the parasite from faeces of infected person to food and food products, thereby contaminating them.

15. Consider the following statements and find out the correct option-

STATEMENT 1. *Ascaris*, an intestinal parasite causes **ascariasis**.

STATEMENT 2. Symptoms of **ascariasis** include internal bleeding, muscular pain, fever, anemia and blockage of the intestinal passage.

1. Both are wrong statements

2. Only statement 1 correct

3. Both are correct statements

4. Only statement 2 correct

16. Match the list 1 and 2 -

List1 List2

a. *Plasmodium*	amoebiasis
b. *Wuchereria*	elephantiasis
c. *Trichophyton*	Ringworm
d. Rhino viruses	common cold

How many of them are correctly matched-

1. one

2. two

3. three

4. four

17. Consider the following -

a) *Wuchereria* the filarial worms cause a slowly developing chronic inflammation of the organs in which they live for many years, usually the lymphatic vessels of the lower limbs and the disease is called filariasis.

b) The genital organs are also often affected, resulting in gross deformities in elephantiasis or filariasis.

c) The pathogens are transmitted to a healthy person through the bite by the female mosquito vectors in elephantiasis or filariasis.

d) Many fungi belonging to the genera *Microsporum*, *Trichophyton* and *Epidermophyton* are responsible for ringworms which is one of the most common infectious diseases in man.

Which of the above statements are correct?

1. b and f only

2. c and b only

3. a,b,c only

4. a,b,c,d

18. Match the list 1 and 2-

List 1   List 2

a. Pneumonia	in humans which infects the alveoli (air filled sacs) of the lungs
b. Malignant malaria	the most serious one and can even be fatal.
c. Common cold	nasal congestion and discharge, sore throat, hoarseness, cough, headache, tiredness,
d. Ringworms	Appearance of dry, scaly lesions on various parts of the body such as skin, nails and scalp

How many of them are correctly matched-

1. one

2. two

3. three

4. four

19. Consider the following statements -

I. Many fungi belonging to the genera *Microsporum*, *Trichophyton* and *Epidermophyton* are responsible for **ringworms** which is one of the most common infectious diseases in man.

II. Appearance of dry, scaly lesions on various parts of the body such as skin, nails and scalp are the main symptoms of the disease.

III. The above lesions are accompanied by intense itching.

IV. Heat and moisture help these fungi to grow, which makes them thrive in skin folds such as those in the groin or between the toes.

How many of them are/is correct for ringworms-

1. one

2. two

3. three

4. four

20. Read the following statements-

I. Maintenance of personal and public hygiene is very important for prevention and control of many infectious diseases.

II. Measures for personal hygiene include keeping the body clean; consumption of clean drinking water, food, vegetables, fruits, etc.

III. Public hygiene includes proper disposal of waste and excreta; periodic cleaning and disinfection of water reservoirs, pools, cesspools and tanks and observing standard practices of hygiene in public catering.

IV. These measures are particularly essential where the infectious agents are transmitted through food and water such as typhoid, amoebiasis and ascariasis.

How many of them are/is correct **statements-**

1. two

2. three

3. four

4. one

21. Consider the following statements and find out the correct option –

STATEMENT 1. The diseases such as pneumonia and common cold are air-borne.

STATEMENT 2. Diseases such as malaria and filariasis that are transmitted through insect vectors, the most important measure is to control or eliminate the vectors and their breeding places.

1. Both are wrong statements

2. Only statement 1 correct

3. Both are correct statements

4. Only statement 2 correct

22. Go through the following statement and find out the correct option-

ASSERTION(A). The advancements made in biological science have armed us to effectively deal with many infectious diseases.

REASON(R). The use of vaccines and immunisation programmes have enabled us to completely eradicate a deadly disease common cold.

1. A correct and R is correct explanation of A

2. A correct and R is also correct but R is not correct explanation of A

3. A correct but R incorrect

4. A and R both are incorrect

23. Go through the following statements and find out the correct option-

A. For diseases such as malaria and filariasis that are transmitted through insect vectors, the most important measure is to control or eliminate the vectors and their breeding places.

B. This can be achieved by avoiding stagnation of water in and around residential areas, regular cleaning of household coolers, use of mosquito nets, introducing fishes like *Gambusia* in ponds that feed on mosquito larvae, spraying of insecticides in ditches, drainage areas and swamps, etc.

C. In addition, doors and windows should be provided with wire mesh to prevent the entry of mosquitoes.

D. Such precautions have become all the more important especially in the light of recent widespread incidences of the vector-borne (*Aedes* mosquitoes) diseases like dengue and chikungunya in many parts of India.

Which of the above statements are correct -

1. A and C only

2. C and D only

3. D, C, A only

4. All are correct

24. Read the statements given below-

A. Everyday we are exposed to large number of infectious agents. But only a few of these exposures result in disease.

B. The overall ability of the host to fight the disease-causing organisms, conferred by the immune system is called immunity.

C. Immunity is of two types - Innate immunity and Acquired immunity.

D. Innate immunity is a specific type of defence, that is present at the time of birth.

E. Innate immunity provide different types of barriers to the entry of the foreign agents into our body.

Which of the above statements are correct?

1. A and C only

2. B only

3. D,B,C only

4. A,B,C,E

25. Read the following statements-

A. Acquired immunity is pathogen specific.

B. Acquired immunity is characterised by memory.

C. Our body when encounters with a pathogen for the first time produces a response called primary response which is of low intensity.

D. Subsequent encounter with the same pathogen elicits a highly intensified secondary or anamnestic response.

E. Secondary response is ascribed to the fact that our body appears to have memory of the first encounter.

Which above statements are correct?

1. A and C only

2. A,B,C,D only

3. D and C only

4. A,B,C,D,E

26. Consider the following statements-

A. The primary and secondary immune responses are carried out with the help of two special types of lymphocytes present in our blood, i.e., **B**-lymphocytes and **T**-lymphocytes.

B. The B-lymphocytes produce an army of proteins in response to pathogens into our blood to fight with them.

C. Army of proteins are called antibodies.

D. The T-cells themselves do not secrete antibodies but help B cells to produce antibodies.

E. Each antibody molecule has two peptide chains, two small called **light chains** and two longer called **heavy chains**.

How many of them are/is incorrect-

1. one

2. two

3. three

4. four

27. Match the list 1 and 2-

List 1   List 2

A. *Physical barriers*	Skin on our body is the main barrier which prevents entry of the micro-organisms.
B. *Physiological barriers*	Acid in the stomach, saliva in the mouth, tears from eyes–all prevent microbial growth.
C. *Cellular barriers*	Virus-infected cells secrete proteins called **interferons** which protect non-infected cells from further viral infection.

Which of them are correctly matched-

1. A

2. A and B

3. A and B

4. A, B, C

28. Read the following statements-

a) Our body produces IgA, IgM only.

b) Various antibodies are found in the blood and this immune response is also called as **humoral immune response**.

c) Humoral immunity is antibody mediated.

d) T cell-mediated immune response called **cell-mediated immunity** (CMI).

e) CMI shows important role in organ transplantation.

Which above statements are/is incorrect-

1. a and c only

2. a only

3. d and c only

4. a,b,c,d

29. Consider the following statements and find out incorrect one-

1. Grafts from just any source – an animal, another primate, or any human beings cannot be made since the grafts would be rejected sooner or later.

2. Tissue matching, blood group matching are essential before undertaking any graft/transplant and even after this the patient has to take immuno–suppresants all his/her life.

3. The humoral immune response is responsible for the graft rejection.

4. An antibody is represented as H_2L_2.

30. Read the following statements -

I. When a host is exposed to antigens, which may be in the form of living or dead microbes or other proteins, antibodies are produced in the host body. This type of immunity is called **active immunity.**

II. Active immunity is slow and takes time to give its full effective response.

III. Smoking also paves the way to hard drugs.

IV. Tobacco has been used by human beings for more than 400 years.

V. It is smoked, chewed or used as a snuff.

How many of them are/is correct –

1. five

2. two

3. three

4. one

31. Read the following statements and find out the correct option-

STATEMENT 1. When ready-made antibodies are directly given to protect the body against foreign agents, it is called **active immunity**.

STATEMENT 2. The yellowish fluid **colostrum** secreted by mother during the initial days of lactation has abundant antibodies (IgA) to protect the infant.

1. Both are wrong statements

2. Both are correct statements

3. Only statement 1 correct

4. Only statement 2 correct

32. Go through the following statement and find out the correct option-

ASSERTION(A). The foetus also receives some antibodies from their mother, through the placenta during pregnancy an examples of passive immunity.

REASON(R). When ready-made antibodies are directly given to protect the body against foreign agents, it is called **passive immunity**.

1. A correct and R is correct explanation of A

2. A correct and R is also correct but R is not correct explanation of A

3. A correct but R incorrect

4. A and R both are incorrect

33. Find out the incorrect option-

1. The principle of immunisation or vaccination is based on the property of 'memory' of the immune system.

2. In vaccination, a preparation of antigenic proteins of pathogen or inactivated/weakened pathogen (vaccine) are introduced into the body.

3. The antibodies produced in the body against antigens neutralise the pathogenic agents during actual infection.

4. The vaccines do not generate memory – B and T-cells that recognize the pathogen quickly on subsequent exposure and overwhelm the invaders with a massive production of antibodies.

34. Read the following statements-

a) If a person is infected with some deadly microbes to which quick immune response is required as in tetanus, we need to directly inject the preformed antibodies, or antitoxin (a preparation containing antibodies to the toxin).

b) Even in cases of snakebites, the injection which is given to the patients, contain preformed antibodies against the snake venom. This type of immunisation is called passive immunisation.

c) Recombinant DNA technology has allowed the production of antigenic polypeptides of pathogen in bacteria or yeast.

Which of the above statements is/are correct-

1. a only

2. b only

3. c, a only

4. a,b,c

35. Consider the following statements -

I. The exaggerated response of the immune system to certain antigens present in the environment is called **allergy**.

II. The substances to which such an immune response is produced are called allergens.

III. The antibodies produced to allergens are of IgE type.

IV. Common examples of allergens are mites in dust, pollens, animal dander, etc.

How many of above are/is correct-

1. three

2. four

3. two

4. one

36. Consider the following statements -

i. Symptoms of allergic reactions include sneezing, watery eyes, running nose and difficulty in breathing.

ii. Allergy is due to the release of chemicals like histamine and serotonin from the mast cells. For determining the cause of allergy, the patient is exposed to or injected with very small doses of possible allergens, and the reactions studied.

iii. The use of drugs like anti-histamine, adrenalin and steroids quickly not reduce the symptoms of allergy.

iv. The modern-day life style has resulted in lowering of immunity and more sensitivity to allergens – more and more children in metro cities of India suffer from allergies and asthma due to sensitivity to the environment.

Which above statements are correct-

1. i,ii only

2. i, ii,iv only

3. i,ii,iii only

4. all are correct

37. Read the following statements-

i. Coca alkaloid or **cocaine** is obtained from coca plant *Erythroxylum coca*, native to South America.

ii. It interferes with the transport of the neuro-transmitter dopamine.

iii. Cocaine, commonly called **coke** or **crack** is usually snorted.

iv. **Cocaine** has a potent stimulating action on **central nervous system**, producing a sense of euphoria and increased energy.

Which of the above statements is/are correct-

1. i and ii only

2. ii only

3. i and iii only

4. All are correct

38. Consider the following statements-

I. The human immune system consists of lymphoid organs, tissues, cells and soluble molecules like antibodies.

II. The immune system is unique in the sense that it recognises foreign antigens, responds to these and remembers them.

III. The immune system also plays an important role in allergic reactions, auto-immune diseases and organ transplantation.

IV. **In Lymphoid organs** origin and/or maturation and proliferation of lymphocytes occur.

V. The primary lymphoid organs are **bone marrow** and **thymus** where immature lymphocytes differentiate into antigen-sensitive lymphocytes.

VI. After maturation the lymphocytes migrate to secondary lymphoid organs like spleen, lymph nodes, tonsils, Peyer's patches of small intestine and appendix.

How many of above are/is correct-

1. three

2. four

3. two

4. six

39. Read the following statements and find out the correct option-

STATEMENT 1. Rheumatoid arthritis which affects many people in our society is an auto-immune disease.

STATEMENT 2. The immune system also plays an important role in allergic reactions, auto-immune diseases and organ transplantation.

1. Both are wrong statements

2. Both are correct statements

3. Only statement 1 correct

4. Only statement 2 correct

40. Read the following statements-

a) The primary lymphoid organs are **bone marrow** and **thymus** where immature lymphocytes differentiate into antigen-sensitive lymphocytes.

b) The secondary lymphoid organs provide the sites for interaction of lymphocytes with the antigen, which then proliferate to become effector cells.

c) The location of various lymphoid organs in the human body are different.

d) The bone marrow is the main lymphoid organ where all blood cells including lymphocytes are produced.

Which of the following are correct?

1. a and b only

2. b and c only

3. c and d only

4. a,b,c,d

41. Go through the following statements and find out the correct option-

ASSERTION(A). The thymus is quite large at the time of birth but keeps reducing in size with age and by the time puberty is attained it reduces to a very small size.

REASON(R). Both bone-marrow and thymus provide micro-environments for the development and maturation of T-lymphocytes.

1. A correct and R is correct explanation of A

2. A correct and R is also correct but R is not correct explanation of A

3. A correct but R incorrect

4. A and R both are incorrect

42. Read the following statements -

   I. The spleen is a large bean shaped organ.

   II. The spleen contains lymphocytes and phagocytes.

   III. The spleen acts as a filter of the blood by trapping blood-borne microorganisms.

   IV. Spleen also has a large reservoir of erythrocytes.

How many of above are/is correct-

1. three

2. four

3. two

4. one

43. Consider the following statements-

   I. The lymph nodes are small solid structures located at different points along the lymphatic system.

   II. Lymph nodes serve to trap the micro-organisms or other antigens, which happen to get into the lymph and tissue fluid.

   III. Antigens trapped in the lymph nodes are responsible for the activation of lymphocytes present there and cause the immune response.

   IV. The lymphoid tissues is also located within the lining of the major tracts (respiratory, digestive and urogenital tracts) called **mucosal associated lymphoid tissue** (MALT).

How many of them are/is correct-

1. one

2. three

3. four

4. two

44. Read the following statements and find out the correct option with respect to AIDS-

STATEMENT 1. AIDS was first reported in 1981 and in the last twenty-five years or so, it has spread all over the world killing more than 25 million persons.

STATEMENT 2. AIDS is caused by the Human Immuno deficiency Virus (HIV), a member of a group of viruses called **retrovirus**, which have an envelope enclosing the RNA genome.

1. Both are correct statements

2. Both are wrong statements

3. Only statement 1 correct

4. Only statement 2 correct

45. Which statements is incorrect -

1. **Opioids** are the drugs, which bind to specific opioid receptors present in our central nervous system only.

2. Morphine is a very effective sedative and painkiller, and given after surgery.

3. Heroin commonly called *smack* is chemically diacetylmorphine which is a white, odourless, bitter crystalline compound.

4. This is obtained by acetylation of morphine, which is extracted from the latex of poppy plant *Papaver somniferum.*

46. Read the following statements and find out the correct option

STATEMENT 1. Natural cannabinoids are obtained from the inflorescences of the plant *Cannabis sativa.*

STATEMENT 2. The flower tops, leaves and the resin of cannabis plant are used in various combinations to produce marijuana, hashish, charas and ganja.

1. Both are correct statements

2. Both are wrong statements.

3. Only statement 1 correct

4. Only statement 2 correct

47. Go through the following statement and find out the correct option-

ASSERTION(A). A widely used diagnostic test for AIDS is **enzyme linked immuno-sorbent assay** (ELISA).

REASON(R). In AIDS due to decrease in the number of helper T lymphocytes so the person starts suffering from infections due to bacteria especially *Mycobacterium*, viruses, fungi and even parasites like *Toxoplasma.*

1. A correct and R is correct explanation of A

2. A correct and R is also correct but R is not correct explanation of A

3. A. correct but R incorrect

4. A and R both are incorrect

48. Transmission of HIV-infection can occurs by-

(a) sexual contact with infected person,

(b) by transfusion of contaminated blood and blood products,

(c) by sharing infected needles as in the case of intravenous drug abusers

(d) from infected mother to her child through placenta.

How many of them are/is correct-

1. one

2. two

3. three

4. four

49. Consider the following statements -

A. AIDS has cure, but prevention is the best option.

B. The HIV infection, more often, spreads due to conscious behavior patterns and is not something that happens inadvertently, like pneumonia or typhoid.

C. Of course, infection in blood transfusion patients, new-borns (from mother) etc., may take place due to poor monitoring.

D. The only excuse may be ignorance and it has been rightly said – "don't die of ignorance".

E. In our country the National AIDS Control Organisation (NACO) and other non-governmental organisation (NGOs) are doing a lot to educate people about AIDS.

Which above statements are/is incorrect-

1. A only

2. D and E only

3. B and D only

4. All are correct

50. Read the following statements-

A. **Cancer** is one of the most dreaded diseases of human beings and is a major cause of death all over the globe.

B. More than a million Indians suffer from cancer and a large number of them die from it annually.

C. The mechanisms that underlie development of cancer or oncogenic transformation of cells, its treatment and control have been some of the most intense areas of research in biology and medicine.

D. In our body, cell growth and differentiation is highly controlled and regulated.

E. In cancer cells, there is breakdown of these regulatory mechanisms.

Which above statements are/is correct-

1. A and C only

2. D and A only

3. A,B,C,D only

4. A,**B**,C,D,E

MICROBES IN HUMAN WELFARE

14.1 Microbes in Household Products

14.2 Microbes in Industrial Products

14.3 Microbes in Sewage Treatment

14.4 Microbes in Production of Biogas

14.5 Microbes as Biocontrol Agents

14.6 Microbes as Biofertilisers

- **Microbes** are a very important component of life on earth.
- Not all microbes are **pathogenic**.
- **Many microbes** are very useful to human beings.

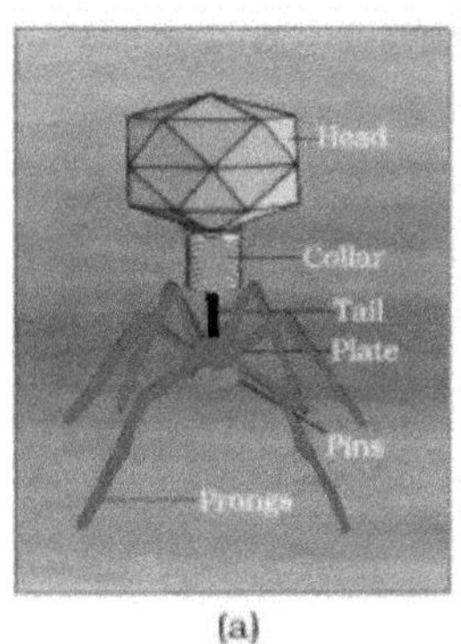

(a)

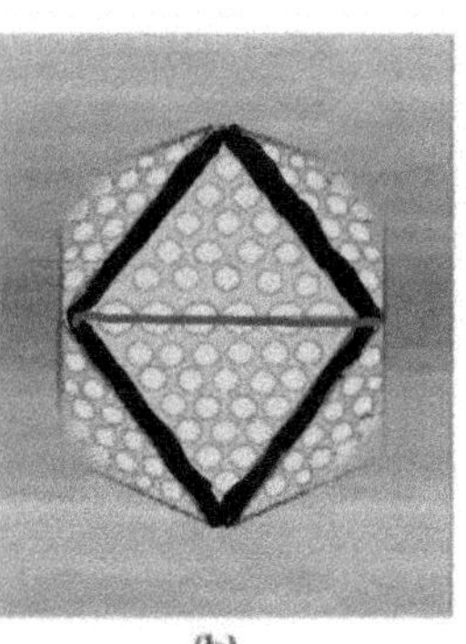
(b)

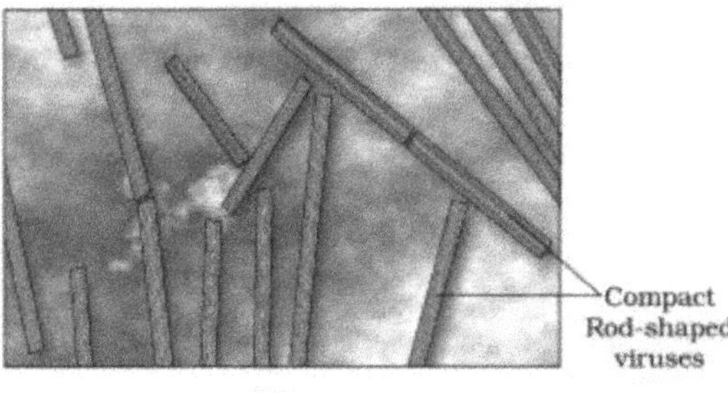

(c)

Viruses: (a) A bacteriophage; (b) Adenovirus which causes respiratory infections; (c) Rod-shaped Tobacco Mosaic Virus (TMV). Magnified about 1,00,000–1,50,000X

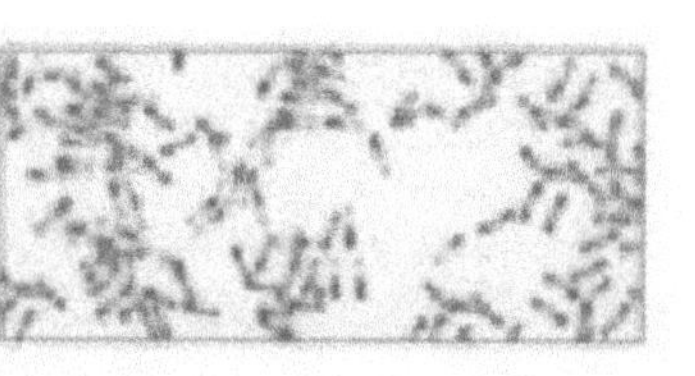
(a)

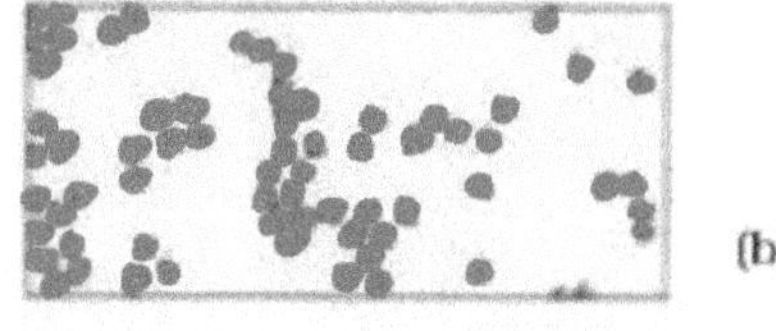
(b)

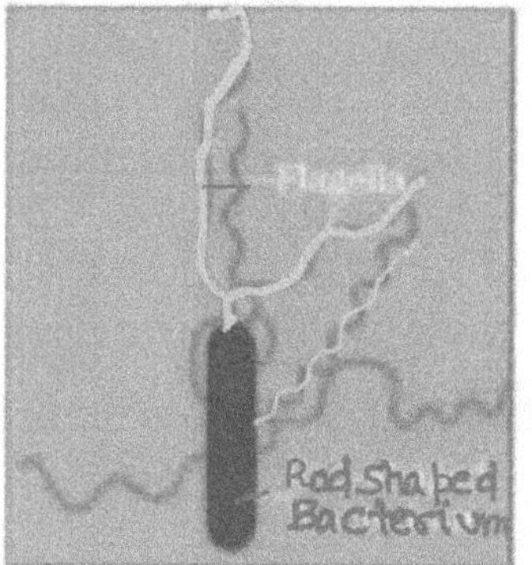

(c)

Bacteria: (a) Rod-shaped, magnified 1500X; (b) Spherical shaped, magnified 1500X; (c) A rod-shaped bacterium showing flagella, magnified 50,000X

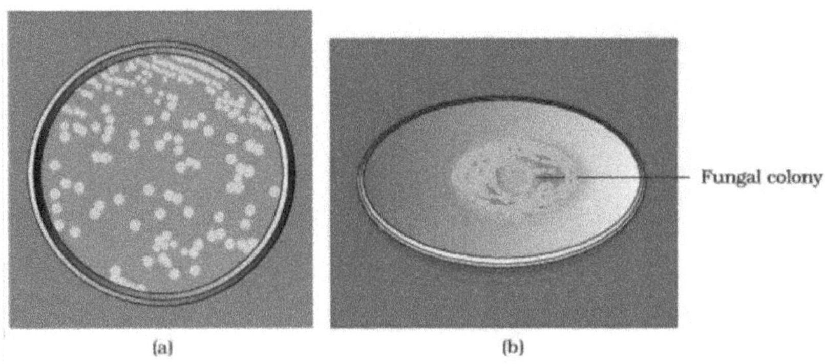

(a) Colonies of bacteria growing in a petri dish;
(b) Fungal colony growing in a petri dish

14.1 MICROBES IN HOUSEHOLD PRODUCTS

- We use microbes or products derived from them everyday.
- A common example is the production of curd from milk.

Lactic acid bacteria (LAB)

- Bacteria such as *Lactobacillus* and others commonly called **lactic acid bacteria (LAB)** grow in milk and convert it to curd.
- During growth, the LAB produce acids that coagulate and partially digest the milk proteins.
- A small amount of curd added to the fresh milk as inoculum or starter which contain millions of LAB.
- At suitable temperature LAB multiply so convert milk to curd.
- LAB improves nutritional quality of milk by increasing **vitamin B$_{12}$**.
- In our stomach too, the **LAB play very beneficial role** in checking disease causing microbes.

Baker's yeast (*Saccharomyces cerevisiae*)

- Similarly the dough, which is used for making bread, is fermented using **baker's yeast (*Saccharomyces cerevisiae*)**.
- The dough, which is used for making foods such as *dosa* and *idli* is also fermented by bacteria.
- The puffed-up appearance of dough is due to the production of CO_2 gas.

Toddy

- A number of traditional drinks and foods are also made by fermentation by the microbes.
- 'Toddy', a traditional drink of some parts of southern India.
- 'Toddy'is made by fermenting sap from palms(**Toddy palm - *Caryota urens***)
- Microbes are also used to ferment fish, **soyabean** and bamboo shoots to make foods.

Cheese

- **Cheese,** is one of the ancient food items in which microbes were used.
- Different varieties of cheese are known by their characteristic texture, flavour and taste, the specificity coming from the microbes used.

- The large holes in **'Swiss cheese'** are due to production of a large amount of CO_2 by a bacterium named ***Propionibacterium sharmanii.***

- **'Swiss cheese' also called hard cheese.**

- The **'Roquefort cheese'** are ripened by growing a specific fungi on them, which gives them a particular flavour.

- Roquefort cheese made with the help of ***Penicillium roqueforti.***

- Roquefort cheese is **semi hard cheese.**

14.2 MICROBES IN INDUSTRIAL PRODUCTS

- Even in industry, microbes are used to synthesise a number of products valuable to human beings. Beverages and antibiotics are some examples.

- Production on an industrial scale, requires growing microbes in very large vessels called **fermentors**.

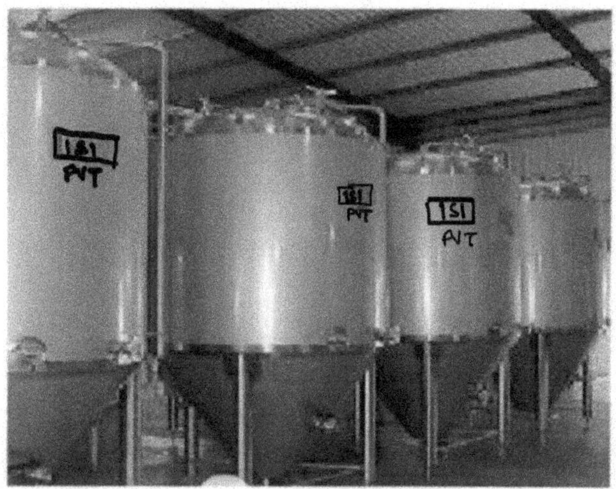

Fermentors

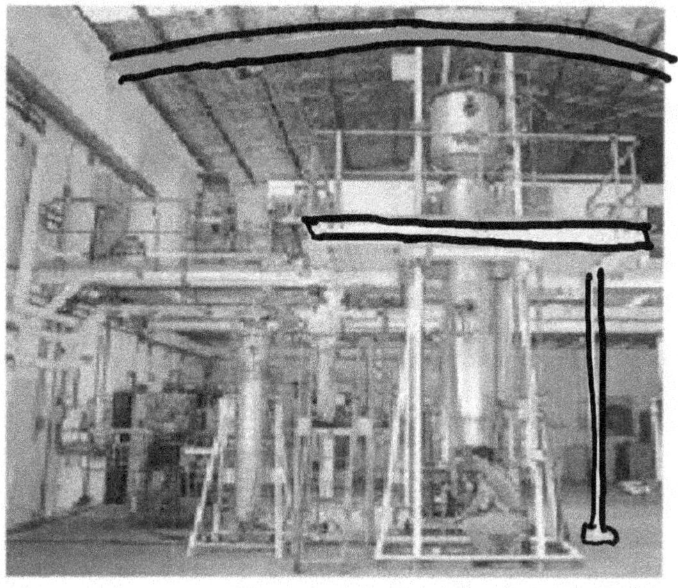

Fermentation Plant

14.2.1 Fermented Beverages

- Microbes, especially yeasts have been used from time immemorial for the production of beverages like **wine, beer, whisky, brandy or rum.**
- Wine contain 10-20% alcohol.
- Beer contain 3-6% alcohol.
- **Whisky, brandy or rum** contain higher percentage of alcohol (40-60%)
- For making fermented beverages **yeast *Saccharomyces cerevisiae* /brewer's yeast**, is used for fermenting malted cereals and fruit juices, to produce ethanol
- Depending on the type of the raw material used for fermentation and the type of processing (with or without distillation) different types of alcoholic drinks are obtained.
- **Wine and beer** are produced **without distillation.**
- **Whisky, brandy and rum** are produced **by distillation** of the fermented broth.

14.2.2 Antibiotics

- **Antibiotics** produced by microbes.
- Antibiotics term given by **Waksman(1942)**
- Antibiotics are regarded as one of the most significant discoveries of the twentieth century.
- Antibiotics gives great contribution in the welfare of the human society.
- ***Anti* is a Greek word** that means 'against', and *bio* means 'life', together they mean 'against life' (in the context of disease causing organisms); whereas with reference to human beings, they are 'pro life' and not against.
- Antibiotics are chemical substances, which are produced by some microbes and can kill or retard the growth of other (disease-causing) microbes.
- **The commonly used antibiotics are - Penicillin, Tetracycline etc.**

Discovery of Penicillin.

- **Penicillin** was the first antibiotic to be discovered, and it was a chance discovery.
- **Alexander Fleming** while working on *Staphylococci* bacteria, once observed a mould growing in one of his unwashed culture plates around which *Staphylococci* could not grow.
- **Alexander Fleming** found out that it was due to a chemical produced by the mould and he named it Penicillin after the mould *Penicillium notatum.*
- The full potential as an effective antibiotic was established much later by **Ernest Chain and Howard Florey.**
- This antibiotic was extensively used to treat American soldiers wounded in **World War II.**

The Nobel Prize

- Fleming, Chain and Florey were awarded the Nobel Prize in 1945, for the discovery of **Penicillin.**

Points to remember-

- After Penicillin, other antibiotics were also purified from other microbes.

- Antibiotics have greatly improved our capacity to treat deadly diseases such as **plague, whooping cough (*kali khansi*), diphtheria (*gal ghotu*) and leprosy (*kusht rog*)** etc.

14.2.3 Chemicals, Enzymes and other Bioactive Molecules

- Microbes are also used for commercial and industrial production of certain chemicals like organic acids, alcohols and enzymes.

I. Chemicals

- Examples of acid producers fungi and bacteria are-
  - ➢ *Aspergillus niger* **(a fungus) of citric acid**
  - ➢ *Acetobacter aceti* **(a bacterium) of acetic acid**
  - ➢ *Clostridium butylicum* **(a bacterium) of butyric acid**
  - ➢ *Lactobacillus* **(a bacterium) of lactic acid.**
- **Yeast (*Saccharomyces cerevisiae*)** is used for commercial production of ethanol.

II. Enzymes

- Microbes are also used for production of enzymes.

a. Lipases

- **Lipases** are used in detergent formulations.
- **Lipases** are helpful in **removing oily stains** from the laundry.

b. Pectinases and **proteases.**

- **The bottled fruit juices** bought from the market are clearer as compared to those made at home.
- **The bottled juices** are clarified by the use of **pectinases** and **proteases.**

c. Streptokinase

- **Streptokinase** produced by the bacterium *Streptococcus.*
- The bacterium *Streptococcus* modified by genetic engineering is used as a 'clot buster' for removing clots from the blood vessels of patients.
- **Streptokinase used to treat** myocardial infraction leading to heart attack.

III. Bioactive Molecules

a. Cyclosporin A

- **Cyclosporin A**, used in organ-transplant patients, is produced by the fungus *Trichoderma polysporum.*
- **Cyclosporin A**,that is used as an immunosuppressive agent.

b. Statins

- **Statins** produced by the yeast *Monascus purpureus.*
- **Statins** have been commercialised as blood-cholesterol lowering agents.
- **Statins** acts by competitively inhibiting the enzyme responsible for synthesis of cholesterol.
- **Statins** acts by competitively inhibiting to the enzyme HMG CoA reductase.

14.3 MICROBES IN SEWAGE TREATMENT

- **The large quantities** of waste water are generated everyday in cities and towns.
- A major component of this waste water is human excreta.
- **This municipal waste-water** is also called sewage.
- Sewage contains large amounts of organic matter and microbes.
- Many microbes are pathogenic found in sewage.
- This cannot be discharged into natural water bodies like rivers and streams directly.
- Before disposal, hence, sewage is treated in sewage treatment plants (STPs) to make it less polluting.
- Treatment of waste water is done by the heterotrophic microbes naturally present in the sewage.

Stages in sewage treatment

- The sewage treatment is carried out in two stages:

  i.Primary treatment

  ii.Secondary treatment / Biological treatment

i.Primary treatment:

- These treatment steps basically involve physical removal of particles – large and small – from the sewage through filtration and sedimentation.
- These are removed in stages; initially, floating debris is removed by sequential filtration.
- Then the **grit (soil and small pebbles)** are removed by sedimentation.
- All solids that settle form the **primary sludge,** and the supernatant forms the effluent.
- The effluent from the **primary settling tank** is taken for secondary treatment.

ii.Secondary treatment (Biological treatment):

- **The primary effluent** is passed into large aeration tanks where it is constantly agitated mechanically and air is pumped into it.
- This allows vigorous growth of useful aerobic microbes into **flocs** (masses of bacteria associated with fungal filaments to form mesh like structures).
- While growing, these microbes consume the major part of the organic matter in the effluent.
- This significantly reduces the **BOD (biochemical oxygen demand)** of the effluent.

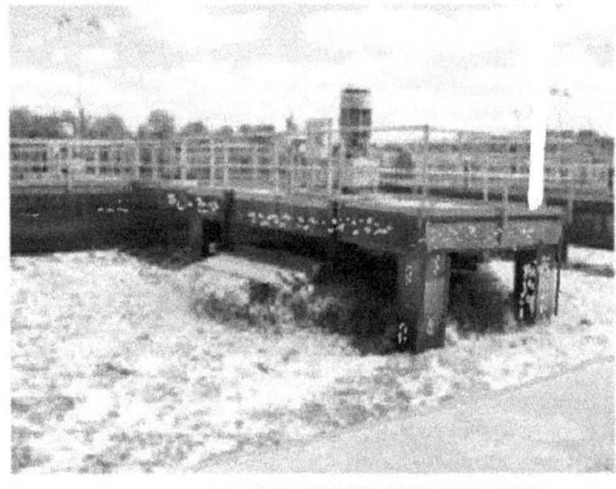

Secondary treatment

BOD (biochemical oxygen demand)

- **BOD** refers to the amount of the oxygen that would be consumed if all the organic matter in one liter of water were oxidised by bacteria.

- The sewage water is treated till the BOD is reduced.

- The **BOD** test measures the rate of uptake of oxygen by micro-organisms in a sample of water.

- Indirectly, **BOD** is a measure of the organic matter present in the water.

- The greater the **BOD** of waste water, more is its polluting potential.

- If the **BOD** of sewage or waste water is reduced significantly, the effluent is then passed into a settling tank where **the bacterial 'flocs'** are allowed to sediment.

- This sediment is called **activated sludge**.

Activated sludge

- A small part of the activated sludge is pumped back into the aeration tank to serve as the inoculum.

- The remaining major part of the sludge is pumped into large tanks called **anaerobic sludge digesters**. Here, other kinds of bacteria, which grow **anaerobically,** digest the bacteria and the fungi in the sludge.

- During this digestion, bacteria produce a mixture of gases such as **methane, hydrogen sulphide and carbon dioxide**.

Biogas/Gobar gas

- The mixture of gases such as **methane, hydrogen sulphide and carbon dioxide** called as biogas.

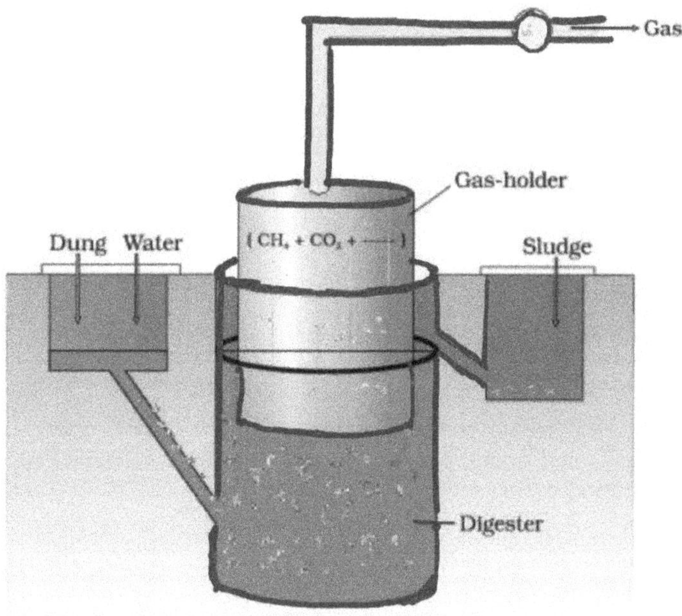

A typical biogas plant

- The **biogas** and can be used as source of energy as it is inflammable.

- **The effluent from the secondary treatment** plant is generally released into natural water bodies like rivers and streams.

- **The microbes play** a major role in treating millions of gallons of waste water everyday across the globe.

- **This methodology to produce biogas** has been practiced for more than a century now, in almost all parts of the world.
- **Till date, no manmade technology** has been able to rival the microbial treatment of sewage.
- Due to increasing urbanisation, sewage is being produced in much larger quantities than ever before.
- **The number of sewage treatment plants** has not increased enough to treat such large quantities.
- So the untreated sewage is often discharged directly into rivers leading to their pollution and increase in **water-borne diseases.**

Ganga Action Plan and Yamuna Action Plan

- The Ministry of Environment and Forests has initiated **Ganga Action Plan** and **Yamuna Action Plan** to save these major rivers of our country from pollution.
- **Ganga Action Plan launched by former P.M. Rajiv Gandhi in 1986 to reduce the pollution load in River.**
- Under these plans, it is proposed to build a large number of sewage treatment plants so that only treated sewage may be discharged in the rivers.

14.4 Microbes in Production of Biogas

Compostion of Biogas

- **Biogas is a mixture of gases (containing predominantly methane)** produced by the microbial activity and which may be used as fuel.
- The microbes produce different types of gaseous end-products during growth and metabolism.
- The main gas produced is **CO_2.**
- Some bacteria, which grow anaerobically on cellulosic material, produce large amount of methane along with **CO_2 and H_2.**

Bacteria involved in Biogas Production

- These anaerobically growing bacteria are collectively called **methanogens**, and one such common bacterium is *Methanobacterium.*
- *Methanobacterium* commonly found in the anaerobic sludge during sewage treatment.
- These bacteria are also present in the rumen (a part of stomach) of cattle.
- **A lot of cellulosic material present** in the food of cattle is also present in the rumen.
- In rumen, these bacteria help in the breakdown of cellulose and play an important role in the nutrition of cattle.
- Thus, the excreta (dung) of cattle, commonly called *gobar*, is rich in these bacteria.
- Dung can be used for generation of biogas, commonly **called *gobar gas.***

Structure of Biogas Plant

- The **biogas** plant consists of a concrete tank (**10-15 feet deep**) in which bio-wastes are collected and a slurry of dung is fed.

- **A floating cover** is placed over the slurry, which keeps on rising as the gas is produced in the tank due to the microbial activity.

- **The biogas plant** has an outlet, which is connected to a pipe to supply biogas to nearby houses.

- The spent slurry is removed through another outlet and may be used as fertiliser.

Biogas Plant Found in Rural Areas

- **Cattle dung is available** in large quantities in rural areas where cattle are used for a variety of purposes.

- So biogas plants are mostly build in **rural areas.**

- The biogas thus produced is used for **cooking and lighting.**

Development of Biogas

- The technology of biogas production was developed in India mainly due to the efforts of **Indian Agricultural Research Institute (IARI)** and **Khadi and Village Industries Commission (KVIC).**

14.5 MICROBES AS BIOCONTROL AGENTS

- **Biocontrol** refers to the use of biological methods for controlling plant diseases and pests.

- In modern society, these problems have been tackled increasingly by the use of chemicals – by use of **insecticides and pesticides.**

- **These chemicals are toxic** and extremely harmful, to human beings and animals alike, and have been polluting our environment (soil, ground water), fruits, vegetables and crop plants.

- **Our soil is also polluted through** our use of weedicides to remove weeds.

Biological control of pests and diseases:

- **In agriculture,** there is a method of controlling pests that relies on natural predation rather than introduced chemicals.

- **A key belief** of the organic farmer is that biodiversity furthers health.

- **The organic farmer,** therefore, works to create a system where the insects that are sometimes called pests are not eradicated, but instead are kept at manageable levels by a complex system of checks and balances within a **living and vibrant ecosystem.**

- **Contrary to the** 'conventional' farming practices which often use chemical methods to kill both useful and harmful life forms indiscriminately, this is a **holistic approach** that seeks to develop an understanding of the webs of interaction between the myriad of organisms that constitute the field fauna and flora.

- **The organic farmer holds** the view that the eradication of the creatures that are often described as pests is not only possible, but also undesirable, for without them the **beneficial predatory and parasitic insects** which depend upon them as food or hosts would not be able to survive.

- **The use of biocontrol** measures will greatly reduce our dependence on toxic chemicals and pesticides.

- **An important part** of the biological farming approach is to become familiar with the various life forms that inhabit the field, predators as well as pests, and also their life cycles, patterns of feeding and the habitats that they prefer will help develop appropriate means of biocontrol.

a. Bacillus thuringiensis

- An example of microbial biocontrol agents that can be introduced in order to control butterfly caterpillars is the bacteria *Bacillus thuringiensis* **(often written as *Bt*).**
- **These are available** in sachets as dried spores which are mixed with water and sprayed onto vulnerable plants such as brassicas and fruit trees, where these are eaten by the insect larvae.
- **In the gut of the larvae,** the toxin is released and the larvae get killed.
- **The bacterial disease** will kill the caterpillars, but leave other insects unharmed.
- Because of the development of methods of genetic engineering in the last decade or so, the scientists have introduced *B. thuringiensis* **toxin genes** into plants. Such plants are resistant to attack by insect pests.
- **Bt-cotton** is one such example, which is being cultivated in some states of our country.

b. The Ladybird, and Dragonflies

- The very familiar beetle with red and black markings – **the Ladybird, and Dragonflies** are useful to get rid of **aphids and mosquitoes**, respectively.

c. Trichoderma

- A biological control being developed for use in the treatment of plant disease is the fungus *Trichoderma.*
- *Trichoderma* species are free-living fungi that are very common in the root ecosystems.
- They are effective biocontrol agents of several plant pathogens.

d. Baculoviruses

- **Baculoviruses** are pathogens that attack insects and other arthropods.
- The majority of baculoviruses used as biological control agents are in the genus *Nucleopolyhedrovirus.*
- **Baculoviruses** viruses are excellent candidates for species-specific, narrow spectrum insecticidal applications.
- **Baculoviruses** shows no negative impacts on plants, mammals, birds, fish or even on non-target insects.
- **Baculoviruses** is especially desirable when beneficial insects are being conserved to aid in an overall **integrated pest management (IPM) programme**, or when an ecologically sensitive area is being treated.

14.6 Microbes as Biofertilisers

- **The use of the chemical fertilisers** to meet the ever-increasing demand of agricultural produce has contributed significantly causes pollution.
- The problems associated with the over use of chemical fertilisers creates a large pressure to switch to **organic farming** – by the use of **biofertilisers.**
- **Biofertilisers** are organisms that enrich the nutrient quality of the soil.
- The main sources of biofertilisers are **bacteria, fungi and cyanobacteria.**

a. Bacteria

- **The root nodules of leguminous plants** form symbiotic association with *Rhizobium* bacteria has nitrogen fixating ability.

- **They converts atmospheric nitrogen** into organic forms, which is used by the plant as nutrient.

- Other bacteria can fix atmospheric nitrogen while free-living in the soil (examples *Azospirillum, Azotobacter*), thus enriching the nitrogen content of the soil.

b. Fungi

- Fungi are also known to form symbiotic associations with plants called **mycorrhiza**.

- Many members of the genus *Glomus* form mycorrhiza.

- **The fungal symbiont** helps to absorb phosphorus from soil and passes it to the plant.

- Plants having such associations show other benefits also, such as resistance to **root-borne pathogens, tolerance to salinity and drought,** and an overall increase in plant growth and development.

c. Cyanobacteria

- *The* **cyanobacteria** are autotrophic microbes widely distributed in aquatic and terrestrial environments many of which can fix atmospheric nitrogen, e.g. *Anabaena, Nostoc, Oscillatoria,* etc.

- In paddy fields, cyanobacteria serve as an **important biofertiliser.**

- Blue green algae increases organic matter **so increase fertility of the soil.**

- Presently, in our country, a number of **biofertilisers** are available commercially in the market and farmers use these regularly in their fields to replenish soil nutrients and to reduce dependence on chemical fertilisers.

1. Consider the following statements and find out the correct option-

A. Micro-organisms such as *Lactobacillus* and others commonly called **lactic acid bacteria (LAB)** grow in milk and convert it to curd.

B. During growth, the LAB produce acids that coagulate and partially digest the milk proteins.

C. A small amount of curd added to the fresh milk as inoculum or starter contain millions of LAB, which at suitable temperatures multiply, thus converting milk to curd, which also improves its nutritional quality by increasing vitamin B_{12}.

D. In our stomach the LAB play very beneficial role in checking disease causing microbes.

Which of the above are correct -

1. A,B,C

2. B,C

3. D,B,A

4. B,C,D

2. Match the list 1 and 2-

List 1   List 2

List 1	List 2
a. Aspergillus niger	j. bread making
b. Saccharomyces cerevisiae	k. statin
c. Monascus purpureus	l. citric acid
d. *Trichoderma polysporum.*	m. immunosupreesive

Find out the correct option –

1. a.k, b.j, c.l, d.m

2. a.k,b.l,c.j,d.m

3. a.l,b.j,c.k,d.m

4. a.l,b.j,c.m,d.k

3. Consider the following statements-

a) BOD refers to the amount of the oxygen that would be consumed if all the organic matter in one liter of water were oxidised by bacteria.

b) The sewage water is treated till the BOD is reduced.

c) The BOD test measures the rate of uptake of oxygen by micro-organisms in a sample of water and thus, indirectly, BOD is a measure of the organic matter present in the water.

d) The greater the BOD of waste water, more is its polluting potential.

e) Once the BOD of sewage or waste water is reduced significantly, the effluent is then passed into a settling tank where the bacterial 'flocs' are allowed to sediment.

Which of the above are/is correct -

1. only a and d

2. a,b,c,e

3. only c and d

4. all are correct

4. Consider the following statements-

a) A small part of the activated sludge is pumped back into the aeration tank to serve as the inoculum.

b) The remaining major part of the sludge is pumped into large tanks called **anaerobic sludge digesters**. Here, other kinds of bacteria, which grow anaerobically, digest the bacteria and the fungi in the sludge.

c) During this digestion, bacteria produce a mixture of gases such as methane, hydrogen sulphide and carbon dioxide.

d) These gases form **biogas** and can be used as source of energy as it is non inflammable.

e) The effluent from the secondary treatment plant is generally released into natural water bodies like rivers and streams.

Which of the above are/is incorrect -

1. d

2. a,b

3. b,d

4. e

5. Consider the following statements and find out the correct option-

STATEMENT 1. A number of traditional drinks and foods are made by fermentation by the microbes. 'Toddy', a traditional drink of some parts of southern India is made by fermenting sap from palms.

STATEMENT 2. Microbes are also used to ferment fish, soyabean and bamboo shoots to make foods.

1. Both are correct statements

2. Only Statement 1 correct

3. Both are wrong statements

4. Only statement 2 correct

6. Go through the following statements-

ASSERTION(A). The large holes in 'Swiss cheese' are due to production of a large amount of CO_2 by a bacterium named *Propionibacterium sharmanii*.

REASON(R). *Propionibacterium sharmanii* generally enter the small intestine through food and water contaminated with them and migrate to other organs through blood.

1. A correct and R is correct explanation of A

2. A correct and R is also correct but R is not correct explanation of A

3. A correct but R incorrect

4. A and R both are incorrect

7. Find out the incorrect statement-

1. A small amount of curd added to the fresh milk as inoculum or starter contain millions of LAB, which at suitable temperatures multiply, thus converting milk to curd, which also improves its nutritional quality by increasing vitamin B_{12}.

2. In our stomach the LAB play very beneficial role in checking diseasecausing microbes.

3. The dough, which is used for making foods such as *dosa* and *idli* is also fermented by bacteria.

4. The puffed-up appearance of dough is due to the production of O_2 gas.

8. Go through the following statements-

I. The dough, which is used for making bread, is fermented using baker's yeast (*Saccharomyces cerevisiae*).

II. A number of traditional drinks and foods are also made by fermentation by the microbes. 'Toddy', a traditional drink of some parts of southern India is made by fermenting sap from palms.

III. Microbes are also used to ferment fish, soyabean and bamboos hoots to make foods.

IV. Cheese, is one of the old food items in which microbes were used.

V. Different varieties of cheese are known by their characteristic texture, flavour and taste, the specificity coming from the microbes used.

How many of them are correct -

1. two

2. three

3. four

4. five

9. Match the list 1 and 2-

List 1　　　　　　　　List 2

a. Streptokinase	produced by the bacterium *Streptococcus* and modified by genetic engineering is used as a 'clot buster' for removing clots from the blood vessels of patients who have undergone myocardial infraction leading to heart attack.
b. Flocs	masses of bacteria associated with fungal filaments to form mesh like structures

c. Baculoviruses	are pathogens that attack insects and other arthropods.
d. *Trichoderma*	species are free-living fungi that are very common in the root ecosystems.

How many of them are correctly matched–

1. one

2. two

3. three

4. four

10. Consider the following statements and find out the correct option

STATEMENT 1. The 'Roquefort cheese' are ripened by growing a specific fungi on them, which gives them a particular flavour.

STATEMENT 2. Production on an industrial scale, requires growing microbes in very large vessels called **fermentors**

1. Both are wrong statements

2. Only Statement 1 correct

3. Both are correct statements

4. Only statement 2 correct

11. Read the following statements very carefully and find out the correct-

a) Microbes especially yeasts have been used from time immemorial for the production of beverages like wine, beer, whisky, brandy or rum.

b) For this purpose the yeast *Saccharomyces cerevisiae* used for bread-making and commonly called brewer's yeast, is used for fermenting malted cereals and fruit juices, to produce ethanol

c) Depending on the type of the raw material used for fermentation and the type of processing (with or without distillation) different types of alcoholic drinks are obtained.

d) Wine and beer are produced without distillation whereas whisky, brandy and rum are produced by distillation of the fermented broth.

Which of the above statements is/are correct?

1. a and c both

2. b only

3. a,b,c,d

4. b and c only

12. Go through the following statements-

ASSERTION(A). Antibiotics produced by microbes are regarded as one of the most significant discoveries of the twentieth century and have greatly contributed towards the welfare of the human society.

REASON(R). *Anti* is a Latin word that means 'against', and *bio* means 'life', together they mean 'against life' (in the context of disease causing organisms); whereas with reference to human beings, they are 'pro life' and not against.

1. A correct and R is correct explanation of A

2. A correct and R is also correct but R is not correct explanation of A

3. A correct but R incorrect

4. A and R both are incorrect

13. Find out incorrect statement -

1. Antibiotics are chemical substances, which are produced by some microbes and can kill or retard the growth of other (disease-causing) microbes.

2. Alexander Fleming while working on *Staphylococci* fungus, once observed a mould growing in one of his unwashed culture plates around which *Staphylococci* could not grow.

3. Alexander Fleming found out that it was due to a chemical produced by the mould and he named it Penicillin after the mould *Penicillium notatum.*

4. However, its full potential as an effective antibiotic was established much later by Ernest Chain and Howard Florey.

14. Find out incorrect statement –

1. Antibiotic was extensively used to treat American soldiers wounded in World War II.

2. Fleming, Chain and Florey were awarded the Nobel Prize in 1745.

3. After Penicillin, other antibiotics were also purified from other microbe.

4. Antibiotics have greatly improved our capacity to treat deadly diseases such as plague, whooping cough (*kali khansi*), diphtheria (*gal ghotu*) and leprosy (*kusht rog*), which used to kill millions all over the globe.

15. Consider the following statements and find out the correct option

STATEMENT 1. Lipases are used in detergent formulations and are helpful in removing oily stains from the laundry.

STATEMENT 2. The bottled fruit juices bought from the market are clearer as compared to those made at home.

1. Both are wrong statements

2. Only statement 1 correct

3. Both are correct statements

4. Only statement 2 correct

16. Consider the following -

a) Streptokinase produced by the bacterium *Streptococcus* and modified by genetic engineering is used as a 'clot buster' for removing clots from the blood vessels of patients who have undergone myocardial infraction leading to heart attack.

b) A bioactive molecule, cyclosporin A, that is used as an immunosuppressive agent in organ-transplant patients, is produced by the fungus *Trichoderma polysporum.*

c) Yeast (*Saccharomyces cerevisiae*) is used for commercial production of ethanol.

d) Lipases are not used in detergent formulations and are helpful in removing oily stains from the laundry.

Which of the above statement are/is incorrect?

1. b and d only

2. c and d only

3. d only

4. a,b,c

17. Consider the following -

a) The bottled fruit juices bought from the market are clearer as compared to those made at home.

b) The bottled juices are clarified by the use of pectinases and proteases.

c) Streptokinase produced by the bacterium *Streptococcus* and modified by genetic engineering is used as a 'clot buster' for removing clots from the blood vessels of patients who have undergone myocardial infraction leading to heart attack.

d) A bioactive molecule, cyclosporin A, that is used as an immunosuppressive agent in organ-transplant patients, is produced by the fungus *Trichoderma polysporum*.

Which of the above statements are/is correct?

1. b and a only

2. c and b only

3. d and a only

4. a,b,c,d

18. Consider the following statements -

I. A number of traditional drinks and foods are also made by fermentation by the microbes. 'Toddy', a traditional drink of some parts of southern India is made by fermenting sap from palms.

II. Microbes are also used to ferment fish, soyabean and bambooshoots to make foods.

III. Cheese, is one of the oldest food items in which microbes were used.

IV. Different varieties of cheese are known by their characteristic texture, flavour and taste, the specificity coming from the microbes used.

V. The large holes in 'Swiss cheese' are due to production of a large amount of CO_2 by a bacterium named *Propionibacterium sharmanii*

VI. The 'Roquefort cheese' are ripened by growing a specific fungi on them, which gives them a particular flavour.

How many of them is/are correct-

1. one

2. two

3. three

4. six

19. Consider the following statements -

I. BOD refers to the amount of the oxygen that would be consumed if all the organic matter in one liter of water were oxidised by bacteria.

II. The sewage water is treated till the BOD is reduced.

III. The BOD test measures the rate of uptake of oxygen by micro-organisms in a sample of water and thus, indirectly, BOD is a measure of the organic matter present in the water.

IV. The greater the BOD of waste water, more is its polluting potential.

How many of them are/is correct -

1. one

2. two

3. three

4. four

20. Read the following statements-

a) The primary effluent is passed into large aeration tanks where it is constantly agitated mechanically and air is pumped into it.

b) This allows vigorous growth of useful aerobic microbes into **flocs** (masses of bacteria associated with fungal filaments to form mesh like structures).

c) While growing, these microbes consume the major part of the organic matter in the effluent.

d) This significantly reduces the **BOD (biochemical oxygen demand)** of the effluent.

How many of them are/is correct **statements-**

1. two

2. three

3. four

4. one

21. Consider the following statements and find out the correct option -

STATEMENT 1. This municipal waste-water is also called sewage. It contains large amounts of organic matter and microbes. Many of which are pathogenic.

STATEMENT 2. Before disposal sewage is treated in sewage treatment plants (STPs) to make it less polluting.

1. Both are wrong statements

2. Only Statement 1 correct

3. Both are correct statements

4. Only statement 2 correct

22. Go through the following statements and find out the correct option-

ASSERTION(A). Statins produced by the yeast *Monascus purpureus* have been commercialised as blood-cholesterol lowering agents.

REASON(R). It acts by competitively inhibiting the enzyme responsible for synthesis of cholesterol.

1. A correct and R is correct explanation of A

2. A correct and R is also correct but R is not correct explanation of A

3. A. correct but R incorrect

4. A and R both are incorrect

23. **Go through the following statements and find out the correct option-**

    A. A small part of the activated sludge is pumped back into the aeration tank to serve as the inoculum.

    B. The remaining major part of the sludge is pumped into large tanks called **anaerobic sludge digesters**. Here, other kinds of bacteria, which grow anaerobically, digest the bacteria and the fungi in the sludge.

    C. During this digestion, bacteria produce a mixture of gases such as methane, hydrogen sulphide and carbon dioxide.

    D. These above gases form **biogas** and can be used as source of energy as it is inflammable.

    Which of the above statement are correct -

    1. A,B,C only

    2. C and D only

    3. D and A only

    4. All are correct

24. **Read the statements given below-**

    A. In the examples cited in relation to fermentation of dough, cheese making and production of beverages, the main gas produced was CO_2.. However, certain bacteria, which grow anaerobically on cellulosic material, produce large amount of methane along with CO_2 and H_2.

    B. These bacteria are collectively called **methanogens**, and one such common bacterium is *Methanobacterium*.

    C. *Methanobacterium* bacteria are commonly found in the aerobic sludge during sewage treatment.

    D. *Methanobacterium* bacteria are also present in the rumen (a part of stomach) of cattle.

    Which of the above statement are/is incorrect?

    1. A and C only

    2. C only

    3. D and A only

    4. A,B,C,D

25. **Read the statements given below-**

    A. The biogas plant has an outlet, which is connected to a pipe to supply biogas to nearby houses.

    B. The spent slurry is removed through another outlet and may be used as fertiliser.

    C. Cattle dung is available in large quantities in rural areas where cattle are used for a variety of purposes.

    D. Biogas plants are build in rural areas.

    E. The biogas is used for cooking and lighting.

Which of the above statement are/is correct?

1. A and C only

2. A,B,C,D

3. D and C only

4. A,B,C,D,E

26. Consider the following statements-

I. Biocontrol refers to the use of biological methods for controlling plant diseases and pests.

II. In modern society, these problems have been increasingly by the use of chemicals – by use of insecticides and pesticides.

III. These chemicals are toxic and extremely harmful, to human beings and animals alike, and have been polluting our environment (soil, ground water), fruits, vegetables and crop plants.

IV. Our soil is also polluted through our use of chemical weedicides to remove weeds.

How many of them are/is correct-

1. one

2. two

3. three

4. four

27. Match the list 1 and 2-

List 1   List 2

A. The example of methanogens	*Methanobacterium.*
B. The biogas plant	consists of a concrete tank (10-15 cm deep) in which bio-wastes are collected and a slurry of dung is fed.
C. Mycorrhiza	symbiotic associations with plant roots

Which of them are/is correctly matched-

1. A

2. A and B

3. A and C

4. A, B, C

28. Read the following statements-

a) The municipal waste-water is also called sewage.

b) It contains large amounts of organic matter and microbes.

c) Many of microbes in sewage are pathogenic.

d) Before disposal sewage is treated in sewage treatment plants (STPs) to make it less polluting.

Which of the above statements are/is correct-

1. a and c only

2. a only

3. d and c only

4. a,b,c,d

29. Consider the following statements and find out incorrect one-

1. The organic farmer works to create a system where the insects that are sometimes called pests are not eradicated, but instead are kept at manageable levels by a complex system of checks and balances within a living and vibrant ecosystem.

2. Contrary to the 'conventional' farming practices which often use chemical methods to kill both useful and harmful life forms indiscriminately, this is a holistic approach that seeks to develop an understanding of the webs of interaction between the myriad of organisms that constitute the field fauna and flora.

3. The organic farmer holds the view that the eradication of the creatures that are often described as pests is not only possible, but also undesirable, for without them the beneficial predatory and parasitic insects which depend upon them as food or hosts would not be able to survive.

4. The use of biocontrol measures will greatly increases our dependence on toxic chemicals and pesticides.

30. Read the following -

I. An important part of the biological farming approach is to become familiar with the various life forms that inhabit the field, predators as well as pests, and also their life cycles, patterns of feeding and the habitats that they prefer.

II. The above point will help develop appropriate means of biocontrol.

III. The very familiar beetle with red and black markings – the Ladybird, and Dragonflies are useful to get rid of aphids and mosquitoes, respectively.

IV. An example of microbial biocontrol agents that can be introduced in order to control butterfly caterpillars is the bacteria *Bacillus thuringiensis* (often written as *Bt*).

How many of them are/is correct –

1. four

2. two

3. three

4. one

31. Read the following statements and find out the correct option-

STATEMENT 1. *Bacillus thuringiensis* are available in sachets as dried spores which are mixed with water and sprayed onto vulnerable plants such as brassicas and fruit trees, where these are eaten by the insect larvae.

STATEMENT 2. When the spore are eaten by insect larvae, the toxin is released and the larvae become resistant.

1. Both are wrong statements

2. Both are correct statements

3. Only statement 1 correct

4. Only statement 2 correct

32. Go through the following statements and find out the correct option-

ASSERTION(A). A biological control being developed for use in the treatment of plant disease is the fungus *Trichoderma.*

REASON(R). *Trichoderma* species are free-living fungi that are very common in the root ecosystems.

1. A correct and R is correct explanation of A

2. A correct and R is also correct but R is not correct explanation of A

3. A correct but R incorrect

4. A and R both are incorrect

33. Find out the incorrect option-

1. *Trichoderma* species are free-living fungi that are very common in the root ecosystems.

2. They are effective biocontrol agents of several plant pathogens.

3. Baculoviruses are pathogens that attack insects and other arthropods.

4. The majority of baculoviruses used as biological control agents are in the genus *Trichoderma.*

34. Read the following statements-

a) The use of the chemical fertilisers to meet the ever-increasing demand of agricultural produce has contributed significantly to this pollution.

b) There are problems associated with the overuse of chemical fertilisers and there is a large pressure to switch to **organic farming** – to use of **biofertilisers.**

c) Biofertilisers are organisms that enrich the nutrient quality of the soil.

Which of the above statements is/are correct-

1. a only

2. b only

3. c, a only

4. a,b,c

35. Consider the following statements -

I. The main sources of biofertilisers are bacteria, fungi and cyanobacteria.

II. The nodules on the roots of leguminous plants formed by the symbiotic association of *Rhizobium.*

III. *Rhizobium* bacteria fix atmospheric nitrogen into organic forms, which is used by the plant as nutrient. Other bacteria can fix atmospheric nitrogen while free-living in the soil (examples *Azospirillum* and *Azotobacter*), thus enriching the nitrogen content of the soil.

IV. Fungi are also known to form symbiotic associations with plants (**mycorrhiza**).

How many of above are/is correct-

1. three

2. four

3. two

4. one

36. Consider the following statements -

i. Many members of the genus *Glomus* form mycorrhiza.

ii. The fungal symbiont in these associations absorbs phosphorus from soil and passes it to the plant.

iii. Plants having such associations show other benefits also, such as resistance to root-borne pathogens, tolerance to salinity and drought, and an overall increase in plant growth and development.

iv. Cyanobacteria are autotrophic microbes widely distributed in aquatic and terrestrial environments many of which can fix atmospheric nitrogen, e.g. *Anabaena, Nostoc, Oscillatoria,* etc.

v. In paddy fields, cyanobacteria serve as an important biofertiliser.

vi. Blue green algae also add organic matter to the soil and increase its fertility.

Which above statements are correct-

1. i,ii only

2. i, ii,iv only

3. i,ii,iii only

4 all are correct

37. Read the following statements-

i. Microbes are a very important component of life on earth. Not all microbes are pathogenic.

ii. Many microbes are very useful to human beings.

iii. We use microbes and microbially derived products almost every day.

iv. Bacteria called lactic acid bacteria (LAB) grow in milk to convert it into curd.

Which above statements is/are correct-

1. i and ii only

2. ii only

3. i and iii only

4. All are correct

38. Consider the following statements-

i. The dough, which is used to make bread, is fermented by yeast called *Saccharomyces cerevisiae.*

ii. Bacteria and fungi are used to impart particular texture, taste and flavor to cheese.

iii. Microbes are used to produce industrial products like lactic acid, acetic acid and alcohol, which are used in a variety of processes in the industry.

iv. Antibiotics like penicillins produced by useful microbes are used to kill disease-causing harmful microbes.

v. Antibiotics have played a major role in controlling infectious diseases like diphtheria,and whooping cough etc.

How many of above are/is correct-

1. three

2. four

3. two

4. five

39. Read the following statements and find out the correct option-

STATEMENT 1. Plants having symbiotic associations show other benefits also, such as resistance to root-borne pathogens, tolerance to salinity and drought, and an overall increase in plant growth and development.

STATEMENT 2. Blue green algae not add organic matter to the soil and increase its fertility.

1. Both are wrong statements

2. Both are correct statements

3. Only statement 1 correct

4. Only statement 2 correct

40. Read the following statements-

a) *Trichoderma* species are free-living fungi that are very common in the root ecosystems.

b) *Trichoderma* are effective biocontrol agents of several plant pathogens.

c) Baculoviruses are pathogens that attack insects and other arthropods.

d) The majority of baculoviruses used as biological control agents are in the genus *Nucleopolyhedrovirus*.

e) Baculoviruses are excellent candidates for species-specific, narrow spectrum insecticidal applications.

f) Baculoviruses shows negative impacts on plants, mammals, birds, fish or even on non-target insects.

Which of the following are correct?

1. a and b only

2. b and c only

3. a,b,c,d only

4. a,b,c,d,e,f

BIOTECHNOLOGY: PRINCIPLES AND PROCESSES

15.1 Principles of Biotechnology

15.2 Tools of Recombinant DNA Technology

15.3 Processes of RecombinantDNA Technology

- **Biotechnology** deals with large scale production and marketing of products and processes using live organisms, cells or enzymes.

- **Biotechnology** is technology that utilize biological system, living organism or parts of this to develop or make different products.

- Modern biotechnology using genetically modified organisms was made possible only when man learnt to alter the chemistry of DNA and construct recombinant DNA.

- This key process is called recombinant DNA technology or genetic engineering.

- The European Federation of Biotechnology (EFB) has given a definition of biotechnology that encompasses both traditional view and modern molecular biotechnology.

- The definition given by **EFB is** as follows: **'The integration of natural science and organisms, cells, parts thereof, and molecular analogues for products and services'.**

15.1 PRINCIPLES OF BIOTECHNOLOGY

The two core techniques that enabled birth of modern biotechnology

- The two core techniques that enabled birth of modern biotechnology are:

(i) Genetic engineering: Techniques to alter the chemistry of genetic material to introduce these into host organisms and thus change the phenotype of the host organism.

(ii) Maintenance of sterile (microbial contamination-free) ambience in chemical engineering processes to enable growth of only the desired microbe/eukaryotic cell in large quantities for the manufacture of biotechnological products like antibiotics, vaccines, enzymes, etc.

- The biotech provides opportunities for variations and formulation of unique combinations of genetic setup, some of which may be beneficial to the organism as well as the population.

- **Asexual reproduction preserves the genetic information,** while sexual reproduction permits variation.

- **Traditional hybridization that means animal and plant breeding** procedures used in plant and animal breeding, very often lead to inclusion and multiplication of undesirable genes along with the desired genes.

- The techniques of genetic engineering which include creation of **recombinant DNA**, use of **gene cloning** and **gene transfer**, overcome this limitation and allows us to isolate and introduce only one or a set of desirable genes without introducing undesirable genes into the target organism.

Gene cloning

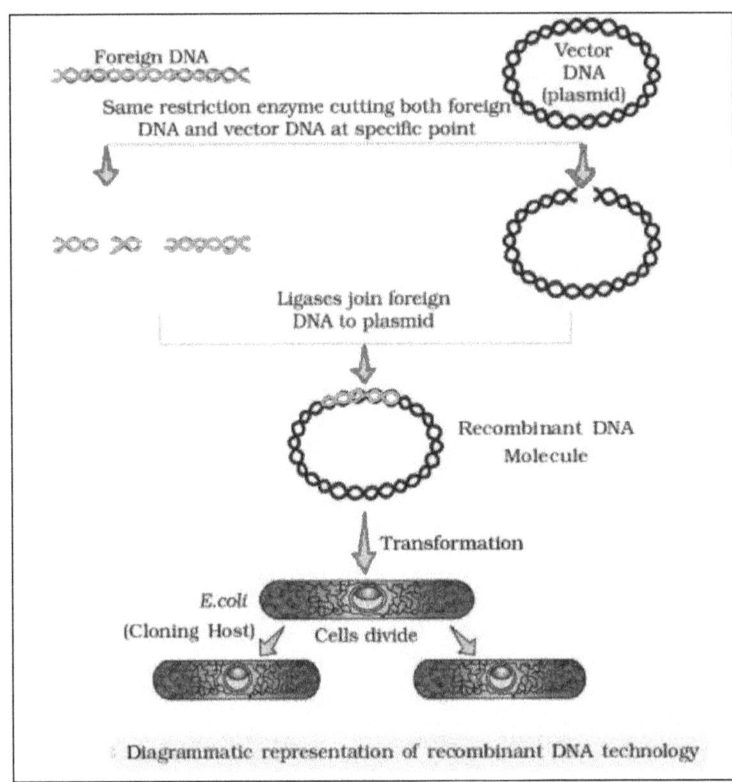

Diagrammatic representation of recombinant DNA technology

- Most likely, this piece of DNA would not be able to multiply itself in the progeny cells of the organism.

- But, when it gets integrated into the genome of the recipient, it may multiply and be inherited along with the host DNA.

- This is because the alien piece of DNA has become part of a chromosome, which has the ability to replicate.

- In a chromosome there is a specific DNA sequence called the **origin of replication,** which is responsible for initiating replication.

- Therefore, for the multiplication of any alien piece of DNA in an organism it needs to be a part of a chromosome(s) which has a specific sequence known as 'origin of replication'.

- Thus, an alien DNA is linked with the origin of replication, so that, this alien piece of DNA can replicate and multiply itself in the host organism.

Discovery of cloning

- This can also be called as **cloning** or making multiple identical copies of any template DNA.

- The DNA emerged from the possibility of linking a gene encoding antibiotic resistance with a native **plasmid** (autonomously replicating circular extra-chromosomal DNA) of *Salmonella typhimurium.*

- **Stanley Cohen and Herbert Boyer** accomplished this in **1972** by isolating the antibiotic resistance gene by cutting out a piece of DNA from a plasmid which was responsible for conferring antibiotic resistance.

Molecular scissors

- The cutting of DNA at specific locations became possible with the discovery of the so-called 'molecular scissors'– **restriction enzymes**.

- The cut piece of DNA was then linked with the plasmid DNA.

Molecular glue

- **DNA ligase join two individual fragment of ds DNA by forming phosphodiester bonds between them.**

Vector

- These plasmid DNA act as **vectors** to transfer the piece of DNA attached to it.

- As we know that mosquito acts as an insect vector to transfer the malarial parasite into human body.

- In the same way, a plasmid can be used as vector to deliver an alien piece of DNA into the host organism.

- The linking of antibiotic resistance gene with the plasmid vector became possible with the enzyme **DNA ligase, which acts on cut DNA** molecules and joins their ends.

- This makes a new combination of circular autonomously replicating DNA created *in vitro* and is known as recombinant DNA.

Note-

- When this **DNA is transferred into *Escherichia coli*,** a bacterium closely related to *Salmonella*, it could replicate using the new host's DNA polymerase enzyme and make multiple copies.

- The ability to multiply copies of antibiotic resistance gene in *E. coli* was called **cloning** of antibiotic resistance gene in *E. coli*.

- There **are three basic steps** in genetically modifying an organism —

(i) identification of DNA with desirable genes;

(ii) introduction of the identified DNA into the host

(iii) maintenance of introduced DNA in the host and transfer of the DNA to its progeny.

15.2 TOOLS OF RECOMBINANT DNA TECHNOLOGY

- The that genetic engineering or recombinant DNA technology can be accomplished only if we have five tools, i.e., **restriction enzymes, polymerase enzymes, ligases, vectors** and **the host organism.**

15.2.1 Restriction Enzymes

a. Discovery and naming

- In 1963, **the two enzymes** responsible for restricting the growth of bacteriophage in *Escherichia coli* were isolated.

- **One of these** added methyl groups to DNA, while the other cut DNA.

- The **2nd enzyme** was called **restriction endonuclease**.
- The **first restriction endonuclease–*Hind II***, whose functioning depended on a specific DNA nucleotide sequence was isolated and characterised five years later.
- It was found that *Hind II* **always cut DNA molecules at a particular point by recognising a specific sequence of six base pairs.**
- This specific base sequence is known as the **recognition sequence** for *Hind II*.
- *Hind I* and *Hind II* isolated from ***Haemophilus influenzae.***

b. Isolation

- Besides *Hind II*, today we know more than **900** restriction enzymes that have been isolated from over **230** strains of bacteria each of which recognise different recognition sequences.
- The convention for naming these enzymes is the first letter of the name comes from the genes and the second two letters come from the species of the prokaryotic cell from which they were isolated, e.g., **EcoRI** comes from *Escherichia coli* **RY 13.**
- In **EcoRI**, the letter 'R' is derived from the name of resistant strain.
- **Roman numbers** following the names indicate the order in which the enzymes were isolated from that strain of bacteria.
- Restriction enzymes belong to a larger class of enzymes called **nucleases**.

c. Types of nucleases.

- These are of two kinds; **exonucleases** and **endonucleases**.

I. Exonucleases

- Exonucleases remove nucleotides from the ends of the DNA.

II. Endonucleases

- Endonucleases make cuts at specific positions within the DNA.
- Each restriction endonuclease functions by 'inspecting' the length of a DNA sequence.

III. Restriction endonuclease

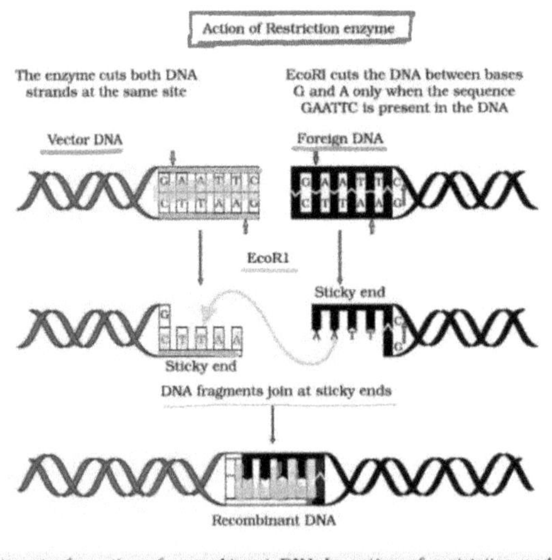

Steps in formation of recombinant DNA by action of restriction endonuclease enzyme - EcoRI

- Once it finds its specific recognition sequence, it will bind to the DNA and cut each of the two strands of the double helix at specific points in their sugar - phosphate backbones.

- RE are 3 types – **Type I, Type II, Type III**

- Type II RE are mostly used RE in Biotechnology.

- Each restriction endonuclease recognises a specific **palindromic nucleotide sequences** in the DNA.

- These are groups of letters that form the same words when read both forward and backward, e.g., "MALAYALAM".

- As against a word-palindrome where the same word is read in both directions, the palindrome in DNA is a sequence of base pairs that reads same on the two strands when orientation of reading is kept the same.

- For example, the following sequences reads the same on the two strands in 5' *to* 3' direction.

- This is also true if read in the 3' *to* 5' direction.

  5' —— GAATTC —— 3'

  3' —— CTTAAG —— 5'

- **Restriction enzymes** cut the strand of DNA a little away from the centre of the palindrome sites, but between the same two bases on the opposite strands.

- This leaves single stranded portions at the ends.

  There are overhanging stretches called **sticky ends** on each strand.

- These are named so because they form hydrogen bonds with their complementary cut counterparts.

- **This stickiness of the ends facilitates the action of the enzyme DNA ligase.**

- **Sticky end cutting RE are – *BamH I, Cla I, EcoR I, Hind III, Pst I***

- **Blunt end cutting RE – *Sma I, EcoR V***

- Restriction endonucleases are used in genetic engineering to form 'recombinant' molecules of DNA, which are composed of DNA from different sources/genomes.

- When cut by the same restriction enzyme, the resultant DNA fragments have the same kind of **'sticky-ends'** and, these can be joined together (end-to-end) using DNA ligases.

- Normally, unless one cuts the vector and the source DNA with the same restriction enzyme, the recombinant vector molecule cannot be created.

Separation and isolation of DNA fragments(By gel electrophoresis)

- The cutting of DNA by restriction endonucleases results in the fragmentes of DNA.

a. Gel electrophoresis.

- DNA fragments can be separated by a technique known as **gel electrophoresis**.

- Since DNA fragments are negatively charged molecules they can be separated by forcing them to move towards the anode under an **electric field through a medium/matrix.**

- The most commonly used **matrix is agarose** which is a natural polymer extracted from sea weeds.

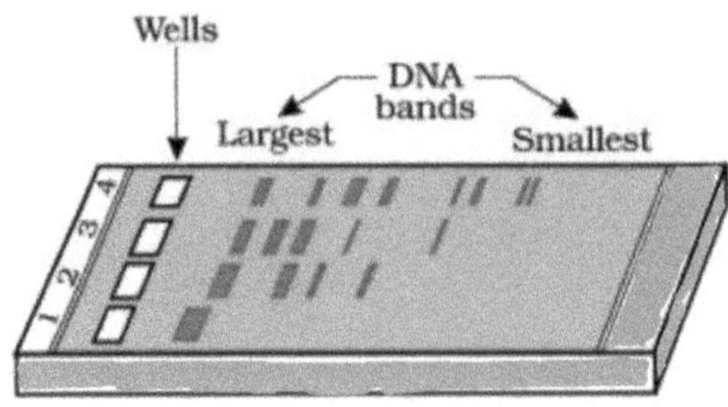

A typical agarose gel electrophoresis showing migration of undigested (lane 1) and digested set of DNA fragments (lane 2 to 4)

b. DNA fragments separate (resolve) according to their size

- The **DNA fragments separate (resolve) according to their size** through sieving effect provided by the agarose gel.

- The smaller the DNA fragment size, it moves more faster.

- The separated DNA fragments can be **visualised** only after staining the DNA with a compound known as **ethidium bromide** followed by exposure to UV radiation.

- We cannot see pure DNA fragments in the visible light and without staining.

c. Bright orange coloured bands of DNA

- We can see **bright orange coloured bands of DNA in** a ethidium bromide stained gel exposed to UV light.

d. Elution

- The separated bands of DNA are cut out from the **agarose gel** and extracted from the gel piece.

- This step extraction is known as **elution.**

Points to remember-

The DNA fragments purified in this way are used in constructing recombinant DNA by joining them with cloning vectors.

15.2.2 Cloning Vectors

- The plasmids and bacteriophages have the ability to replicate within bacterial cells independent of the control of chromosomal DNA.

Very high copy numbers

- **Bacteriophages** because of their high number per cell, have very high copy numbers of their genome within the bacterial cells.

- Some plasmids may have only **one or two copies** per cell whereas others may have **15-100 copies** per cell.

- Their numbers can go even higher.

Link an alien piece of DNA with bacteriophage or plasmid DNA

- If we are able to link an alien piece of DNA with bacteriophage or plasmid DNA, we can multiply its numbers equal to the copy number of the **plasmid or bacteriophage.**

- Vectors used at present, are engineered in such way that they help easy linking of foreign DNA and selection of recombinants from non-recombinants.

Features cloning vector.

The following are the features that are required to facilitate cloning into a vector.

(i) *Origin of replication (ori):*

- This is a sequence from where **replication starts** and **any piece of DNA** when linked to this sequence can be made to replicate within the host cells.

- **This sequence** is also responsible for controlling the copy number of the **linked DNA.**

- So, if one wants to recover many copies of the target DNA it should be cloned in a vector whose origin support **high copy number.**

(ii) *Selectable marker:*

- In addition to 'ori', **the vector requires a selectable marker,** which helps in identifying and eliminating nontransformants and selectively permitting the growth of the transformants.

- Transformation is a procedure through which a piece of DNA is introduced in a host bacterium.

- The genes encoding resistance to antibiotics such as **ampicillin, chloramphenicol, tetracycline or kanamycin, etc.,** are considered useful selectable markers for *E. coli.*

- The normal *E. coli* cells do not carry resistance against any of these antibiotics.

(iii) *Cloning sites:*

- In order to link the alien DNA, the vector needs to have very few, preferably single, **recognition sites** for the commonly used restriction enzymes.

- Presence of more than one recognition sites within the vector will generate several fragments, which will complicate the gene cloning.

- The ligation of alien DNA is carried out at a restriction site present in one of the two **antibiotic resistance** genes.

- For example, you can ligate a foreign DNA at the Bam H I site of tetracycline resistance gene in the vector pBR322.

- The recombinant plasmids will lose tetracycline resistance due to insertion of foreign DNA but can still be selected out from non-recombinant ones by plating the **transformants on ampicillin** containing medium.

- The transformants growing on **ampicillin containing medium** are then transferred on a medium containing tetracycline.

- **The recombinants** will grow in ampicillin containing medium but not on that containing tetracycline.

- But, **non recombinants will grow** on the medium containing both the antibiotics.

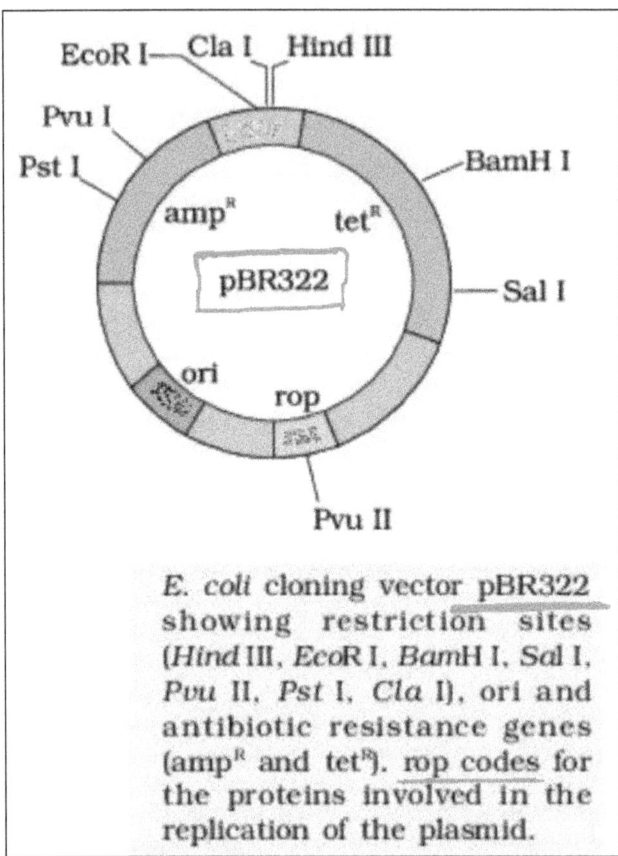

E. coli cloning vector pBR322 showing restriction sites (*Hind* III, *EcoR* I, *BamH* I, *Sal* I, *Pvu* II, *Pst* I, *Cla* I), ori and antibiotic resistance genes (amp^R and tet^R). rop codes for the proteins involved in the replication of the plasmid.

- ➢ In this case, one antibiotic resistance gene helps in electing the transformants, whereas the other **antibiotic resistance gene gets 'inactivated due to insertion'** of alien DNA, and helps in selection of recombinants.

- ➢ **Selection of recombinants due to inactivation of antibiotics** is a cumbersome procedure because it requires simultaneous plating on two plates having different antibiotics.

- ➢ Therefore, alternative selectable markers have been developed which differentiate recombinants **from non-recombinants** on the basis of their ability to produce colour in the presence of a chromogenic substrate.

- ➢ In this, a recombinant DNA is inserted within the coding sequence of an enzyme, **beta-galactosidase.**

- ➢ So **beta - galactosidase become inactivated,** which is referred to as **insertional inactivation**.

- ➢ The presence of a chromogenic substrate gives blue coloured colonies if the plasmid in the bacteria does not have an insert.

- ➢ Presence of insert results into insertional inactivation of the **alpha-galactosidase** and the colonies do not produce any colour, these are identified as recombinant colonies.

(iv) *Vectors for cloning genes in plants and animals:*

- ➢ You may be surprised to know that we have learnt the lesson of transferring genes into plants and animals from bacteria and viruses which have known this for ages – how to deliver genes to transform eukaryotic cells and force them to do what the bacteria or viruses want.

- ➢ The *Agrobacterium tumifaciens,* a pathogen of several dicot plants is able to deliver a piece of DNA known as 'T-DNA' to transform normal plant cells into a **tumor** and direct these tumor cells to produce the chemicals required by the pathogen.

➢ The retroviruses in animals have the ability to transform normal cells into **cancerous** cells.

➢ A better understanding of the art of delivering genes by pathogens in their eukaryotic hosts has generated knowledge to transform these tools of pathogens into useful vectors for delivering genes of interest to humans.

➢ **The tumor inducing (Ti) plasmid of *Agrobacterium tumifaciens*** has now been modified into a cloning vector which is no more pathogenic to the plants but is still able to use the mechanisms to deliver genes of our interest into a variety of plants.

➢ Similarly, **retroviruses have also been disarmed** and are now used to **deliver desirable genes into** animal cells.

➢ So, once a gene or a DNA fragment has been ligated into a suitable vector it is transferred into a bacterial, plant or animal host (where it multiplies).

15.2.3 Competent Host (For Transformation with Recombinant DNA)

• DNA is a hydrophilic molecule, it cannot pass through cell membranes.

a. Force bacteria to take up the plasmid/ Gene transfer

• In order to force bacteria to take up **the plasmid, the bacterial cells** must first be made 'competent' to take up DNA.

• This is done by treating them with a **specific concentration of a divalent cation, such as calcium,** which increases the efficiency with which DNA enters the bacterium through pores in its cell wall.

• Recombinant DNA can then be forced into such cells by incubating the cells with recombinant DNA on ice, followed by placing them briefly **at 42⁰C (heat shock),** and then putting them back on ice.

• This enables the bacteria to take up the **recombinant DNA.**

• This is not the only way to introduce alien **DNA into host cells.**

b. Micro-injection

• In a method known as **micro-injection,** recombinant DNA is directly injected into the nucleus of an animal cell.

c. Biolistics or **gene gun.**

• In another method, suitable for plants, cells are bombarded with high velocity micro-particles of gold or tungsten coated with DNA in a method known as **biolistics** or **gene gun.**

Point to remember-

And the last method uses 'disarmed pathogen' vectors, which when allowed to infect the cell, transfer the recombinant DNA into the host.

15.3 PROCESSES OF RECOMBINANT DNA TECHNOLOGY

• Recombinant DNA technology involves several steps in specific sequence such as-

➢ isolation of DNA,

➢ fragmentation of DNA by restriction endonucleases

➢ isolation of a desired DNA fragment,

➢ ligation of the DNA fragment into a vector,

➢ transferring the recombinant DNA into the host,

➢ culturing the host cells in a medium at large scale

➢ extraction of the desired product.

15.3.1 Isolation of the Genetic Material (DNA)

- The nucleic acid is the genetic material of all organisms without exception.

- In majority of organisms this is **deoxyribonucleic acid or DNA.**

- In order to cut the DNA with **restriction enzymes**, it needs to be in pure form, free from other macro-molecules.

- The DNA is enclosed within the membranes, so to break the cell open to release DNA along with other macromolecules such as **RNA, proteins, polysaccharides and also lipids.**

- This can be achieved by treating the bacterial cells/plant or animal tissue with enzymes such as **lysozyme** (bacteria), **cellulase** (plant cells), **chitinase** (fungus).

- The genes are located on long molecules of DNA interwined with proteins such as histones.

- **The RNA** can be removed by treatment with ribonuclease whereas proteins can be removed by treatment with protease.

- **The purified DNA ultimately precipitates** out after the addition of chilled ethanol.

- This can be seen as collection of fine threads in the suspension.

- **DNA that separates out can be removed by spooling.**

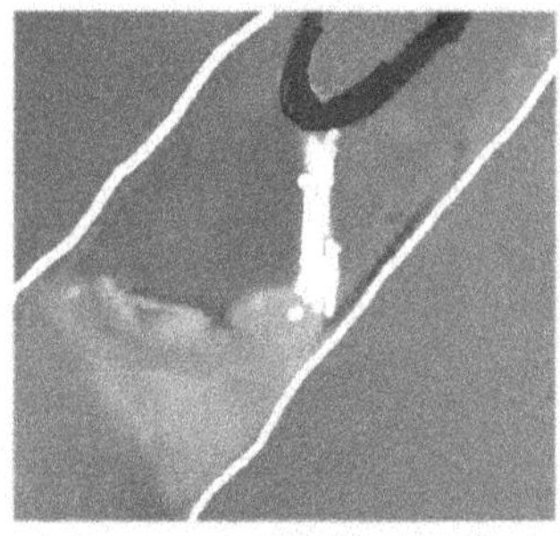

DNA that separates out can be removed by spooling

15.3.2 Cutting of DNA at Specific Locations

- **Restriction enzyme digestions** are performed by incubating purified DNA molecules with the restriction enzyme, at the optimal conditions for that specific enzyme.

- **Agarose gel electrophoresis** is employed to check the progression of a restriction enzyme digestion.

- **DNA is a negatively charged** molecule, hence it moves towards the positive electrode (anode).

- **The process is repeated** with the vector DNA also.

- **The joining of DNA** involves several processes.

- After having cut the source DNA as well as the vector DNA with a specific restriction enzyme, the cut out **'gene of interest'** from the source DNA and the cut vector with space are mixed and ligase is added.

- This results in the preparation of recombinant DNA.

Amplification of Gene of Interest using PCR

- PCR stands for **Polymerase Chain Reaction.**

- Photocopy of DNA/gene.

- PCR was invented by Kary Mullis in 1983 and got Nobel prize in chemistry 1993.

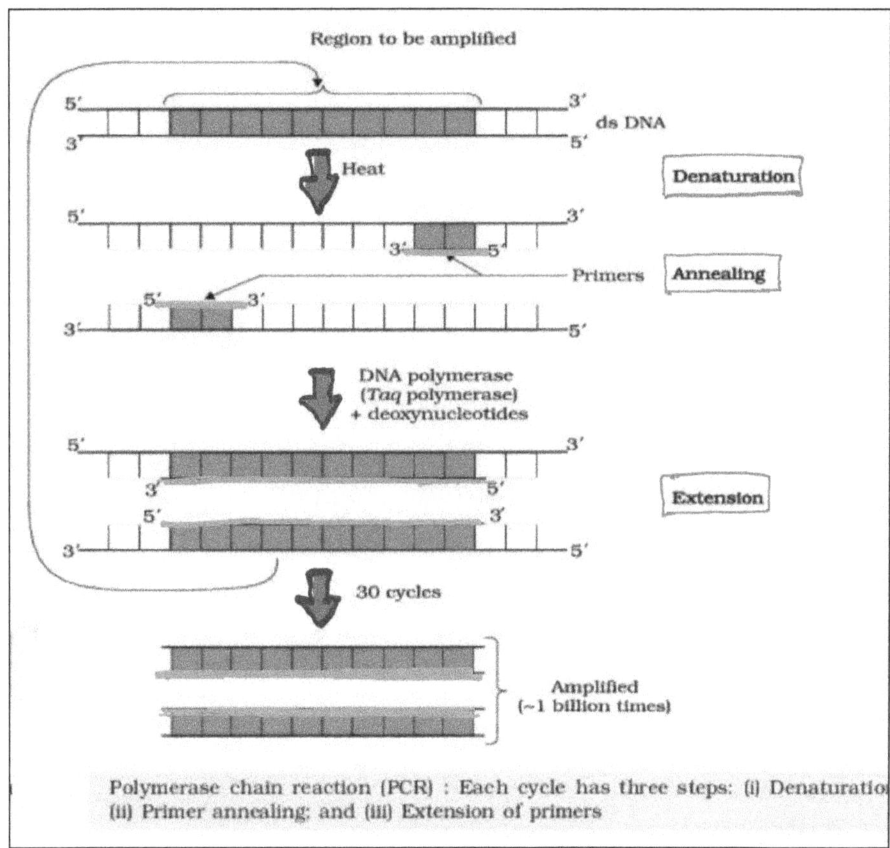

Polymerase chain reaction (PCR) : Each cycle has three steps: (i) Denaturation (ii) Primer annealing; and (iii) Extension of primers

- By using PCR multiple copies of the gene (or DNA) of interest is synthesised *by in vitro* method.

- *in vitro* method we uses two sets of primers (small chemically synthesised oligonucleotides that are complementary to the regions of DNA) and the enzyme DNA polymerase.

- The enzyme extends the primers using the nucleotides provided in the reaction and the genomic DNA as template.

- If the process of replication of DNA is repeated many times, the segment of DNA can be amplified to approximately billion times, i.e., 1 billion copies are made.

- Such repeated amplification is achieved by the use of a thermostable DNA polymerase (isolated from a bacterium, *Thermus aquaticus*), which remain active during the high temperature induced denaturation of double stranded DNA.

- *Thermus aquaticus* bacteria found in yellow stone national park USA.

- The amplified fragment if desired can now be used to ligate with a vector for further cloning.

- RT-PCR used to test covid-19 virus.

15.3.4 Insertion of Recombinant DNA into the Host Cell/Organism

- There are several methods of introducing the **ligated DNA** into recipient cells.

- Recipient cells after making them 'competent' to receive, take up DNA present in its surrounding.

- So, if a recombinant DNA bearing gene for resistance to an antibiotic (**e.g., ampicillin**) is transferred into *E. coli* cells, the host cells become transformed into ampicillin-resistant cells.

- If we spread the transformed cells on agar plates containing ampicillin, only transformants will grow, untransformed recipient cells will die.

- Since, due to **ampicillin resistance gene**, one is able to select a transformed cell in the presence of ampicillin.

- The ampicillin resistance gene in this case is called a **selectable marker**.

15.3.5 Obtaining the Foreign Gene Product

- When we insert a piece of alien DNA into a cloning vector and transfer it into a bacterial, plant or animal cell, the alien DNA gets multiplied.

- In most of recombinant technologies, the ultimate aim is to produce a desirable protein.

- Hence, there is a need for the recombinant DNA to be expressed.

- **The foreign gene gets** expressed under appropriate conditions.

- The expression of foreign genes in host cells involve understanding many technical details. After having cloned the gene of interest and having optimised the conditions to induce the expression of the target protein, one has to consider producing it on a large scale.

- If any protein encoding gene is expressed in a heterologous host, is called a **recombinant protein**. The cells harbouring cloned genes of interest may be grown on a small scale in the laboratory.

- The cultures may be used for extracting the **desired protein and then purifying** it by using different separation techniques.

- The cells can also be **multiplied in a continuous culture system** wherein the used medium is drained out from one side while fresh medium is added.

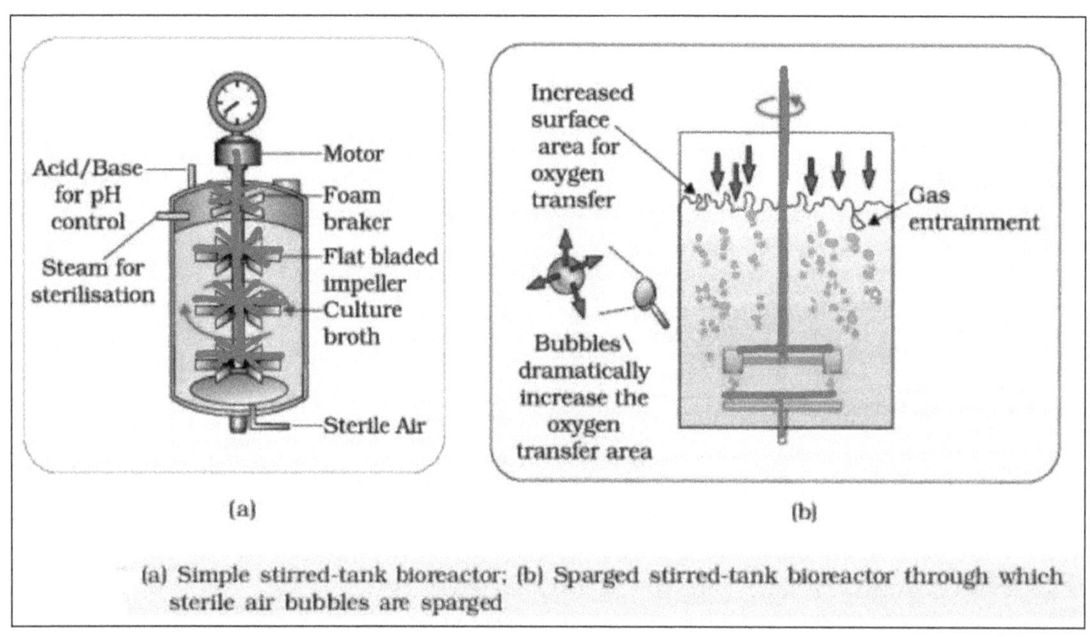

(a) Simple stirred-tank bioreactor; (b) Sparged stirred-tank bioreactor through which sterile air bubbles are sparged

- **A stirred-tank reactor** is usually cylindrical or with a curved base to facilitate the mixing of the reactor contents.

- The **stirrer facilitates** even mixing and oxygen availability throughout the bioreactor.

- The air can be **bubbled through** the reactor.

- The bioreactor has-
  - an agitator system
  - an oxygen delivery system and a foam control system
  - a temperature control system
  - pH control system and sampling ports so that small volumes of the culture can be withdrawn periodically

- To produce in large quantities, the development of **bioreactors**, where large volumes **(100-1000 litres)** of culture can be processed, was required.

- **Bioreactors** can be thought of as vessels in which raw materials are biologically converted into specific products, individual enzymes, etc., using microbial plant, animal or human cells.

- **A bioreactor provides** the optimal conditions for achieving the desired product.

- **A bioreactor provides** optimum growth conditions (temperature, pH, substrate, salts, vitamins, oxygen).

- The most commonly used **bioreacters are of stirring type.**

15.3.6 Downstream Processing

- After completion of the biosynthetic stage, the product has to be subjected through a series of processes before it is ready for marketing as a finished **active log/exponential phase.**

- It refers to the **recovery and purification** of biosynthetic products.

- The processes include separation and purification, which are collectively referred to as **downstream processing.**

- The product has to be **formulated with suitable preservatives.**

- Such formulation has to undergo thorough clinical trials as in case of drugs.

- **Strict quality control testing** for each product is also required.

- The downstream processing and quality control testing vary from product to product.

1. Consider the following statements and find out the correct option-

   A. DNA emerged from the possibility of linking a gene encoding antibiotic resistance with a native **plasmid** (autonomously replicating circular extra-chromosomal DNA) of *Salmonella typhimurium*.

   B. Stanley Cohen and Herbert Boyer accomplished this in 1972 by isolating the antibiotic resistance gene by cutting out a piece of DNA from a plasmid which was responsible for conferring antibiotic resistance.

   C. The cutting of DNA at specific locations became possible with the discovery of the so-called 'molecular scissors'– **restriction enzymes**.

   D. The cut piece of DNA was then linked with the plasmid DNA.

   E. These plasmid DNA act as **vectors** to transfer the piece of DNA attached to it.

   Which of the above are correct -

   1. A,E,C

   2. B,C

   3. D,E,A

   4. A,B,C,D,E

2. **Consider the following statements and find out the correct option-**

   STATEMENT 1. The linking of antibiotic resistance gene with the plasmid vector became possible with the enzyme DNA ligase, which acts on cut DNA molecules and joins their ends.

   STATEMENT 2. When this DNA is transferred into *Escherichia coli*, a bacterium closely related to *Salmonella*, it could replicate using the new host's DNA polymerase enzyme and make multiple copies.

   1. Both are correct statements

   2. Only Statement 1 correct

   3. Both are wrong statements

   4. Only statement 2 correct

3. **Consider the following statements-**

   a) The linking of antibiotic resistance gene with the plasmid vector became possible with the enzyme DNA ligase, which acts on cut DNA molecules and joins their ends.

   b) This makes a new combination of circular autonomously replicating DNA created *in vitro* and is known as recombinant DNA.

   c) When this DNA is transferred into *Escherichia coli*, a bacterium closely related to *Salmonella,* it could replicate using the new host's DNA polymerase enzyme and make multiple copies.

   d) The ability to multiply copies of antibiotic resistance gene in *E. coli* was called **cloning** of antibiotic resistance gene in *E. coli.*

   Which of the above are/is correct -

   1. only a and d

   2. a,b,c only

   3. only c and d

   4. all are correct

4. **Consider the following statements-**

   a) In the year 1963, the two enzymes responsible for restricting the growth of bacteriophage in *Escherichia coli* were isolated.

   b) One of these added methyl groups to DNA, while the other cut DNA.

   c) The later was called **restriction endonuclease**.

   d) The first restriction endonuclease–*Hind II*, whose functioning depended on a specific DNA nucleotide sequence was isolated and characterised five years later.

   Which of the above are/is correct -

   1. d,b,c

   2. a,b

   3. b,d

   4. a,b,c,d

5. **Consider the following statements and find out the correct option-**

   STATEMENT 1. The *Hind II* always cut DNA molecules at a particular point by recognising a specific sequence of six base pairs.

   STATEMENT 2. Besides *Hind II*, today we know more than 900 restriction enzymes that have been isolated from over 230 strains of bacteria each of which recognise different recognition sequences.

   1. Both are correct statements

   2. Only Statement 1 correct

   3. Both are wrong statements

   4. Only statement 2 correct

6. Go through the following statement-

ASSERTION(A). Restriction enzymes belong to a larger class of enzymes called **nucleases**.

REASON(R). Endonucleases remove nucleotides from the ends of the DNA whereas, exonucleases make cuts at specific positions within the DNA.

1. A correct and R is correct explanation of A

2. A correct and R is also correct but R is not correct explanation of A

3. A correct but R incorrect

4. A and R both are incorrect

7. Which statement is incorrect -

1. More than 900 restriction enzymes that have been isolated from over 230 strains of protozoa each of which recognise different recognition sequences.

2. The convention for naming these enzymes is the first letter of the name comes from the genes and the second two letters come from the species of the prokaryotic cell from which they were isolated, e.g., EcoRI comes from *Escherichia coli* RY 13.

3. In EcoRI, the letter 'R' is derived from the name of strain.

4. Roman numbers following the names indicate the order in which the enzymes were isolated from that strain of bacteria.

8. Go through the following statements-

A. The exonucleases remove nucleotides from the ends of the DNA whereas, endonucleases make cuts at specific positions within the DNA.

B. Each restriction endonuclease functions by 'inspecting' the length of a DNA sequence.

C. Once it finds its specific recognition sequence, it will bind to the DNA and cut each of the two strands of the double helix at specific points in their sugar - phosphate backbones.

D. Each restriction endonuclease recognises a specific **palindromic nucleotide sequences** in the DNA.

How many of them are correct -

1. two

2. three

3. four

4. one

9. Read the following statements and find out the correct option-

STATEMENT 1. In PCR repeated amplification is achieved by the use of a thermostable DNA polymerase (isolated from a bacterium, *Thermus aquaticus*), which remain active during the high temperature induced denaturation of double stranded DNA.

STATEMENT 2. The separated DNA fragments can not be visualised after staining the DNA with a compound known as ethidium bromide.

1. Both are wrong statements

2. Both are correct statements

3. Only statement 1 correct

4. Only statement 2 correct

10. Consider the following statements and find out the correct option

STATEMENT 1. Each restriction endonuclease recognises a specific **palindromic nucleotide sequences** in the DNA.

STATEMENT 2. Each restriction endonuclease functions by 'inspecting' the length of a DNA sequence.

1. Both are wrong statements

2. Only Statement 1 correct

3. Both are correct statements

4. Only statement 2 correct

11. Read the following statements very carefully and find out the correct-

a) The cutting of DNA by restriction endonucleases results in the fragmentes of DNA.

b) These fragments can be separated by a technique known as **gel electrophoresis**.

c) DNA fragments are negatively charged molecules they can be separated by forcing them to move towards the anode under an electric field through a medium/matrix.

d) The most commonly used matrix is agarose which is a natural polymer extracted from sea weeds.

e) The DNA fragments separate (resolve) according to their size through sieving effect provided by the agarose gel.

Which of the above statement are/is correct?

1. a and c both

2. b only

3. a,b,c,d only

4. all are correct

12. Go through the following statement-

ASSERTION(A). The separated DNA fragments can be visualised only after staining the DNA with a compound known as ethidium bromide followed by exposure to UV radiation.

REASON(R). We can see black coloured bands of DNA in a ethidium bromide stained gel exposed to UV light.

1. A correct and R is correct explanation of A

2. A correct and R is also correct but R is not correct explanation of A

3. A correct but R incorrect

4. A and R both are incorrect

13. Find out incorrect statement -

1. The DNA fragments not separate (resolve) according to their size through sieving effect provided by the agarose gel.

2. The separated bands of DNA are cut out from the agarose gel and extracted from the gel piece.

3. The cutting of DNA band from gel is known as elution.

4. pBR322 is not a cloning vector.

14. **Find out incorrect statement –**

    1. Bacteriophages have very high copy numbers of their genome within the bacterial cells.

    2. Some plasmids may have only one or two copies per cell whereas others may have 15-100 copies per cell.

    3. The copy numbers can go even higher.

    4. If we are able to link an alien piece of DNA with bacteriophage or plasmid DNA, we can never multiply its numbers equal to the copy number of the plasmid or bacteriophage.

15. **Consider the following statements and find out the correct option**

    STATEMENT 1. Vectors used at present, are engineered in such way that they help easy linking of foreign DNA and selection of recombinants from non-recombinants.

    STATEMENT 2. In order to link the alien DNA, the vector needs to have very few, preferably single, **recognition sites** for the commonly used restriction enzymes.

    1. Both are wrong statements

    2. Only Statement 1 correct

    3. Both are correct statements

    4. Only statement 2 correct

16 **Consider the following statements-**

    a) The ligation of alien DNA is carried out at a restriction site present in one of the two **antibiotic resistance** genes.

    b) We can ligate a foreign DNA at the Bam H I site of tetracycline resistance gene in the vector pBR322.

    c) The recombinant plasmids will lose tetracycline resistance due to insertion of foreign DNA but can still be selected out from non-recombinant ones by plating the transformants on ampicillin containing medium.

    d) The transformants growing on ampicillin containing medium are then transferred on a medium containing tetracycline.

    e) The recombinants will grow in ampicillin containing medium but not on that containing tetracycline.

    f) The nonrecombinants will grow on the medium containing both the antibiotics.

    Which above statement are/is correct?

    1. b and f only

    2. c and e only

    3. a,b,c,d only

    4. all are correct

17. **Consider the following statements-**

    a) Selection of recombinants due to inactivation of antibiotics is a cumbersome procedure because it requires simultaneous plating on two plates having different antibiotics.

    b) Therefore, alternative selectable markers have been developed which differentiate recombinants from non-recombinants on the basis of their ability to produce colour in the presence of a chromogenic substrate.

c) In this, a recombinant DNA is inserted within the coding sequence of an enzyme, **beta**-galactosidase.

d) This results into inactivation of the Enzyme, which is referred to as **insertional inactivation**.

e) The presence of a chromogenic substrate gives blue coloured colonies if the plasmid in the bacteria does not have recombinant gene.

Which above statement are correct?

1. b and f only

2. a,b,c,d only

3. d and e only

4. a,b,c,d,e

18. **Consider the following statements -**

i. You may be surprised to know that we have learnt the lesson of transferring genes into plants and animals from bacteria and viruses which have known this for ages – how to deliver genes to transform eukaryotic cells and force them to do what the bacteria or viruses want.

ii. For example, *Agrobacterioum tumifaciens*, a pathogen of several dicot plants is able to deliver a piece of DNA known as 'T-DNA' to transform normal plant cells into a **tumor** and direct these tumor cells to produce the chemicals required by the pathogen.

iii. Similarly, retroviruses in animals have the ability to transform normal cells into **cancerous** cells.

iv. A better understanding of the art of delivering genes by pathogens in their eukaryotic hosts has generated knowledge to transform these tools of pathogens into useful vectors for delivering genes of interest to humans.

How many of them are correct-

1. one

2. two

3. three

4. four

19. **Consider the following statements -**

i. In a method known as **micro-injection**, recombinant DNA is directly injected into the nucleus of an animal cell.

ii. In another method, suitable for plants, cells are bombarded with high velocity micro-particles of gold or tungsten coated with DNA in a method known as **biolistics** or **gene gun**.

iii. We also uses 'disarmed pathogen' vectors, which when allowed to infect the cell, transfer the recombinant DNA into the host.

iv. Recombinant DNA can then be forced into such cells by incubating the cells with recombinant DNA on ice, followed by placing them briefly at 42^0C (heat shock), and then putting them back on ice.

v. Heat and shock method enables the bacteria to take up the recombinant DNA.

How many of them are/is correct -

1. one

2. two

3. three

4. five

20. **Recombinant DNA technology involves several steps in specific sequence such-**

    I.   as isolation of DNA, fragmentation of DNA by restriction endonucleases,

    II.   isolation of a desired DNA fragment,

    III.   ligation of the DNA fragment into a vector,

    IV.   transferring the recombinant DNA into the host,

    V.   culturing the host cells in a medium at large scale and extraction of the desired product.

Arrange them in ascending order -

1. II,I,IV,V,III

2. I,IV,II,III,V

3. I,II,III,IV,V

4. II,I,V,IV,III

21. **Consider the following statements and find out the correct option -**

STATEMENT 1. Restriction enzyme digestions are performed by incubating purified DNA molecules with the restriction enzyme, at the optimal conditions for that specific enzyme.

STATEMENT 2. Agarose gel electrophoresis is employed to check the progression of a restriction enzyme digestion.

1. Both are wrong statements

2. Only Statement 1 correct

3. Both are correct statements

4. Only statement 2 correct

22. **Go through the following statement and find out the correct option-**

ASSERTION(A). After having cut the source DNA as well as the vector DNA with a specific restriction enzyme, the cut out 'gene of interest' from the source DNA by using Restriction Enzyme.

REASON(R). Restriction endonuclease helps in the preparation of recombinant DNA.

1. A correct and R is correct explanation of A

2. A correct and R is also correct but R is not correct explanation of A

3. A. correct but R incorrect

4. A and R both are incorrect

23. **Go through the following statement and find out the correct option-**

    A.   Restriction enzyme digestions are performed by incubating purified DNA molecules with the restriction enzyme, at the optimal conditions for that specific enzyme.

    B.   Agarose gel electrophoresis is employed to check the progression of a restriction enzyme digestion. DNA is a negatively charged molecule, hence it moves towards the positive electrode (anode).

    C.   The above process is repeated with the vector DNA.

    D.   After having cut the source DNA as well as the vector DNA with a specific restriction enzyme, the cut out 'gene of interest' from the source DNA and the cut vector with space are mixed and ligase is added.

Which of the above statements are correct -

1. A,B,C only

2. C and D only

3. D and A only

4. All are correct

24. **Read the statements given below-**

A. A better understanding of the art of delivering genes by pathogens in their eukaryotic hosts has generated knowledge to transform these tools of pathogens into useful vectors for delivering genes of interest to humans.

B. The tumor inducing (Ti) plasmid of *Agrobacterium tumifaciens* uses as a cloning vector which is never pathogenic to the plants but is still able to use the mechanisms to deliver genes of our interest into a variety of animals only.

C. Retroviruses have also been disarmed and are now used to deliver desirable genes into animal cells.

D. A gene or a DNA fragment has been ligated into a suitable vector it is transferred into a bacterial, plant or animal host (where it multiplies).

Whichof the above statement are/is incorrect -

1. A only

2. B only

3. D and E only

4. A,B,C,D

25. **Consider the following statements -**

A. The nucleic acid is the genetic material of all organisms without exception.

B. In majority of organisms this is deoxyribonucleic acid or DNA.

C. In order to cut the DNA with restriction enzymes, it needs to be in pure form, free from other macro-molecules.

D. DNA is a macromolecule.

E. **Lysozyme** is used to digest bacterial cell wall.

Which of the above statement are/is correct?

1. A and C only

2. A only

3. D and C only

4. A,B,C,D,E

26. **Consider the following statements with respect to downstream processing-**

I. After completion of the biosynthetic stage, the product has to be subjected through a series of processes before it is ready for marketing as a finished active log/exponential phase.

II. It includes separation and purification.

III.   The product has to be formulated with suitable preservatives.

IV.   Such formulation has to undergo thorough clinical trials as in case of drugs.

V.   Strict quality control testing for each product is not required.

How many of them are/is incorrect-

1. five

2. two

3. three

4. one

27. **Read the following statements and find out the correct option**

STATEMENT 1. The bioreactors can be thought of as vessels in which raw materials are biologically converted into specific products, individual enzymes, etc., using microbial plant, animal or human cells.

STATEMENT 2. A bioreactor do not provide the optimal conditions for achieving the desired product by providing optimum growth conditions (temperature, pH, substrate, salts, vitamins, oxygen).

1. Both are wrong statements

2. Both are correct statements

3. Only statement 1 correct

4. Only statement 2 correct

28. **Read the following statements -**

a)   When insert a piece of alien DNA into a cloning vector and transfer it into a bacterial, plant or animal cell, the alien DNA gets multiplied.

b)   In almost all recombinant technologies, the ultimate aim is to produce a desirable protein.

c)   In recombinant technologies there is a need for the recombinant DNA to be expressed.

d)   The foreign gene gets expressed under appropriate conditions.

e)   The expression of foreign genes in host cells involve understanding many technical details. After having cloned the gene of interest and having optimised the conditions to induce the expression of the target protein, one has to consider producing it on a large scale.

Which above statements are/is correct-

1. a and c only

2. a only

3. a,b,c only

4. a,b,c,d,e

29. **Consider the following statements and find out an incorrect one-**

1.   If any protein encoding gene is expressed in a heterologous host, is called a non-**recombinant protein**.

2.   The cells harbouring cloned genes of interest may be grown on a small scale in the laboratory.

3.   The cultures may be used for extracting the desired protein and then purifying it by using different separation techniques.

4. The cells can also be multiplied in a continuous culture system wherein the used medium is drained out from one side while fresh medium is added from the other to maintain the cells in their physiologically most

30. Read the following statements -

I.   A stirred-tank bioreactor is usually cylindrical or with a curved base to facilitate the mixing of the reactor contents.

II.   The stirrer facilitates even mixing and oxygen availability throughout the bioreactor.

III. Alternatively air can be bubbled through the reactor.

IV.   If you look at the figure closely you will see that the bioreactor has an agitator system, an oxygen delivery system and a foam control system, a temperature control system, pH control system and sampling ports so that small volumes of the culture can be withdrawn periodically.

V.   To produce in large quantities, the development of **bioreactors**, where small volumes 100-1000 ml of culture can be processed, was required.

How many of them are/is incorrect –

1. four

2. two

3. three

4. one

31. Read the following statements and find out the correct option

STATEMENT 1. The bioreactors used to form specific products, individual enzymes by using microbial plant, animal or human cells.

STATEMENT 2. A bioreactor provides the optimal conditions for achieving the desired product.

1. Both are wrong statements

2. Both are correct statements

3. Only statement 1 correct

4.Only statement 2 correct

32. Go through the following statement and find out the correct option w.r.t. downstream processing-

ASSERTION(A). After completion of the biosynthetic stage, the product has to be subjected through a series of processes before it is ready for marketing as a finished active log/exponential phase.

REASON(R). The processes include separation and purification, which are collectively referred to as downstream processing.

1. A correct and R is correct explanation of A

2. A correct and R is also correct but R is not correct explanation of A

3. A correct but R incorrect

4. A and R both are incorrect

33. **Find out the incorrect option-**

   1. There are several methods of introducing the ligated DNA into recipient cells.

   2. Recipient cells after making them 'competent' to receive, take up DNA present in its surrounding.

   3. So, if a recombinant DNA bearing gene for resistance to an antibiotic (e.g., ampicillin) is transferred into *E. coli* cells, the host cells become transformed into ampicillin-resistant cells.

   4. If we spread the transformed cells with ampicillin resistance gene than cells shows resistant against all antibiotics.

34. **Read the following statements-**

   a) If a recombinant DNA bearing gene for resistance to an antibiotic (e.g., ampicillin) is transferred into *E. coli* cells, the host cells become transformed into ampicillin-resistant cells.

   b) If we spread the transformed cells on agar plates containing ampicillin, only transformants will grow, untransformed recipient cells will die.

   c) Since, due to ampicillin resistance gene, one is able to select a transformed cell in the presence of ampicillin.

   d) The ampicillin resistance gene in this case is called a **selectable marker**.

   Which of the above statements is/are correct-

   1. a only

   2. b only

   3. c, a only

   4. a,b,c,d

35. **Consider the following statements -**

   I.   Agarose gel electrophoresis uses to separate DNA fragment.

   II.   DNA is a negatively charged molecule, hence it moves towards the positive electrode (anode).

   III.   After having cut the source DNA as well as the vector DNA with a specific restriction enzyme, the cut out 'gene of interest' from the source DNA and the cut vector with space are mixed and ligase is added.

   IV.   Restriction enzymes obtained by protozons.

   How many of above are/is correct-

   1. three

   2. four

   3. two

   4. one

36. **Consider the following statements -**

   i.   The DNA is enclosed within the membranes, we have to break the cell open to release DNA.

   ii.   This can be achieved by treating the bacterial cells/plant or animal tissue with enzymes such as **lysozyme** (bacteria), **cellulase** (plant cells), **chitinase** (fungus).

iii. The genes are located on long molecules of DNA interwined with proteins such as histones.

iv. The RNA can be removed by treatment with ribonuclease whereas proteins can be removed by treatment with protease.

v. The purified DNA ultimately precipitates out after the addition of chilled ethanol.

Which of the above statements are correct-

1. i,ii only

2. i, ii,iv only

3. i,ii,iii only

4. all are correct

37. **Read the following statements-**

i. The plants, cells are bombarded with high velocity micro-particles of gold or tungsten coated with DNA in a method known as **biolistics** or **gene gun**.

ii. The 'disarmed pathogen' vectors, which when allowed to infect the cell can be use to transfer the recombinant DNA into the host.

iii. Ligase also known as molecular glue.

Which of the above statements is/are correct-

1. i and ii only

2. ii only

3. i and iii only

4. All are correct

38. **Consider the following statements-**

i. Biotechnology deals with large scale production and marketing of products and processes using live organisms, cells or enzymes.

ii. Modern biotechnology using genetically modified organisms was made possible only when man learnt to alter the chemistry of DNA and construct recombinant DNA.

iii. Construction of new type of DNA is called recombinant DNA technology or genetic engineering.

iv. Recombinant DNA technology involves the use of restriction endonucleases, DNA ligase only.

How many of above are/is correct-

1. three

2. four

3. two

4. one

39. **Read the following statements and find out the correct option-**

STATEMENT 1. PCR multiple copies of the gene (or DNA) of interest is synthesised *in vitro by* using two sets of primers (small chemically synthesised oligonucleotides that are complementary to the regions of DNA) and the enzyme DNA polymerase.

STATEMENT 2. The enzyme extends the primers using the nucleotides provided in the PCR and the genomic DNA as template.

1. Both are wrong statements

2. Both are correct statements

3. Only statement 1 correct

4. Only statement 2 correct

40. **Read the following statements-**

   a) In almost all recominant technologies, the ultimate aim is to produce a desirable protein.

   b) Hence, there is a need for the recombinant DNA to be expressed.

   c) The foreign gene gets expressed under appropriate conditions.

   d) The expression of foreign genes in host cells involve understanding many technical details. After having cloned the gene of interest and having optimised the conditions to induce the expression of the target protein, one has to consider producing it on a large scale.

   Which of the following are/is correct?

   1. a and b only

   2. b and c only

   3. c,b,d only

   4. a,b,c,d

Biotechnology and its Applications

- **Biotechnology** has given to humans several useful products by using microbes, plant, animals and their metabolic machinery.

- **Recombinant DNA technology** has made it possible to engineer microbes, plants and animals such that they have novel capabilities.

- **Genetically Modified Organisms** have been created by using methods other than natural methods to transfer one or more genes from one organism to another, generally using techniques such as recombinant DNA technology.

16.1 Biotechnological Applications in Agriculture

Green Revolution/Third Agricultural Revolution

- The **Green Revolution** succeeded in tripling the food supply but yet it was not enough to feed the growing human population.

- Father of green revolution was **Norman Borlaug.**

- Father of Indian green revolution **is Dr M.S. Swaminathan.**

- Increased yields have partly been due to the use of improved crop varieties, but mainly due to the use of better management practices and use of agrochemicals (fertilisers and pesticides).

- The farmers in the developing world, agrochemicals are often too expensive, and further increases in yield with existing varieties are not possible using conventional breeding.

- Our understanding of genetics can show so that farmers may obtain maximum yield from their fields.

- By the study of genetics the use of fertilisers and chemicals can be reduced.

- Use of genetically modified crops is a possible solution.

- As traditional breeding techniques failed to keep pace with demand and to provide sufficiently fast and efficient systems for crop improvement, another technology called tissue culture got developed.

Tissue culture

- **As traditional breeding techniques** failed to keep pace with demand and to provide sufficiently fast and efficient systems for crop improvement, another technology called tissue culture got developed.

- **During 1950s,** that whole plants could be regenerated from explants, i.e., any part of a plant taken out and grown in a test tube, under sterile conditions in special nutrient media.

Totipotency

- **The capacity to generate** a whole plant from any cell/explant is called **totipotency.**

- It is important to stress here that the nutrient medium must provide a carbon source such as sucrose and also inorganic **salts, vitamins, amino acids and growth** regulators **like auxins, cytokinins** etc.

- **By application of these methods** it is possible to achieve propagation of a large number of plants in very short durations.

Micro-propagation

- The method of producing thousands of plants through tissue culture is **called micro-propagation.**

Somaclones

- Each of these plants will be genetically identical to the original plant from which they were grown, i.e., they are **somaclones.**

- **Many important food plants** like tomato, banana, apple, etc., have been produced on commercial scale using this method.

Recovery of healthy plants from diseased plants

- Even if the plant is infected with a virus, the meristem **(apical and axillary)** is free of virus.

- We can remove the meristem and grow it in vitro to **obtain virus-free plants.**

- Scientists have succeeded in culturing meristems of **banana, sugarcane, potato,** etc.

- Scientists have even isolated single cells from plants and after digesting their cell walls have been able to isolate naked protoplasts (surrounded by **plasma membranes**).

Somatic hybrids

- Isolated protoplasts from two different varieties of plants – each having a desirable character – can be fused to get hybrid protoplasts, which can be further grown to form a new plant.

- These hybrids are called **somatic hybrids** while the process is called somatic hybridisation.

- When a protoplast of tomato is fused with that of potato, and then they are grown – to form new hybrid plants combining tomato and potato characteristics.

Pomato

- Well, this has been achieved – resulting in formation of **pomato;** unfortunately this plant did not have all the desired combination of characteristics for **its commercial utilisation.**

- Our understanding of genetics can show so that farmers may obtain maximum yield from their fields.

- There a way to minimise the use of fertilisers and chemicals so that their harmful effects on the environment are reduced.

- Use of genetically modified crops is a possible solution.

Genetically Modified Organisms (GMO).

- Plants, bacteria, fungi and animals whose genes have been altered by manipulation are called **Genetically Modified Organisms (GMO)**.

- GM plants have been useful in many ways.

- **Genetic modification** can- a. made crops more tolerant to abiotic stresses (cold, drought, salt, heat).

b. reduced reliance on chemical pesticides (pest-resistant crops).

c. helped to reduce post harvest losses.

d. increased efficiency of mineral usage by plants

(this prevents early exhaustion of fertility of soil).

e. enhanced nutritional value of food, e.g., Vitamin 'A' enriched rice.

- **GM has been used to create tailor-made** plants to supply alternative resources to industries, in the form of starches, fuels and pharmaceuticals.

- **Tailor-made plants means** genotype of plant altered by Human for welfare of biosphere.

- Some of the applications of biotechnology in agriculture that you will study in detail are the production of pest resistant plants, which could decrease the amount of pesticide used.

Bt toxin

- **Bt toxin** is produced by a bacterium called *Bacillus thuringiensis* **(Bt for short)**.

- *Bacillus thuringiensis* is gram positive bacteria.

- Bt toxin gene has been cloned from the bacteria and been expressed in plants to provide resistance to insects without the need for insecticides; in effect created a bio-pesticide. Examples are Bt cotton, Bt corn, rice, tomato, potato and soyabean etc.

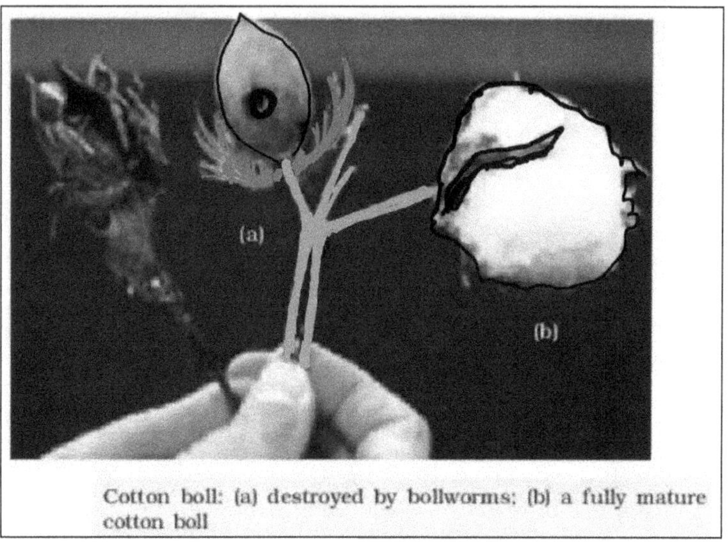

Cotton boll: (a) destroyed by bollworms; (b) a fully mature cotton boll

Bt Cotton

- **Bt Cotton:** Some strains of *Bacillus thuringiensis* produce proteins that kill certain insects.

- **Bt Cotton** provide resistant against insects such as lepidopterans (tobacco budworm, armyworm), coleopterans (beetles) and dipterans (flies, mosquitoes).

- *B. thuringiensis* forms protein crystals during a particular phase of their growth.
- These crystals contain a toxic **insecticidal protein**.

Why does this toxin not kill the Bacillus?

- The Bt toxin protein exist as **inactive *protoxins*** but once an insect ingest the inactive toxin, it is converted into an active form of toxin due to the alkaline pH of the gut which solubilise the crystals.
- The activated toxin binds to the **surface of midgut epithelial cells** and create pores that cause cell swelling and lysis and eventually cause death of the insect.

Specific Bt toxin genes

- **Specific Bt toxin genes** were isolated from *Bacillus thuringiensis* and incorporated into the several crop plants such as cotton.
- The choice of genes depends upon the crop and the targeted pest, as most Bt toxins are insect-group specific.
- The toxin is coded by a gene named **cry**.
- **Examples of cry gene** - the proteins encoded by **the genes *cryIAc* and *cryIIAb*** control the cotton bollworms, that of *cryIAb* controls corn borer.

Pest Resistant Plants

- **Pest Resistant Plants**: Several nematodes parasitise a wide variety of plants and animals including human beings.
- A nematode *Meloidegyne incognitia* infects the roots of tobacco plants and causes a great reduction in yield.
- A novel strategy was adopted to prevent this infestation which was based on the process of **RNA interference** (RNAi).

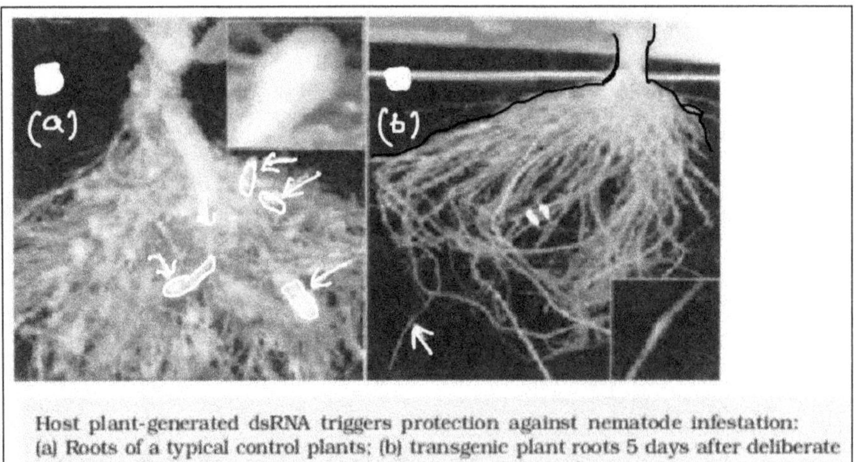

Host plant-generated dsRNA triggers protection against nematode infestation: (a) Roots of a typical control plants; (b) transgenic plant roots 5 days after deliberate infection of nematode but protected through novel mechanism.

RNA interference (RNAi)

- **RNAi takes place** in all eukaryotic organisms as a method of cellular defense.
- **RNAi** involves silencing of a specific mRNA due to a **complementary dsRNA** molecule that binds to and prevents translation of the mRNA (silencing).

- The source of this **complementary RNA** could be from an infection by viruses having RNA genomes or mobile genetic elements (transposons) that replicate via an RNA intermediate.

- Using *Agrobacterium* vectors, **nematode-specific genes were introduced into the host plant**.

- The introduction of DNA was such that it produced both **sense and anti-sense RNA** in the host cells.

- These two RNA's being complementary to each other formed a **double stranded (dsRNA) that initiated RNAi** and thus, silenced the specific mRNA of the nematode.

- The consequence was that the parasite could not survive in a transgenic host expressing **specific interfering RNA.**

- The transgenic plant therefore got **itself protected from the parasite**.

16.2 BIOTECHNOLOGICAL APPLICATIONS IN MEDICINE

- The recombinant DNA technological processes have made immense impact in the area of healthcare by enabling mass production of safe and more effective therapeutic drugs.

- The recombinant therapeutics do not induce unwanted immunological responses as is common in case of similar products isolated from non-human sources.

- At present, about **30 recombinant therapeutics** have been approved for human-use the world over.

- In India, **12 recombinant therapeutics** of these are presently being marketed.

16.2.1 Genetically Engineered Insulin

Insulin from an animal source

- **Insulin used for diabetes** was earlier extracted from pancreas of slaughtered cattle and pigs.

- **Insulin** from an animal source, though caused some patients to develop allergy or other types of reactions to the foreign protein.

Insulin consists of

- Insulin consists of **two short polypeptide chains: chain A and chain B**, that are linked together by disulphide bridges.

Genetically Engineered Insulin

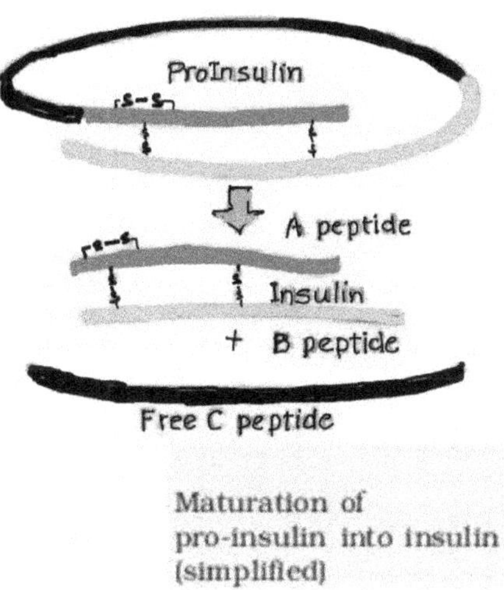

Maturation of
pro-insulin into insulin
(simplified)

- In mammals, including humans, **insulin is synthesised** as a prohormone (like a pro-enzyme, the pro-hormone also needs to be processed before it becomes a fully mature and functional hormone) which contains an extra stretch called the **C peptide**.

- **The C peptide** is not present in the mature insulin and is removed during maturation into insulin.

- The main challenge for production of insulin **using rDNA techniques** was getting insulin assembled into a mature form.

Eli Lilly an American company

- **In 1983, Eli Lilly an American company** prepared two DNA sequences corresponding to A and B, chains of human insulin and introduced them in plasmids of *E. coli* to produce insulin chains.

Bonds involved to make insulin

- **Chains A and B** were produced separately, extracted and combined by creating disulfide bonds to form human insulin.

16.2.2 GENE THERAPY

- **Gene therapy** is a collection of methods that allows correction of a gene defect that has been diagnosed in a child/embryo.

- **Gene therapy** is the insertion of genes into an individual's cells and tissues to treat diseases especially hereditary diseases.

- It does so by replacing a defective mutant allele with a functional one or gene targeting which **involves gene amplification.**

- **Viruses that attack their hosts** and introduce their genetic material into the host cell as part of their replication cycle are used as vectors to transfer healthy genes or more recently portions of genes.

- Here genes are inserted into a person's cells and tissues to treat a disease.

- Correction of a **genetic defect involves delivery** of a normal gene into the individual or embryo to take over the function of and compensate for the non-functional gene.

Case study of gene therapy

- The first clinical gene therapy was given in **1990 to a 4-year old girl** with **adenosine deaminase (ADA) deficiency.**

- **Adenosine deaminase (ADA)** enzyme is crucial for the immune system to function.

- The disorder is caused due to the deletion of the gene for adenosine deaminase.

- In some children ADA deficiency can be cured by bone marrow transplantation; in others it can be treated by enzyme replacement therapy, in which functional ADA is given to the patient by injection. But the problem with both of these approaches that they are not completely curative.

- The first step towards gene therapy, lymphocytes from the blood of the patient are grown in a culture outside the body.

- A functional **ADA cDNA (using a retroviral vector)** is then introduced into these lymphocytes, which are subsequently returned to the patient.

Points to remember-

- As these cells are not immortal, the patient requires periodic infusion of such genetically engineered lymphocytes.

- If the gene isolate from marrow cells producing ADA is introduced into cells at early embryonic stages, it could be a permanent cure.

16.2.3 Molecular Diagnosis

- It includes Recombinant DNA technology, Polymerase Chain Reaction **(PCR)** and Enzyme Linked Immuno-sorbent Assay **(ELISA)** etc.

- For the effective treatment of a disease, early diagnosis and understanding its pathophysiology is very important.

- By using conventional methods of diagnosis **(serum and urine analysis, etc.)** early detection is not possible.

- Presence of a pathogen **(bacteria, viruses, etc.)** is normally suspected only when the pathogen has produced a disease symptom.

- By this time the concentration of pathogen is already very high in the body.

The techniques that serve the purpose of early diagnosis

- Recombinant DNA technology, Polymerase Chain Reaction (PCR) and Enzyme Linked Immuno-sorbent Assay (ELISA) are some of the techniques that serve the purpose of early diagnosis.

a. PCR

- The very low concentration of a bacteria or virus (at a time when the symptoms of the disease are not yet visible) can be detected by amplification of their **nucleic acid by PCR.**

- **PCR** is now routinely used to detect HIV in suspected AIDS patients.

- **PCR** is being used to detect mutations in genes in suspected cancer patients too.

- **PCR** is a powerful technique to identify many other genetic disorders.

- **RT-PCR used to detect Covid-19 in early stages.**

b. ELISA

- **ELISA** is based on the principle of antigen-antibody interaction.

- Infection by pathogen can be detected by the presence of antigens (proteins, glycoproteins, etc.) or by detecting the antibodies synthesized against the pathogen.

Points to remember-

Radioactive molecule (probe)

- A single stranded DNA or RNA, tagged with a **radioactive molecule (probe)** is allowed to hybridise to its complementary DNA in a clone of cells followed by detection using **autoradiography.**

- **The clone having the mutated gene** will hence not appear on the photographic film, because the probe will not have complementarity with the mutated gene.

16.3 Transgenic Animals

- Animals that have had their DNA manipulated to possess and express an extra (foreign) gene are known as **transgenic animals**.

- **Transgenic rats, rabbits, pigs, sheep, cows and fish** have been produced, although over 95 per cent of all existing transgenic animals are mice.

- The transgenic animals are used for study-

(i) *Normal physiology and development:*

   ➢ **Transgenic animals** can be specifically designed to allow the study of how genes are regulated, and how they affect the normal functions of the body and its development, e.g., study of complex factors involved in growth such as insulin-like growth factor.

   ➢ **By introducing genes** from other species that alter the formation of this factor and studying the biological effects that result, information is obtained about the biological role of the factor in the body.

(ii) *Study of disease:*

   ➢ **Many transgenic animals** are designed to increase our understanding of how genes contribute to the development of disease.

   ➢ **Transgenic animals** serve as models for human diseases so that investigation of new treatments for diseases is made possible.

   ➢ **The transgenic models exist** for many human diseases such as **cancer, cystic fibrosis, rheumatoid arthritis and Alzheimer's**.

(iii) *Biological products:*

   ➢ Medicines required to treat certain human diseases can contain biological products, but such products are often expensive to make.

   ➢ Transgenic animals that produce useful biological products can be created by the introduction of the portion of DNA (or genes) which codes for a particular product such as human protein **alpha -1- antitrypsin** used to treat emphysema.

   ➢ Transgenic animals are being made for treatment of phenylketonuria (PKU) and cystic fibrosis.

   ➢ In 1997, the first transgenic cow, Rosie, produced human protein-enriched milk (2.4 grams per litre).

   ➢ The milk contained the human alpha-lactalbumin and was nutritionally a more balanced product for human babies than natural cow-milk.

(iv) *Vaccine safety:*

   ➢ **Transgenic mice** are being developed for use in testing the safety of vaccines before they are used on humans.

   ➢ **Transgenic mice** are being used to test the safety of the polio vaccine.

   ➢ If successful and found to be reliable, than we use **monkeys to test the safety** of batches of the vaccine.

(v) *Chemical safety testing:*

   ➢ **Transgenic animals** are made that carry genes which make them more sensitive to toxic substances than non-transgenic animals.

- ➤ This is known as **toxicity/safety testing.**
- ➤ The procedure is the same as that used for **testing toxicity of drugs.**
- ➤ **Transgenic animals** are made that carry genes which make them more sensitive to toxic substances than non-transgenic animals.
- ➤ They are then exposed **to the toxic substances** and the effects studied.
- ➤ **Toxicity testing in such animals** will allow us to obtain results in less time.

16.4 ETHICAL ISSUES

- **Genetic modification of organisms can have unpredicatable** results when such organisms are introduced into the ecosystem.
- Going beyond the morality of such issues, the biological significance of such things is also important.
- The genetical change in living organisms by the human race regulated. Some ethical standards are required to evaluate the morality of all human activities that might help or harm living organisms.

GEAC (Genetic Engineering Approval Committee)

- The Indian Government has set up organisations such as **GEAC** (Genetic Engineering Approval Committee).
- **GEAC** will make decisions regarding the validity of **GM research** and the safety of introducing **GM-organisms** for public services.
- The modification of living organisms for public services (as food and medicine sources, for example) has also created problems with patents granted for the same.
- There is **growing public anger** that certain companies are being granted patents for products and technologies that make use of the genetic materials, plants and other biological resources that have long been identified, developed and used by farmers and indigenous people of a specific region/country.

Rice

- Rice is an important food grain, the presence of which goes back thousands of years in Asia's agricultural history.
- About **200,000** varieties of rice found in India.
- **The diversity of rice in India is one of the richest in the world.**
- Basmati rice is distinct for its unique aroma and flavour and **27 documented varieties of Basmati are grown in India.**
- There is reference to Basmati in ancient texts, folklore and poetry, as it has been grown for centuries.
- **In 1997, an American company got patent rights on Basmati rice through the US Patent and Trademark Office.**
- This **American** company sell the above variety of Basmati, in the US and abroad.
- This 'new' variety of Basmati had actually been derived from Indian farmer's varieties.
- Indian Basmati was crossed with semi-dwarf varieties and claimed as an invention or a novelty by the **American company**

- The patent extends to functional equivalents, implying that other people selling Basmati rice could be restricted by the patent.
- Several attempts have also been made to patent uses, products and processes based on Indian traditional herbal medicines, e.g., **turmeric, neem.**
- If we are not alert and we do not immediately counter these patent applications, other countries/individuals may encash on our rich legacy.

Biopiracy

- **Biopiracy** is the term used to refer to the use of bio-resources by multinational companies and other organisations without proper authorisation from the countries and people concerned without compensatory payment.
- **Most of the industrialised nations are rich financially** but poor in biodiversity and traditional knowledge.
- **In contrast the developing and the underdeveloped world is rich** in biodiversity and traditional knowledge related to bio-resources.

Traditional knowledge

- **Traditional knowledge related to bio-resources** can be exploited to develop modern applications and can also be used to save time, effort and expenditure during their commercialisation.
- **There has been growing realisation of the injustice, inadequate** compensation and benefit sharing between developed and developing countries.
- Therefore, some nations are developing laws to prevent such unauthorised exploitation of their bio-resources and traditional knowledge.

Indian patent Bill

- The Indian Parliament has recently cleared the second amendment of the Indian Patents Bill, that takes such issues into consideration, including patent terms emergency provisions and research and development.

Fate of Biotechnology

- Biotechnology has given to humans several useful products by using microbes, plant, animals and their metabolic machinery.
- **Recombinant DNA technology** has made it possible to engineer microbes, plants and animals such that they have novel capabilities.
- **Genetically Modified Organisms** have been created by using methods other than natural methods to transfer one or more genes from one organism to another, generally using techniques such as recombinant DNA technology.
- **GM plants** have been useful in increasing crop yields, reduce postharvest losses and make crops more tolerant of stresses.
- There are several **GM crop plants with improved nutritional value of foods** and reduced the reliance on chemical pesticides (pest-resistant crops).

1. Consider the following statements and find out the correct option-

A. The **Green Revolution** succeeded in tripling the food supply but yet it was not enough to feed the growing human population.

B. Increased yields have partly been due to the use of improved crop varieties, but mainly due to the use of better management practices and use of agrochemicals (fertilisers and pesticides).

C. For farmers in the developing world, agrochemicals are often too expensive, and further increases in yield with existing varieties are not possible using conventional breeding.

D. Plants, bacteria, fungi and animals whose genes have been altered by manipulation are called **Genetically Modified Organisms (GMO)**.

E. GM plants have been useful in many ways.

Which of the above are correct -

1. A,E,C only

2. B,C only

3. D,E,A only

4. A,B,C,D,E

2. Consider the following statements and find out the correct option-

STATEMENT 1. Bt toxin gene has been cloned from the bacteria and been expressed in plants to provide resistance to insects without the need for insecticides; in effect created a bio-pesticide.

STATEMENT 2. Some strains of *Bacillus thuringiensis* produce proteins that kill certain insects such as lepidopterans (tobacco budworm, armyworm), coleopterans (beetles) and dipterans (flies, mosquitoes).

1. Both are correct statements

2. Only Statement 1 correct

3. Both are wrong statements

4. Only statement 2 correct

3. Consider the following statements-

a) *B. thuringiensis* forms protein crystals during a particular phase of their growth.

b) These crystals contain a toxic **insecticidal protein**.

c) The Bt toxin protein exist as inactive *protoxins* but once an insect ingest the inactive toxin, it is converted into an active form of toxin due to the alkaline pH of the gut which solubilise the crystals.

d) The activated toxin binds to the surface of midgut epithelial cells and create pores that cause cell swelling and lysis and eventually cause death of the insect.Specific Bt toxin genes were isolated from *Bacillus thuringiensis* and incorporated into the several crop plants such as cotton

Which of the above are/is correct -

1. only a and d

2. a,b,c only

3. only c and d

4. all are correct

4. Consider the following statements-

a) The choice of genes depends upon the crop and the targeted pest, as most Bt toxins are insect-group specific.

b) The toxin is coded by a gene named **cry**.

c) There are a number of them, for example, the proteins encoded by the genes *cryIAc* and *cryIIAb* control the cotton bollworms, that of *cryIAb* controls corn borer.

d) All nematodes are parasitise a wide variety of plants and animals including human beings.

Which of the above are/is incorrect -

1. d

2. a,b

3. b,d

4. a

5.Consider the following statements and find out the correct option-

STATEMENT 1. A nematode *Meloidegyne incognitia* infects the roots of tobacco plants and causes a great reduction in yield.

STATEMENT 2. RNAi takes place in all eukaryotic organisms as a method of cellular defense.

1. Both are correct statements

2. Only Statement 1 correct

3. Both are wrong statements

4. Only statement 2 correct

6. Go through the following statement-

ASSERTION(A). A novel strategy was adopted to prevent this infestation which was based on the process of **RNA interference** (RNAi).

REASON(R). This method involves silencing of a specific mRNA due to a complementary dsRNA molecule that binds to and prevents translation of the mRNA (silencing).

1. A correct and R is correct explanation of A

2. A correct and R is also correct but R is not correct explanation of A

3. A correct but R incorrect

4. A and R both are incorrect

7. Which statement is incorrect -

1. The recombinant DNA technological processes have made immense impact in the area of healthcare by enabling mass production of safe and more effective therapeutic drugs.

2. Further, the recombinant therapeutics do not induce unwanted immunological responses as is common in case of similar products isolated from non-human sources.

3. At present, about 300 recombinant therapeutics have been approved for human-use the world over.

4. In India, 12 recombinant therapeutics are presently being marketed.

8. Go through the following statements-

A. Insulin used for diabetes was earlier extracted from pancreas of slaughtered cattle and pigs.

B. Insulin from an animal source, though caused some patients to develop allergy or other types of reactions to the foreign protein. Insulin consists of two short polypeptide chains: chain A and chain B, that are linked together by disulphide bridges.

C. In mammals, including humans, insulin is synthesised as a prohormone (like a pro-enzyme, the pro-hormone also needs to be processed before it becomes a fully mature and functional hormone) which contains an extra stretch called the **C peptide**.

D. The C peptide is not present in the mature insulin and is removed during maturation into insulin.

How many of them are/is correct -

1. two

2. three

3. four

4. one

9. Read the following statements and find out the correct option-

STATEMENT 1. In 1983, Eli Lilly an American company prepared two DNA sequences corresponding to A and B, chains of human insulin and introduced them in plasmids of *E. coli* to produce insulin chains.

STATEMENT 2. Chains A and C were produced separately, extracted and combined by creating disulfide bonds to form human insulin.

1. Both are wrong statements

2. Both are correct statements

3. Only statement 1 correct

4. Only statement 2 correct

10. Consider the following statements and find out the correct option

STATEMENT 1. Gene therapy is a collection of methods that allows correction of a gene defect that has been diagnosed in a child/embryo.

STATEMENT 2. If a person is born with a hereditary disease, can be corrected by Gene therapy.

1. Both are wrong statements

2. Only Statement 1 correct

3. Both are correct statements

4. Only statement 2 correct

11. Read the following statements very carefully and find out the correct-

a) Gene therapy is a collection of methods that allows correction of a gene defect that has been diagnosed in a child/embryo.

b) Here genes are inserted into a person's cells and tissues to treat a disease.

c) Correction of a genetic defect involves delivery of a normal gene into the individual or embryo to take over the function of and compensate for the non-functional gene.

d) The first clinical gene therapy was given in 1990 to a 4-year old girl with adenosine deaminase (ADA) deficiency.

Which above statement are correct?

1. a and c both

2. b only

3. a,b,c only

4. all are correct

12. Go through the following statement-

ASSERTION(A). In some children ADA deficiency can be cured by bone marrow transplantation; in others it can be treated by enzyme replacement therapy, in which functional ADA is given to the patient by injection.

REASON(R). The advantage with both of above approaches that they are completely curative.

1. A correct and R is correct explanation of A.

2. A correct and R is also correct but R is not correct explanation of A.

3. A correct but R incorrect.

4. A and R both are incorrect

13. Find out incorrect statement -

1. In some children ADA deficiency can be cured by bone marrow transplantation; in others it can be treated by enzyme replacement therapy, in which functional ADA is given to the patient by injection. But the problem with both of these approaches that they are not completely curative.

2. As a first step towards gene therapy, lymphocytes from the blood of the patient are grown in a culture outside the body.

3. A functional ADA cDNA (using a retroviral vector) is then introduced into these lymphocytes, which are subsequently returned to the patient.

4. If the gene isolate from marrow cells producing ADA is introduced into cells at later embryonic stages, it could be a permanent cure.

14. Find out incorrect statement –

1. Polymerase Chain Reaction (PCR) and Enzyme Linked Immuno-sorbent Assay (ELISA) are some of the techniques that serve the purpose of early diagnosis.

2. Presence of a pathogen (bacteria, viruses, etc.) is normally suspected only when the pathogen has produced a disease symptom.

3. By this time the concentration of pathogen is already very high in the body.

4. The very low concentration of a bacteria or virus (at a time when the symptoms of the disease are not yet visible) can be detected by amplification of their nucleic acid by ELISA.

15. Consider the following statements and find out the correct option

STATEMENT 1. PCR is now routinely used to detect HIV in suspected AIDS patients.

STATEMENT 2. ELISA is based on the principle of antigen-antibody interaction.

1. Both are wrong statements

2. Only Statement 1 correct

3. Both are correct statements

4. Only statement 2 correct

16. Consider the following -

a) Polymerase Chain Reaction (PCR) and Enzyme Linked Immuno-sorbent Assay (ELISA) are some of the techniques that serve the purpose of early diagnosis.

b) Presence of a pathogen (bacteria, viruses, etc.) is normally suspected only when the pathogen has produced a disease symptom, at this time the concentration of pathogen is already very high in the body.

c) The very low concentration of a bacteria or virus (at a time when the symptoms of the disease are not yet visible) can be detected by amplification of their nucleic acid by PCR.

d) PCR is now routinely used to detect HIV in suspected AIDS patients.

Which of the above statement are/is correct?

1. b and a only

2. c,b,d only

3. d only

4. all are correct

17. Consider the following statements w.r.t. pBR 322 and pUC 8-

a. Selection of recombinants due to inactivation of antibiotics is a cumbersome procedure in pBR 322 because it requires simultaneous plating on two plates having different antibiotics.

b. In pUC 8 alternative selectable markers have been developed which differentiate recombinants from non-recombinants on the basis of their ability to produce colour in the presence of a chromogenic substrate.

c. In pUC 8 a recombinant DNA is inserted within the coding sequence of an enzyme, **beta**-galactosidase.

d. This results into inactivation of the enzyme **beta**-galactosidase in pUC 8 which is referred to as **insertional inactivation**.

e. The presence of a chromogenic substrate gives blue coloured colonies if the plasmid pUC 8 in the bacteria does not have an insert.

Which above statement are correct?

1. b and c only

2. c and e only

3. a,b.c,d only

4. a,b,c,d,e

18. **Consider the following statements:**

a) PCR is being used to detect mutations in genes in suspected cancer patients too.

b) PCR is a powerful techqnique to identify many other genetic disorders.

c) A single stranded DNA or RNA, tagged with a radioactive molecule (probe) is allowed to hybridise to its complementary DNA in a clone of cells followed by detection using autoradiography.

d) The clone having the mutated gene will hence not appear on the photographic film, because the probe will not have complimentarity with the mutated gene.

How many of them are/is correct-

1. one

2. two

3. three

4. four

19. **Consider the following statements -**

a. Transgenic animals can be specifically designed to allow the study of how genes are regulated, and how they affect the normal functions of the body and its development, e.g., study of complex factors involved in growth such as insulin-like growth factor.

b. By introducing genes from other species that alter the formation of this factor and studying the biological effects that result, information is obtained about the biological role of the factor in the body.

c. Animals that have had their DNA manipulated to possess and express an extra (foreign) gene are known as **transgenic animals**.

d. Transgenic rats, rabbits, pigs, sheep, cows and fish have been produced, although over 5 per cent of all existing transgenic animals are mice.

How many of them are/is correct -

1. one

2. two

3. three

4. four

20. Consider the following statements-

a) Transgenic mice are being developed for use in testing the safety of vaccines before they are used on humans.

b) Transgenic mice are being used to test the safety of the polio vaccine.

c) Transgenic animals are made that carry genes which make them more sensitive to toxic substances than non-transgenic animals.

d) Transgenic animals are used to study the effects toxic substances on animals.

How many of them are/is correct -

1. two

2. three

3. four

4. one

21. Consider the following statements and find out the correct option -

STATEMENT 1. Many transgenic animals are designed to increase our understanding of how genes contribute to the development of disease.

STATEMENT 2. The transgenic models used to study many human diseases such as cancer, cystic fibrosis, rheumatoid arthritis and Alzheimer's.

1. Both are wrong statements

2. Only Statement 1 correct

3. Both are correct statements

4. Only statement 2 correct

22. Go through the following statement and find out the correct option-

ASSERTION(A). Transgenic animals that produce useful biological products can be created by the introduction of the portion of DNA (or genes) which codes for a particular product such as human protein alpha-1-antitrypsin used to treat emphysema.

REASON(R). In 1997, the first transgenic cow, Rosie, produced human protein-enriched milk (2.4 grams per litre).

1. A correct and R is correct explanation of A

2. A correct and R is also correct but R is not correct explanation of A

3. A correct but R incorrect

4. A and R both are incorrect

23. Go through the following statement and find out the correct option for w.r.t. Transgenic animals-

A. The can carry genes which make them more sensitive to toxic substances than non-transgenic animals.

B. The procedure is the same as that used for testing toxicity of drugs.

C. They are then exposed to the toxic substances and the effects studied.

D. Toxicity testing in such animals will allow us to obtain results in less time.

Which of the above statement are correct -

1. A,B, C only

2. C and D only

3. D and A only

4. All are correct

24. Read the statements given below-

A. Transgenic mice are being developed for use in testing the safety of vaccines before they are used on humans.

B. Transgenic mice are never used to test the safety of the polio vaccine.

C. Transgenic monkeys can be used to test the safety of batches of the vaccine.

D. The milk contained the human alpha-lactalbumin and was nutritionally a more balanced product for human babies than natural cow-milk.

Which of the above statement are/is incorrect -

1. A only   2. B only

3. D and E only   4. A,B,C,D

25. Find out the correct statements-

A. The manipulation of living organisms by the human race cannot go on any further, without regulation. Some ethical standards are required to evaluate the morality of all human activities that might help or harm living organisms.

B. Going beyond the morality of such issues, the biological significance of such things is also important.

C. Genetic modification of organisms can have unpredicatable results when such organisms are introduced into the ecosystem.

D. The Indian Government has set up organisations such as **GEAC** (Genetic Engineering Approval Committee), which will make decisions regarding the validity of GM research and the safety of introducing GM-organisms for public services.

Which of the above statement are correct?

1. A and C only

2. A only

3. D and C only

4. A,B,C,D

26. Consider the following statements -

I. The modification/usage of living organisms for public services (as food and medicine sources, for example) has also created problems with patents granted for the same.

II. There is growing public anger that certain companies are being granted patents for products and technologies that make use of the genetic materials, plants and other biological resources that have long been identified, developed and used by farmers and indigenous people of a specific region/country.

III. Rice is an important food grain, the presence of which goes back thousands of years in Asia's agricultural history.

IV. There are an estimated 200 varieties of rice in India alone.

How many of them are/is incorrect-

1. four

2. two

3. three

4. one

27. Read the following statements and find out the correct option-

STATEMENT 1. Rice is an important food grain, the presence of which goes back thousands of years in Asia's agricultural history.

STATEMENT 2. There is no reference of Basmati in ancient texts, folklore and poetry.

1. Both are wrong statements

2. Both are correct statements

3. Only statement 1 correct

4. Only statement 2 correct

28. Read the following statements -

a) In 1997, an American company got patent rights on Basmati rice through the US Patent and Trademark Office.

b) This allowed the company to sell a 'new' variety of Basmati, in the US and abroad.

c) This 'new' variety of Basmati had actually been derived from Indian farmer's varieties. Indian Basmati was crossed with semi-dwarf varieties and claimed as an invention or a novelty.

d) The patent extends to functional equivalents, implying that other people selling Basmati rice could be restricted by the patent.

Which above statements are/is correct-

1. a and c only

2. a only

3. d and c only

4. a,b,c,d

29. Consider the following statements and find out incorrect one-

1. **Biopiracy** is the term used to refer to the use of bio-resources by multinational companies and other organisations without proper authorisation from the countries and people concerned without compensatory payment.

2. Most of the industrialised nations are rich financially but poor in biodiversity and traditional knowledge.

3. In contrast the developing and the underdeveloped world is poor in biodiversity and traditional knowledge related to bio-resources.

4. Traditional knowledge related to bio-resources can be exploited to develop modern applications and can also be used to save time, effort and expenditure during their commercialisation.

30. Read the following -

I. A nematode *Meloidegyne incognitia* infects the roots of tobacco plants and causes a great reduction in yield.

II. A novel strategy was adopted to prevent this infestation which was based on the process of **RNA interference** (RNAi).

III. RNAi takes place in all eukaryotic organisms as a method of cellular defense.

IV. This method involves silencing of a specific mRNA due to a complementary dsRNA molecule that binds to and prevents translation of the mRNA (silencing).

V. The source of this complementary DNA could be from an infection by viruses having DNA genomes or mobile genetic elements (transposons) that replicate via an DNA intermediate.

How many of them are/is incorrect –

1. four

2. two

3. three

4. one

31. Read the following statements and find out the correct option

STATEMENT 1. Increased yields have partly been due to the use of improved crop varieties, but mainly due to the use of better management practices and use of agrochemicals (fertilisers and pesticides).

STATEMENT 2. The **Green Revolution** succeeded in tripling the food supply but yet it was not enough to feed the growing human population.

1. Both are wrong statements

2. Both are correct statements

3. Only statement 1 correct

4. Only statement 2 correct

32. Go through the following statement and find out the correct option-

ASSERTION(A). The activated toxin binds to the surface of midgut epithelial cells and create pores that cause cell swelling and lysis and eventually cause death of the insect.

REASON(R). The Bt toxin protein exist as inactive *protoxins* but once an insect ingest the inactive toxin, it is converted into an active form of toxin due to the alkaline pH of the gut which solubilise the crystals.

1. A correct and R is correct explanation of A

2. A correct and R is also correct but R is not correct explanation of A

3. A correct but R incorrect

4. A and R both are incorrect

33. Find out the incorrect option-

1. Specific Bt toxin genes were isolated from *Bacillus thuringiensis* and incorporated into the cotton only.

2. The choice of genes depends upon the crop and the targeted pest, as most Bt toxins are insect-group specific.

3. The toxin is coded by a gene named **cry**.

4. There are a number of them, for example, the proteins encoded by the genes *cryIAc* and *cryIIAb* control the cotton bollworms, that of *cryIAb* controls corn borer.

34. Read the following statements with respect to RNAi-

a) The introduction of DNA was such that it produced both sense and anti-sense RNA in the host cells.

b) These two RNA's being complementary to each other formed a double stranded (dsRNA) that initiated RNAi and thus, silenced the specific mRNA of the nematode.

c) The consequence was that the parasite could not survive in a transgenic host expressing specific interfering RNA.

d) The transgenic plant therefore got itself protected from the parasite.

Which of the above statements is/are correct-

1. a only

2. b only

3. c, a only

4. a,b,c,d

35. Consider the following statements-

I. In 1983, Eli Lilly an American company prepared two DNA sequences corresponding to A and B, chains of human insulin and introduced them in plasmids of *E. coli* to produce insulin chains.

II. Chains A and B were produced separately, extracted and combined by creating disulfide bonds to form human insulin.

III. If a person is born with a hereditary disease, a corrective therapy known as Gene therapy can use to treat.

IV. Gene therapy is a collection of methods that allows correction of a gene defect that has been diagnosed in a child/embryo.

V. The first clinical gene therapy was given in 1990 to a 4-year old girl with adenosine deaminase (ADA) deficiency.

How many of above are/is correct-

1. three

2. four

3. two

4. five

36. Consider the following statements -

i. As a first step towards gene therapy, lymphocytes from the blood of the patient are grown in a culture outside the body.

ii. A functional ADA cDNA (using a retroviral vector) is then introduced into these lymphocytes, which are subsequently returned to the patient.

iii. However, as these Lymphocytes are not immortal, the patient requires periodic infusion of such genetically engineered lymphocytes.

iv. If the gene isolate from marrow cells producing ADA is introduced into cells at early embryonic stages, it could be a permanent cure.

Which of the above statements are correct-

1. i,ii only

2. i, ii,iv only

3. i,ii,iii only

4. all are correct

37. Read the following statements-

i. Using conventional methods of diagnosis (serum and urine analysis, etc.) early detection is not possible.

ii. Polymerase Chain Reaction (PCR) and Enzyme Linked Immuno-sorbent Assay (ELISA) are some of the techniques that serve the purpose of early diagnosis.

iii. The very low concentration of a bacteria or virus (at a time when the symptoms of the disease are not yet visible) can be detected by amplification of their nucleic acid by PCR.

iv. PCR is never used to detect HIV in suspected AIDS patients.

v. PCR is being used to detect mutations in genes in suspected cancer patients too.

Which above statements is/are incorrect-

1. i and ii only

2. iv only

3. i and iii only

4. All are incorrect

38. Consider the following statements-

I. The manipulation of living organisms by the human race cannot go on any further, without regulation. Some ethical standards are required to evaluate the morality of all human activities that might help or harm living organisms.

II. Going beyond the morality of such issues, the biological significance of such things is also important.

III. Genetic modification of organisms can have unpredicatable results when such organisms are introduced into the ecosystem.

IV. The Indian Government has set up organisations such as **GEAC** (Genetic Engineering Approval Committee), which will make decisions regarding the validity of GM research and the safety of introducing GM-organisms for public services.

How many of above are/is correct-

1. three

2. four

3. two

4. one

39. Read the following statements and find out the correct option-

STATEMENT 1. Transgenic mice are being developed for use in testing the safety of vaccines before they are used on humans.

STATEMENT 2. Transgenic mice are being used to test the safety of the polio vaccine.

1. Both are wrong statements

2. Both are correct statements

3. Only statement 1 correct

4. Only statement 2 correct

40. Read the following statements-

a) **Biopiracy** is the term used to refer to the use of bio-resources by multinational companies and other organisations without proper authorisation from the countries and people concerned without compensatory payment.

b) Most of the industrialised nations are rich financially but poor in biodiversity and traditional knowledge.

c) There has been growing realisation of the injustice, inadequate compensation and benefit sharing between developed and developing countries.

d) The Indian Parliament has recently cleared the second amendment of the Indian Patents Bill, that takes such issues into consideration, including patent terms emergency provisions and research and developmen.

Which of the above are correct?

1. a and b only

2. b and c only

3. c,b,d only

4. a,b,c,d

1. Consider the following statements and find out the correct option:

   (A) A soft and spongy layer of skin forms a mantle over the visceral hump.

   (B) The space between the hump and the mantle is called the mantle cavity in which feather like gills are present.

   (C) Gills have respiratory and excretory functions.

   (D) The anterior head region has sensory tentacles.

   (E) The mouth contains a file-like rasping organ for feeding, called **proboscis**.

   (F) They are usually dioecious and viviparous with indirect development.

   Which of the above are incorrect for Mollusca:

   (1) (A), (E), (C)   (2) (F) (E)

   (3) (D), (E), (A)   (4) (A), (B), (C), (D), (E), (F)

2. Match the **List-I** and **List-II**:

	List-I		List-II
(A)	*Bombyx*	(i)	Garden lizard
(B)	*Calotes*	(ii)	Silk worm
(C)	*Pinctada*	(iii)	Pearl oyster
(D)	*Torpedo*	(iv)	Electric ray

   Find out the correct option:

   (1) (A)-(ii), (B)-(i), (C)-(iii), (D)-(iv)

   (2) (A)-(ii), (B)-(iii), (C)-(i), (D)-(iv)

   (3) (A)-(iii), (B)-(i), (C)-(ii), (D)-(iv)

   (4) (A)-(iii), (B)-(i), (C)-(iv), (D)-(ii)

3. Consider the following features:

   (A) Hemichordata was earlier considered as a sub-phylum under phylum Chordata. But now it is placed as a separate phylum under non-chordata.

(B) This phylum consists of a small group of **worm-like** marine animals with organ-system level of organization.

(C) They are bilaterally symmetrial, triploblastic and coelomate animals.

(D) The body is cylindrical and is composed of an anterior **proboscis**, a **collar** and a long **trunk**.

(E) Circulatory system is of closed type.

Which above features are found in Hemichordates:

(1) Only (A) and (D)

(2) (A), (B), (C), (D)

(3) Only (C) and (D)

(4) (A), (E), (C)

4. Read the following statement carefully with respect to Cyclostomata:

(i) All living members of the class Cyclostomata are endoparasites on some fishes.

(ii) They have an elongated body bearing 6-15 pairs of **gill slits** for respiration.

(iii) Cyclostomes have a sucking and circular mouth without jaws.

(iv) Their body is devoid of scales and paired fins.

(v) Cranium and vertebral column are cartilaginous.

How many of them are correct:

(1) Three

(2) Four

(3) Five

(4) Two

5. Consider the following statements and find out the correct option:

Statement-I: Gapjunctions facilitate the cells to communicate with each other by connecting the cytoplasm of adjoining cells, for rapid transfer of ions, small molecules and sometimes big molecules.

Statement-II: Tight junctions do not help to stop substances from leaking across a tissue.

(1) Both are correct statements

(2) Only Statement-I correct

(3) Both are wrong statements

(4) Only statement-II correct

6. Go through the following statement:

Assertion-A: The development of *P. americana* is holometabolous, meaning there is development through nymphal stage.

Reason-R: The nymph grows by moulting about 50 times to reach the adult form.

(1) **A** correct and **R** is correct explanation of **A**

(2) **A** correct and **R** is also correct but **R** is not correct explanation of **A**

(3) **A** correct but **R** incorrect

(4) **A** and **R** both are incorrect

7. Which statement is incorrect for Cockroach:

(1) The respiratory system consists of a network of trachea, that open through 10 pairs of small holes called spiracles present on the lateral side of the body

(2) Thin branching tubes (tracheal tubes subdivided into tracheoles) carry oxygen from the air to all the parts

(3) The opening of the spiracles is regulated by the sphincters

(4) Exchange of gases take place at the tracheoles by Osmosis.

8. Go through the following matchings:

(i) **Expiratory Reserve Volume (ERV): 1000 mL to 1100 mL**
(ii) **Residual Volume (RV):** 5100 mL to 5200 mL
(iii) **Inspiratory Capacity (IC):** TV+IRV
(iv) **Expiratory Capacity (EC):** TV+ERV How many of them is/are correct:

(1) Two   (2) Three

(3) Four   (4) One

9. Go through the following statement and find out the correct option:

(A) A protein is imagined as a line, the left end represented by the first amino acid and the right end represented by the last amino acid.

(B) The first amino acid is also called as N-terminal amino acid.

(C) The last amino acid is called the C-terminal amino acid.

Which of the above statement are/is correct?

(1) (A) and (C) only   (2) (C) and (B) only

(3) (D) only   (4) (A), (B), (C)

10. Read the statements given below:

(A) Organic chemists always write a two dimensional view of the molecules while representing the structure of the molecules (e.g., benzene, naphthalene, etc.).

(B) Physicists conjure up the three dimensional views of molecular structures while biologists describe the protein structure at four levels.

(C) The sequence of amino acids i.e., the positional information in a protein-which is the first amino acid, which is second, and so on-is called the primary structure of a protein.

Which above statement are/is correct?

(1) (A) and (C) only   (2) (B) only

(3) (B) and (C) only   (4) (A), (B), (C)

11. Read the following statements very carefully and find out the correct:

(A) Alveoli are the primary sites of exchange of gases

(B) Exchange of gases also occur between blood and tissues

(C) O_2 and CO_2 are exchanged in these sites by simple diffusion mainly based on pressure/concentration gradient

(D) Solubility of the gases as well as the thickness of the membranes involved in diffusion are also some important factors that can affect the rate of diffusion

(E) Pressure contributed by an individual gas in a mixture of gases is called partial pressure and is represented as pO_2 for oxygen and pCO_2 for carbon dioxide.

Which of the above statements are correct?

(1) (A) and (C) both

(2) (D) only

(3) (A), (B), (C), (D), (E)

(4) (B) and (E) both

12. Go through the following statement:

Assertion-A: Heart, the mesodermally derived organ, is situated in the thoracic cavity, in between the two lungs, slightly tilted to the left.

Reason-R: It is protected by a double walled membranous bag, **pericardium,** enclosing the pleural fluid.

(1) **A** correct and **R** is correct explanation of **A**

(2) **A** correct and **R** is also correct but **R** is not correct explanation of **A**

(3) **A** correct but **R** incorrect

(4) **A** and **R** both are incorrect

13. Find out incorrect statement with respect to Human:

(1) During a cardiac cycle, each ventricle pumps out approximately 70 mL of blood which is called the stroke volume

(2) The stroke volume multiplied by the heart rate (no. of beats per min.) gives the cardiac output.

(3) The cardiac output can be defined as the volume of blood pumped out by each ventricle per second and averages 5000 mL or 5 litres in a healthy individual

(4) The body has the ability to alter the stroke volume as well as the heart rate and thereby the cardiac output.

14. Read the following statements and find out correct option:

(A) The dietary proteins are the source of essential amino acids

(B) The amino acids can be essential or nonessential.

(C) The latter are those which our body can make, while we get essential amino acids through our diet/ food

(D) Proteins carry out many functions in living organisms, some transport nutrients across cell membrane, some fight infectious organisms, some are hormones, some are enzymes

(E) Collagen is the most abundant protein in plant world.

How many of them are correct:

(1) Four

(2) Five

(3) Two

(4) Three

15. Consider the following statements and find out the correct option:

Statement-I: A nucleotide has three chemically distinct components.

Statement-II: One is a heterocyclic compound, the second is a monosaccharide and the third a phosphoric acid or phosphate

(1) Both are wrong statements

(2) Only Statement-I correct

(3) Both are correct statements

(4) Only statement-II correct

16. Match the List-I and List-II with respect to % of the total cellular mass:

	List-I	List-II
(A)	Water	70-90%
(B)	Protein	10-15%
(C)	Lipid	2%
(D)	Ions	1%

How many of them are correctly matched:

(1) One

(2) Two

(3) Three

(4) Four

17. Consider the following:

(A) The outer layer of kidney is a loose capsule.

(B) Inside the kidney, there are two zones, an outer *cortex* and an inner *medulla*

(C) The medulla is divided into a few conical masses (medullary pyramids) projecting into the calyces (sing.: calyx)

(D) The cortex extends in between the duct and tubule medullary pyramids as renal columns called **Columns of Bertini**

(E) Each kidney has nearly two million complex tubular structures called **nephrons**, which are the functional units Which above statement are correct?

(1) (B) and (F) only

(2) (B), (C), (D), (E)

(3) (D) and (E) only

(4) (B), (C), (D)

18. Match the List-I and List-II:

	List-I	List-II
(A)	Malfunctioning of kidneys can lead to accumulation of urea in blood	Transplantation
(B)	The largest gland in our body, secretes bile-containing substances like bilirubin, biliverdin, cholesterol, degraded steroid hormones, vitamins and drugs	Liver
(C)	Stone or insoluble mass of crystallised salts (oxalates, etc.) formed within the kidney	Renal calculi
(D)	the ultimate method in the correction of acute **renal failures**	Uremia

How many of them are correctly matched:

(1) One   (2) Two

(3) Three   (4) Four

19. Consider the following statements with respect to humans:

(A) Muscle is a specialised tissue of endodermal origin

(B) About 4-5 per cent of the body weight of a human adult is contributed by muscles

(C) They have special properties like excitability,

contractility, extensibility and elasticity

(D) Muscles have been classified using different criteria, namely location, appearance and nature of regulation of their activities.

How many of them are correct:

(1) One   (2) Two

(3) Three   (4) Four

20. Read the following statements:

(A) Muscle contains a red coloured oxygen storing pigment called haemoglobin

(B) Myoglobin content is high in some of the muscles which gives a reddish appearance.

(C) These muscles also contain plenty of mitochondria which can utilise the large amount of oxygen stored in them for ATP production.

(D) Red fibre muscles, therefore, can also be called aerobic muscles. On the other hand, some of the muscles possess very less quantity of myoglobin and therefore, appear pale or whitish

How many of them is/are correct **statements**:

(1) Two   (2) Three

(3) Four   (4) One

21. Consider the following statements and find out the correct option for frog:

Statement-I: In frog has 2 chambered heart present like fishes.

Statement-II: Frog has single circulation.

(1) Both are wrong statements

(2) Only Statement-I correct

(3) Both are correct statements

(4) Only statement-II correct

22. Go through the following statement and find out the correct option:

Assertion-A: The forebrain consist of pons and cerebellum. **Reason-R:** It controls circadian (24-hour) rhythms of our body.

(1) **A** correct and **R** is correct explanation of **A**

(2) **A** correct and **R** is also correct but **R** is not correct explanation of **A**

(3) **A** correct but **R** incorrect

(4) **A** and **R** both are incorrect

23. **Match the List-I and List-II**

	List-I		List-I
(A)	GFR	(i)	6.0
(B)	The pH of urine	(ii)	18-20%
(C)	Filtration fraction	(iii)	180 liter
(D)	Presence of ketone bodies in urine	(iv)	Ketoneuria

Find out the correct option:

(1) (A)-(ii), (B)-(i), (C)-(iii), (D)-(iv)

(2) (A)-(ii), (B)-(iii), (C)-(i), (D)-(iv)

(3) (A)-(iii), (B)-(i), (C)-(ii), (D)-(iv)

(4) (A)-(iii), (B)-(i), (C)-(iv), (D)-(ii)

24. **Read the statements given below:**

(A) The adrenal medulla secretes many hormones, commonly called as **corticoids**.

(B) The corticoids, which are involved in carbohydrate metabolism are called glucocorticoids.

(C) In our body, insulin is the main glucocorticoid.

(D) Corticoids, which regulate the balance of water and electrolytes in our body are called mineralocorticoids.

(E) Aldosterone is the main glucocorticoid in our body.

(F) Glucocorticoids stimulate, gluconeogenesis, lipolysis and proteolysis; and inhibit cellular uptake and utilisation of amino acids.

Which of the above statement are incorrect?

(1) (A),(C),(E) only   (2) (E) only

(3) (D) and (E) only   (4) (D), (E), (F) only

25. **Which statement are correct:**

(A) Thyroid hormones control the metabolism of carbohydrates, proteins and fats.

(B) Maintenance of water and electrolyte balance is also influenced by thyroid hormones.

(C) Thyroid gland also secretes a protein hormone called thyrocalcitonin (TCT) which regulates the blood calcium levels.

(D) Thymus gland is degenerated in old individuals resulting in a decreased production of FSH.

Which of the above statement are/is correct?

(1) (A) and (C) only   (2) (A) only

(3) (D) and (C) only   (4) (A), (B), (C)

26. Go through the following Statement:

Assertion-A: Each ovary is about 2 to 4 cm in length and is connected to the pelvic wall and uterus by ligaments.

Reason-R: Each ovary is covered by a thick epithelium which encloses the ovarian cortex only.

(1) **A** correct and **R** is correct explanation of **A**.

(2) **A** correct and **R** is also correct but **R** is not correct explanation of **A**.

(3) **A** correct but **R** incorrect.

(4) **A** and **R** both are incorrect.

27. Go through the following statement and find out the correct option:

Assertion-A: The advancements in biological science have armed us to effectively deal with many infectious diseases.

Reason-R: The use of vaccines and immunisation programmes uses to completely eradicate a deadly disease like smallpox.

(1) **A** correct and **R** is correct explanation of **A**.

(2) **A** correct and **R** is also correct but **R** is not correct explanation of **A**.

(3) **A** correct but **R** incorrect.

(4) **A** and **R** both are incorrect.

28. Read the following statements:

(A) Ovaries are the female secondary sex organs that produce the female gamete (ovum) and several steroid hormones (ovarian hormones).

(B) The ovaries are located one on each side of the upper abdomen.

(C) Each oviduct is about 20 to 40 cm in length and is connected to the pelvic wall and uterus by ligaments.

(D) Each ovary is covered by a thin epithelium which encloses the ovarian stroma.

(E) The stroma is divided into two zones – a peripheral cortex and an inner medulla.

Which above statements are incorrect:

(1) (A) and (C) only　　　　　　(2) (A) & (B) only

(3) (D) and (C) only　　　　　　(4) (A), (B), (C)

29. Consider the following statements and find out incorrect one:

(1) In testis, the immature male germ cells (spermatogonia) produce sperms by **spermatogenesis** that begins at puberty.

(2) The **spermatogonia** (sing. spermatogonium) present on the inside the wall of seminiferous tubules multiply by mitotic division and increase in numbers.

(3) Each spermatogonium is diploid and contains 23 chromosomes.

(4) Some of the spermatogonia called **primary spermatocytes** periodically undergo meiosis.

30. Read the following facts:

(i) The reproductive cycle in the female primates (e.g. monkeys, apes and human beings) is called Oestrus cycle.

(ii) The first menstruation begins at puberty and is called **menarche**.

(iii) In human females, menstruation is repeated at an average interval of about 28/29 days, and the cycle of events starting from one menstruation till the next one is called the **menstrual cycle**.

(iv) One ovum is released (ovulation) during approx the end of each menstrual cycle.

How many of them are correct:

(1) Four   (2) Two

(3) three   (4) Five

31. Read the following statements and find out the correct option w.r.t. humans:

Statement-I: The meiotic division starts as the zygote moves through the isthmus of the oviduct called **cleavage** towards the uterus and forms 2, 4, 8, 16 daughter cells called **blastomeres**.

Statement-II: The morula continues to divide and transforms into blastocyst as it moves further into the uterus.

(1) Both are wrong statements

(2) Both are correct statements

(3) Only statement-I correct

(4) Only statement-II correct

32. Go through the following statement and find out the correct option:

Assertion-A: Diaphragms, cervical caps and **vaults** are also barriers made of rubber that are inserted into the male reproductive tract to cover the cervix during coitus.

Reason-R: They prevent conception by blocking the entry of sperms through the isthmus.

(1) **A** correct and **R** is correct explanation of **A**

(2) **A** correct and **R** is also correct but **R** is not correct explanation of **A**

(3) **A** correct but **R** incorrect

(4) **A** and **R** both are incorrect

33. Find out the incorrect option:

(1) Surgical methods, also called **sterilisation**, are generally advised for the male/female partner as a terminal method to prevent any more pregnancies.

(2) Surgical intervention blocks gamete transport and thereby prevent conception.

(3) Sterilisation procedure in the male is called 'vasectomy' and that in the female, 'tubectomy'.

(4) In vasectomy, a small part of the vasa efferentia is removed or tied up through a large incision on the scrotum whereas in tubectomy, a small part of the cervix is removed or tied up through a small incision in the abdomen or through vagina.

34. Read the following events with respect origin of life:

(i) By the time of 5000 mya, invertebrates were formed and active.

(ii) Jawless fish probably evolved around 350 mya.

(iii) Sea weeds and few plants existed probably around 320 mya.

(iv) About 20 million years ago (mya) the first cellular forms of life appeared on earth.

How many of above are incorrect:

(1) three   (2) four

(3) two   (4) one

35. Which of the following is/are correct with respect to Human evolution:

(i) About 150 bya, primates called *Dryopithecus* and *Ramapithecus* were existing.

(ii) Dryopithecus were hairy and walked like gorillas and chimpanzees.

(iii) *Ramapithecus* was more man-like while *Dryopithecus* was more ape-like.

(iv) Few fossils of man-like bones have been discovered in Ethiopia and Tanzania.

How many of above is/are incorrect:

(1) Three   (2) four

(3) Two   (4) one

36. Consider the following statements:

(i) Five factors are known to affect Hardy-Weinberg equilibrium. These are gene migration or gene flow, genetic drift, mutation, genetic recombination and natural selection.

(ii) When migration of a section of population to another place and population occurs, gene frequencies change in the original as well as in the new population. New genes/alleles are added to the new population and these are lost from the old population.

(iii) There would be a gene flow if this gene migration, happens multiple times.

(iv) If the same change occurs by chance, it is called genetic drift.

Which above statements are correct:

(1) (i), (ii) only   (2) (i), (iii), (iv) only

(3) (i), (ii), (iii) only   (4) All are correct

37. Read the following statements:

(A) Adaptive ability is inherited.

(B) It has genetic basis.

(C) Fitness is the end result of the ability to adapt and get selected by nature.

(D) **Branching descent** and **natural selection** are the two key concepts of Darwinian Theory of Evolution.

(E) Before Darwin, a French naturalist Lamarck had said that evolution of life forms had occurred but driven by use and disuse of organs.

(F) The work of Lamarck on populations influenced Darwin.

Which above statements is/are incorrect:

(1) (E) and (B) only   (2) (F) only

(3) (A) and (B) only   (4) All are correct

38. Consider the following statements:

(A) **Cannabinoids** are a group of chemicals, which interact with cannabinoid receptors present principally in the eye.

(B) Natural cannabinoids are obtained from the inflorescences of the plant *Cannabis sativa.*

(C) The flower tops, **leaves** and the resin of cannabis plant are used in various combinations to produce marijuana, hashish, charas and ganja.

How many of above are correct:

(1) A,B   (2) A,B,C

(3) A,C   (4) A only

39. Read the following statements and find out the correct option:

Statement-I: Those who take drugs intravenously (direct injection into the vein using a needle and syringe), are much more likely to acquire serious infections like AIDS and hepatitis *B*.

Statement-II: AIDS can be transmitted to one's life partner through sexual contact while Hepatitis *B* is transmitted through infected blood.

(1) Both are wrong statements

(2) Both are correct statements

(3) Only statement-I correct

(4) Only statement-II correct

40. Read the following statements:

(A) Adolescence means both 'a period' and 'a process' during which a child becomes mature in terms of his/her attitudes and beliefs for effective participation in society.

(B) The period between 20-28 years of age may be thought of as adolescence period.

(C) In other words, adolescence is a bridge linking old age and adulthood.

(D) Adolescence is accompanied by several biological and behavioural changes. Adolescence, thus is a very vulnerable phase of mental and psychological development of an individual.

(E) Curiosity, need for adventure and excitement, and experimentation, constitute common causes, which motivate youngsters towards drug and alcohol use.

Which of the following are incorrect?

(1) (A) and (B) only   (2) (B) and (C) only

(3) (C) and (D) only   (4) (A), (B), (C), (d), (E)

41. Go through the following statement and find out the correct option:

Assertion-A: The exaggerated response of the immune system to certain antigens present in the environment is called **allergy.**

Reason-R: The antibodies produced to these are of IgE type.

(1) **A** correct and **R** is correct explanation of **A**

(2) **A** correct and **R** is also correct but **R** is not correct explanation of **A**

(3) **A** correct but **R** incorrect

(4) **A** and **R** both are incorrect

42. Read the following statement and find out the suitable option:

(i) Cheese, is one of the ancient food items in which microbes were used.

(ii) Different varieties of cheese are known by their characteristic texture, flavour and taste, the specificity coming from the microbes used.

(iii) The large holes in 'Swiss cheese' are due to production of a large amount of CO_2 by a bacterium named *Clostridium*.

(iv) The 'Roquefort cheese' are ripened by growing a specific virus on them, which gives them a particular flavour.

How many of above are correct:

(1) Three   (2) Four

(3) Two   (4) Five

43. Consider the following statements:

(A) **Biogas** is a mixture of gases (containing predominantly methane) produced by the microbial activity and which may be used as fuel.

(B) These bacteria are collectively called **methanogens**, and one such common bacterium is *Methanobacterium*.

(C) Antibiotics are chemical substances, which are produced by some microbes and can kill or retard the growth of other (disease-causing) microbes.

(D) Watson and Crick while working on *Staphylococci* bacteria, once observed a mould growing in one of his unwashed culture plates around which *Staphylococci* could not grow.

How many of them is/are correct:

(1) One   (2) Three

(3) Four   (4) Two

44. Read the following statements and find out the correct option with respect to sewage treatment:

Statement-I: Primary treatment of sewage basically involve physical removal of particles – large and small – from the sewage through filtration and sedimentation.

Statement-II: All solids that settle during **secondary treatment** form the **primary sludge**, and the supernatant forms the effluent.

(1) Both are correct statements

(2) Both are wrong statements

(3) Only statement-I correct

(4) Only statement-II correct

45. Read the following statements and find out correct option:

   (i) These biochemical similarities point to the same shared ancestry as structural similarities among diverse organisms.

   (ii) Man has bred selected plants and animals for agriculture, horticulture, sport or security.

   (iii) Man has domesticated many wild animals and crops.

   (iv) The intensive breeding programme has created breeds that differ from other breeds (e.g., dogs) but still are of the same group.

   (v) It is argued that if within three of years, man could create new breeds.

How many of them are incorrect:

(1) Four   (2) Five

(3) One   (4) Three

46. Consider the following statements and find out the correct option:

Statement-I: The original drifted population becomes founders and the effect is called founder effect.

Statement-II: Microbial experiments show that pre-existing advantageous mutations when selected will result in observation of new phenotypes.

(1) Both are wrong Statements

(2) Only Statement-I correct

(3) Both are correct Statements

(4) Only Statement-II correct

47. Go through the following statement and find out the correct option:

Assertion-A: *B. thuringiensis* forms protein crystals during a particular phase of their growth. These crystals contain a toxic **insecticidal protein**.

Reason-R: The activated toxin binds to the surface of midgut epithelial cells and create pores that cause cell swelling and lysis and eventually cause death of the insect.

(1) **A** correct and **R** is correct explanation of **A**

(2) **A** correct and **R** is also correct but **R** is not correct explanation of **A**

(3) **A** correct but **R** incorrect

(4) **A** and **R** both are incorrect

48. Read the following statements:

(A) In **micro-injection**, recombinant DNA is directly injected into the nucleus of an animal cell.

(B) In plants, cells are bombarded with high velocity micro-particles of gold or tungsten coated with DNA in a method known as **biolistics** or **gene gun**.

(C) In gel electrophoresis separated DNA fragments can be visualised only after staining the DNA with a compound known as ethidium bromide.

(D) Each restriction endonuclease recognises a specific **non-palindromic nucleotide sequences** in the DNA.

How many of them are correct:

(1) One

(2) Two

(3) Three

(4) Four

49. Consider the following statements:

(A) Restriction enzymes belong to a larger class of enzymes called **nucleases**.

(B) These are of two kinds; **exonucleases** and **endonucleases**.

(C) Exonucleases remove nucleotides from the ends of the DNA whereas, endonucleases make cuts at specific positions within the DNA.

(D) Each restriction endonuclease functions by 'inspecting' the length of a DNA sequence.

Which of the above statements are correct:

(1) (A) and (C) only

(2) (D) and (A) only

(3) (B) and (D) only

(4) All are correct

50. Read the following Statements:

(A) PCR not used to detect HIV in suspected AIDS patients.

(B) PCR can used to detect mutations in genes in suspected cancer patients too.

(C) It is a powerful technique to identify many other genetic disorders.

(D) A single stranded DNA or RNA, tagged with a radioactive molecule (probe) is allowed to hybridise to its complementary DNA in a clone of cells followed by detection using autoradiography.

Which above statements are correct:

(1) (A) and (C) only

(2) (B), (C), (D)

(3) (B) and (D) only

(4) (A), (C), (D)

1. Consider the following Statements and find out the correct option.

(A) Alimentary canal is complete with a well-developed **muscular pharynx.**

(B) An excretory tube removes body wastes from the body cavity through the excretory pore.

(C) Sexes are separate (**dioecious**), i.e., males and females are distinct.

(D) Often males are longer than females.

(E) Fertilisation is internal and development may be direct (the young ones resemble the adult) or indirect.

Which of the above are correct for roundworms:

(1) (A), (E), (C),(B)　　　　　(2) (B), (E), (D)

(3) (D), (E), (A)　　　　　(4) All are correct

2. Match the List-I and List-II:

	List-I		List-II
(A)	*Asterias*	(i)	Angel fish
(B)	*Pterophyl-lum*	(ii)	Limbless amphibian
(C)	*Ichthyophis*	(iii)	Star fish
(D)	*Columba*	(iv)	Pigeon

Find out the correct option:

(1)　(A)-(ii), (B)-(i), (C)-(iii), (D)-(iv)

(2)　(A)-(ii), (B)-(iii), (C)-(i), (D)-(iv)

(3)　(A)-(iii), (B)-(i), (C)-(ii), (D)-(iv)

(4)　(A)-(iii), (B)-(i), (C)-(iv), (D)-(ii)

3. Consider the following features:

(A) Heterodont dentition.

(B) Heart is Three chambered.

(C) They are cold blooded.

(D) Respiration is by lungs.

(E) Sexes are separate and fertilisation is external.

(F) They are viviparous with few exceptions and development is direct.

Which above features is/are not found in class Mammalia?

(1) only (A) and (D)

(2) only (E) and (C)

(3) only (C) and (D)

(4) (B), (C), (E),

4. Read the following statement carefully:

(i) *Ascidia is an* Urochordata.

(ii) *Branchiostoma* called as Amphioxus.

(iii) The members of subphylum Vertebrata possess notochord during the embryonic period.

(iv) In vertebrates notochord is replaced by a cartilaginous or bony **vertebral column** in the adult.

(v) All vertebrates are chordates but all chordates are not vertebrates.

How many of them are correct:

(1) Three

(2) Four

(3) Five

(4) Two

5. Consider the following Statements and find out the correct option-

Statement-I: Insulin is a polymer of fructose.

Statement-II: Starch is a polymeric polysaccharide consisting of only one type of monosaccharide called, pectin.

(1) Both are correct Statements

(2) Only Statement-I correct

(3) Both are wrong Statements

(4) Only Statement-II correct

6. Go through the following statements:

Statement-I: Exoskeletons of arthropods, have a complex polysaccharide called chitin.

Statement-II: In a polysaccharide the individual monosaccharides are linked by **peptide bond**.

(1) Both are correct Statements

(2) Only Statement-I correct

(3) Both are wrong Statements

(4) Only Statement-II correct

7. Which statement is incorrect with respect to enzyme activity:

(1) When the binding of the chemical shuts off enzyme activity, the process is called **inhibition** and the chemical is called an **inhibitor**.

(2) When the inhibitor closely resembles the substrate in its molecular structure and inhibits the activity of the enzyme, it is known as **competitive inhibitor**.

(3) **In competitive inhibitor** there is a close structural similarity with the substrate, the inhibitor competes with the substrate for the substrate binding site of the enzyme.

(4) The inhibition of succinic dehydrogenase by malonate which closely resembles the substrate succinate in structure is an example of non-competitive inhibition.

8. Go through the following Statements:

(A) **Simple epithelium** is made of more than one layer (multi-layered) of cells and thus has a limited role in secretion and absorption.

(B) **Simple epithelium** main function is to provide protection against chemical and mechanical stresses.

(C) **Simple epithelium** cover the dry surface of the skin, the moist surface of buccal cavity, pharynx, inner lining of ducts of salivary glands and of pancreatic ducts.

(D) All cells in epithelium are held together with little intercellular material

Find out the correct statements and choose the suitable option:

(1) (A), (B), (C), (D)   (2) (B), (C), (D) only

(3) (D) only   (4) (C), (D), only

9. Match the List-I and List-II:

	List-I		List-II
(A)	Squamous epithelium	(i)	Lining of Intestine
(B)	Cuboidal epithelium	(ii)	Germinal ET
(C)	Columnar epithelium	(iii)	Alveoli
(D)	Ciliated epithelium	(iv)	Inner surface of hollow organs like bronchioles and fallopian tubes

Find out the correct option:

(1) (A)-(ii), (B)-(i), (C)-(iii), (D)-(iv)

(2) (A)-(ii), (B)-(iii), (C)-(i), (D)-(iv)

(3) (A)-(iii), (B)-(i), (C)-(ii), (D)-(iv)

(4) (A)-(iii), (B)-(ii), (C)-(i), (D)-(iv)

10. Consider the following Statements and find out the correct option:

Statement-I: Each restriction endonuclease recognises a specific non-palindromic nucleotide sequences in the DNA.

Statement-II: Each restriction endonuclease functions by 'inspecting' the length of a DNA sequence.

(1) Both are wrong Statements

(2) Only Statement-I correct

(3) Both are correct Statements

(4) Only Statement-II correct

11. Consider the following Statements and find out the correct option:

Statement-I: Ctenophores, commonly known as sea walnuts or comb jellies are exclusively marine, Asymmetrical, diploblastic organisms with tissue level of organisation.

Statement-II: The body bears eight external rows of ciliated comb plates, which help in locomotion

(1) Both are wrong Statements

(2) Only Statement-I correct

(3) Both are correct Statements

(4) Only Statement-II correct

12. Go through the following statement:

Assertion-A: Trachea helps in transport of the atmospheric air to the alveoli, clears it from foreign particles, humidifies and also brings the air to body temperature.

Reason-R: Exchange part is the site of actual diffusion of O_2 and CO_2 between blood and atmospheric air.

(1) **A** correct and **R** is correct explanation of **A**

(2) **A** correct and **R** is also correct but **R** is not correct explanation of **A**

(3) **A.** correct but **R** incorrect

(4) **A** and **R** both are incorrect

13. Find out incorrect statement with respect to transport of gases:

(1) The 3 per cent of O_2 is carried in a dissolved state through the plasma.

(2) Blood is the medium of transport for O_2 and CO_2, About 97 per cent of O_2 is transported by RBCs in the blood.

(3) Nearly 20-25 per cent of CO_2 is transported by RBCs whereas 2 per cent of it is carried as bicarbonate.

(4) About 7 per cent of CO_2 is carried in a dissolved state through plasma.

14. Read the following Statements and find out correct option:

(i) Normal activities of the heart are regulated intrinsically, i.e., auto regulated by specialised muscles (nodal tissue), hence the heart is called myogenic.

(ii) A special neural centre in the medulla oblangata can moderate the cardiac function through autonomic nervous system (ANS).

(iii) Neural signals through the sympathetic nerves (part of ANS) can increase the rate of heart beat, the strength of ventricular contraction and thereby the cardiac output.

(iv) On the other hand, parasympathetic neural signals (another component of ANS) decrease the rate of heart beat, speed of conduction of action potential and thereby the cardiac output.

(v) Adrenal medullary hormones can also increase the cardiac output.

How many of them are correct:

(1) Four   (2) Two

(3) Five   (4) Three

15. Consider the following Statements and find out the correct option

Statement-I: Angina pectoris, often referred to as **atherosclerosis**, affects the vessels that supply blood to the heart muscle.

Statement-II: Atherosclerosis is caused by deposits of calcium, fat, cholesterol and fibrous tissues, which makes the lumen of arteries narrower.

(1) Both are wrong Statements

(2) Only Statement-I correct

(3) Both are correct Statements

(4) Only Statement-II correct

16. Consider the following Statements

(A) Each nephron has two parts-PCT and the LOH.

(B) Glomerulus is a tuft of capillaries formed by the afferent arteriole a fine branch of renal vein.

(C) Blood from the glomerulus is carried away by an Afferent arteriole.

(D) The renal tubule begins with a double walled cup-like structure called **Bowman's capsule**, which encloses the glomerulus.

(E) Glomerulus alongwith Bowman's capsule, is called the *malpighian body* or *renal corpuscle*.

Which of the above Statements are incorrect:

(1) (A), (C), only

(2) (A), (B), (C), (D), (E)

(3) (A), (B), (D) only

(4) (A), (B), (C) only

17. Consider the following:

(A) Nearly all of the essential nutrients, and 70-80 per cent of electrolytes and water are reabsorbed by this segment.

(B) PCT also helps to maintain the pH and ionic balance of the body fluids by selective secretion of hydrogen ions, ammonia and potassium ions into the filtrate and by absorption of HCO_3^- from it.

(C) Mammals do not have the ability to produce a concentrated urine.

(D) The Henle's loop and *vasa recta* do not play a significant role in to produce a concentrated urine.

Which of the above statement are incorrect?

(1) (A) and (C) only

(2) (A), (B), (C), (D) only

(3) (D) and (E) only

(4) (A), (B), (C), (D), (E)

18. Match the List-I and List-II:

	List-I		List-II
(A)	Ball and socket joint	(i)	between carpal and metacarpal of thumb
(B)	Hinge joint	(ii)	between atlas and axis
(C)	Pivot joint	(iii)	between femur and pelvic girdle
(D)	Saddle joint	(iv)	elbow joint

Find out the correct option

(1) (A)-(ii), (B)-(i), (C)-(iii), (D)-(iv)

(2) (A)-(ii), (B)-(iii), (C)-(i), (D)-(iv)

(3) (A)-(iii), (B)-(iv), (C)-(ii), (D)-(i)

(4) (A)-(iii), (B)-(i), (C)-(iv), (D)-(ii)

19. Consider the following Statements and find out the incorrect one with respect to humans pectoral girdle:

(1) The dorsal, flat, triangular body of scapula has a slightly elevated ridge called the spine which projects as a flat, expanded process called the acromion.

(2) Below the acromion is a depression called the glenoid cavity which articulates with the head of the humerus to form the shoulder joint.

(3) Each clavicle is a long slender bone with five curvatures.

(4) Clavicle is commonly called the collar bone.

20. Read the following Statements:

(i) A neuron is a microscopic structure composed of three major parts, namely, **cell body, dendrites** and **axon.**

(ii) The axon is a long fibre, the distal end of which is branched.

(iii) Each branch terminates as a bulb-like structure called **synaptic knob** which possess synaptic vesicles containing chemicals called **neurotransmitters**.

(iv) The axons transmit nerve impulses away from the cell body to a synapse or to a neuro-muscular junction.

How many of them are/is correct **statements:**

(1) Two   (2) Three

(3) Four   (4) one

21. Consider the following Statements and find out the incorrect one for thyroid gland:

(1) Help to play an important role in the regulation of the basal metabolic rate.

(2) Help to development and maturation of the central neural system.

(3) Play any role in erythropoiesis and metabolism of carbohydrates proteins and fats.

(4) Do not help to regulate menstrual cycle.

22. Consider the following Statements and find out the incorrect one:

(1) The hypothalamus synthesize release antidiuretic hormone (ADH) or vasopressin from the neurohypophysis.

(2) ADH facilitates water reabsorption from latter parts of the tubule, thereby preventing diuresis.

(3) An increase in body fluid volume can switch off the osmoreceptors and suppress the ADH release to complete the feedback.

(4) ADH can also affect the kidney function by its dilatory effects on blood vessels.

23. Which of the following is/are correct:

(i) The exaggerated response of the immune system to certain antigens present in the environment is called allergy.

(ii) The substances to which such an immune response is produced are called allergens.

(iii) The antibodies produced in allergy are of IgA type.

(iv) Common examples of allergens are mites in dust, pollens, animal dander, etc.

How many of above are/is correct:

(1) Three

(2) Four

(3) Two

(4) One

24. Read the Statements given below:

(A) When blood pressure is increased, **ANF** is secreted which causes dilation of the blood vessels.

(B) The **juxtaglomerular cells** of kidney produce a peptide hormone called **erythropoietin.**

(C) **Gastrin** acts on the gastric glands and stimulates the secretion of hydrochloric acid and pepsinogen.

(D) **CCK** acts on both pancreas and gall bladder and stimulates the secretion of pancreatic enzymes and bile juice, respectively.

Which above statement is/are incorrect?

(1) (A) and (C) only

(2) (B) only

(3) (D) only

(4) (A), (B), (C), (D)

25. Which statement is incorrect for Human thyroid Gland:

(1) The thyroid gland is composed of two lobes which are located on either side of the trachea

(2) Both the lobes are interconnected with a thin flap of connective tissue called isthmus.

(3) The thyroid gland is composed of **follicles** and **stromal tissues**. Each thyroid follicle is composed of follicular cells, enclosing a cavity.

(4) These follicular cells synthesise two hormones, **tetraiodothyronine** or **thyroxine** (T_4) and Insulin.

26. Read the following statement:

(i) The spleen is a large bean shaped organ

(ii) It mainly contains lymphocytes and phagocytes (iii) It acts as a filter of the blood by trapping blood-borne microorganisms

(iv) Spleen also has a large reservoir of erythrocytes.

How many of above are/is correct:

(1) Three

(2) Four

(3) Two

(4) One

27. Match the List-I and List-II:

	List-I		List-II
(A)	The process of fusion of a sperm with an ovum is called	(i)	Parturition
(B)	The uterus is single and it is also called	(ii)	Fertilization
(C)	process of delivery of the foetus (childbirth) is called	(iii)	Womb
(D)	tiny finger-like structure which lies at the upper junction of the two labia minora above the urethral opening	(iv)	Clitoris

Find out the correct option:

(1) (A)-(ii), (B)-(i), (C)-(iii), (D)-(iv)

(2) (A)-(ii), (B)-(iii), (C)-(i), (D)-(iv)

(3) (A)-(iii), (B)-(iv), (C)-(ii), (D)-(i)

(4) (A)-(iii), (B)-(i), (C)-(iv), (D)-(ii)

28. Read the following paragraph and find out the X:

- A large number of these follicles degenerate during the phase from birth to puberty.

- The at puberty only X primary follicles are left in each ovary.

(1) 60,000-80,000

(2) 1,60,000-1,80,000

(3) 60,0000-80,0000

(4) 160,0000-180,0000

29. Consider the following Statements and find out incorrect one:

(1) Just after implantation, the inner cell mass (embryo) differentiates into an outer layer called **ectoderm** and an inner layer called **endoderm**.

(2) A **mesoderm** soon appears between the ectoderm and the endoderm.

(3) These above three layers give rise only few tissues (organs) in adults.

(4) It needs to be mentioned here that the inner cell mass contains certain cells called **stem** cells which have the potency to give rise to all the tissues and organs.

30. Read the following facts regarding human female:

(i) The menstrual flow results due to breakdown of endometrial lining of the uterus and its blood vessels which forms liquid that comes out through vagina.

(ii) In the later phase of pregnancy, a hormone called **relaxin** is also secreted by the ovary.

(iii) By the end of nine months of pregnancy, the foetus is fully developed and is ready for delivery.

(iv) Parturition is induced by a neuroendocrine mechanism.

How many of them are correct:

(1) Four   (2) Two

(3) Three   (4) one

31. Read the following Statements and find out the correct option:

Statement-I: Inside the seminiferous tubules **interstitial cells** or **Leydig cells present.**

Statement-II: Leydig cells synthesise and secrete testicular hormones called androgens.

(1) Both are wrong Statements

(2) Both are correct Statements

(3) Only Statement-I correct

(4) Only Statement-II correct

32. Go through the following statement and find out the correct option:

Assertion-A: Labia majora is part of internal genitalia of male.

Reason-R: In a majority of organisms, male gamete is non-motile and the female gamete is stationary.

(1) **A** correct and **R** is correct explanation of **A**

(2) **A** correct and **R** is also correct but **R** is not correct explanation of **A**

(1) **A** correct but **R** incorrect

(4) **A** and **R** both are incorrect

33. Find out the incorrect option with respect to contraceptive:

(1) IUDs increase phagocytosis of sperms within the uterus.

(2) The hormone releasing IUDs, in addition, make the uterus unsuitable for implantation and the cervix hostile to the sperms.

(3) IUDs are ideal contraceptives for the females who want to delay pregnancy and/or space children. It is one of most widely accepted methods of contraception in India.

(4) Oral administration of high doses of either progestogens or progestogen–estrogen combinations is another contraceptive method used by the females.

34. Go through the following statement and find out the correct option:

(i) Except for hepatitis-B, genital herpes and HIV infections, other STDs diseases are completely curable if detected early and treated properly.

(ii) Complications of most STDs include itching, fluid discharge, slight pain, swellings, etc., in the genital region.

(iii) Infected females may often be asymptomatic and hence, may remain undetected for long.

(iv) Absence or less significant symptoms in the early stages of infection and the social stigma attached to the STDs, deter the infected persons from going for timely detection and proper treatment.

How many of the above are correct:

(1) Three   (2) Four

(3) Two   (4) One

35. Which of the following is incorrect:

(1) During his journey Lamarck went to Malay archipelago Islands.

(2) Darwin observed an amazing diversity of creatures of particular interest, small black birds later called Darwin's Finches amazed him.

(3) Darwin realised that there were many varieties of finches in the same island.

(4) All the varieties, Darwin conjectured, evolved on the island itself. From the original seed-eating features, many other forms with altered beaks arose, enabling them to become insectivorous and vegetarian finches

36. Consider the following Statements:

(i) The rate of appearance of new forms is linked to the life cycle or the life span.

(ii) Microbes that divide fast have the ability to multiply and become millions of individuals within hours.

(iii) Nature selects for fitness.

(iv) One must remember that the so-called fitness is based on characteristics which are inherited.

Which above Statements is/are correct:

(1) (i), (ii), (iii), (iv)

(2) (i), (iii), (iv) only

(3) (i), (ii), (iii) only

(4) (ii), (iii), (iv)

37. Read the following Statements:

(i) In 1938, a fish caught in South Africa happened to be a Coelacanth which was thought to be extinct.

(ii) Some of these land reptiles went back into water to evolve into fish like reptiles probably 200 mya (e.g. *Ichthyosaurs*).

(iii) The land reptiles were dinosaurs.

(iv) The biggest of them, i.e., *Tyrannosaurus rex* was about 200 feet in height and had huge fearsome dagger like teeth.

(v) About 650 mya, the dinosaurs suddenly disappeared from the earth.

Which of the above Statements is/are correct:

(1) (v) and (ii) only

(2) (iii) and (ii) only

(3) (i), (ii), (iii)

(4) (vi) and (v) only

38. Which is not true for Hardy-Weinberg principle:

(1) Hardy-Weinberg principle says that allele frequencies in a population are stable and is constant from generation to generation.

(2) The gene pool (total genes and their alleles in a population) remains a constant. This is called genetic equilibrium.

(3) Sum total of all the allelic frequencies is 0.5.

(4) Disturbance in genetic equilibrium, or Hardy - Weinberg equilibrium, i.e., change of frequency of alleles in a population would then be interpreted as resulting in evolution.

39. Read the following Statements and find out the correct option:

Statement-I: *Entamoeba histolytica* is a bacterial parasite in the large intestine of human which causes **amoebiasis (amoebic dysentery).**

Statement-II: Symptoms of **amoebic dysentery** disease include constipation, abdominal pain and cramps, stools with excess mucous and blood clots.

(1) Both are wrong Statements

(2) Both are correct Statements

(3) Only Statement-I correct

(4) Only Statement-II correct

40. **Read the following Statements:**

(A) The *B*-lymphocytes produce an army of proteins in response to pathogens into our blood to fight with them.

(B) These above proteins are called antibodies.

(C) The *T*-cells themselves do not secrete antibodies but help B cells produce them.

(D) Each antibody molecule has four peptide chains, two small called **light chains** and two longer called **heavy chains.**

(E) An antibody is represented as H_2L_2.

(F) Different types of antibodies are produced in our body. IgA, IgM, IgE, IgG are some of them.

Which of the above are correct?

(1) (A) and (B) only

(2) (B) (A) (C) only

(3) (C) (B) (D) only

(4) All are correct

41. **Go through the following statement and find out the correct option:**

Assertion-A: When a host is exposed to antigens, which may be in the form of living or dead microbes or other proteins, antibodies are not produced in the host body. This type of immunity is called **active immunity.**

Reason-R: Active immunity is very fast to give its full effective response.

(1) **A** correct and **R** is correct explanation of **A**

(2) **A** correct and **R** is also correct but **R** is not correct explanation of **A**

(3) **A** correct but **R** incorrect

(4) **A** and **R** both are incorrect

42. **Find out the incorrect statement:**

(i) Memory-based acquired immunity evolved in higher vertebrates based on the ability to differentiate foreign organisms (e.g., pathogens) from selfcells.

(ii) Higher vertebrates can distinguish foreign molecules as well as foreign organisms.

(iii) Due to genetic and other unknown reasons, the body attacks self-cells. This results in damage to the body and is called **auto-immune** disease.

(iv) SLE - Systemic lupus erythematosus is an auto-immune disease.

How many of them are/is correct:

(1) One

(2) Two

(3) Three

(4) Four

43. Consider the following Statements:

(i) Open circulatory system is present in arthropods and molluscs.

(ii) Annelids and chordates have a closed circulatory system. (iii) Closed circulatory system more advantageous as the flow of fluid can be more precisely regulated.

(iv) All vertebrates possess a muscular chambered heart.

(v) Fishes have a 2-chambered heart with an atrium and a ventricle.

How many of them are correct:

(1) Five

(2) Two

(3) Three

(4) Four

44. Read the following statement and find out the X:

X is absolutely necessary for the many biological activities of proteins.

(1) Primary structure

(2) Tertiary structure

(3) Quaternary structure

(4) Secondary structure

45. Consider the following Statements with respect to secondary treatment of sewage:

(A) BOD refers to the amount of the oxygen that would be consumed if all the organic matter in one liter of water were oxidised by bacteria.

(B) The sewage water is treated till the BOD is reduced.

(C) The BOD test measures the rate of uptake of oxygen by micro-organisms in a sample of water and thus, indirectly, BOD is a measure of the organic matter present in the water.

(D) (D) The greater the BOD of waste water, more is its polluting potential.

(E) Once the BOD of sewage or waste water is reduced significantly, the effluent is then passed into a settling tank where the bacterial 'flocs' are allowed to sediments. This sediment is called **activated sludge**.

Which of the above Statements is/are correct:

(1) (A), (B), (C), (D), only

(2) (C) and (E) only

(3) (A), (B), (C), (D), (E)

(4) (E) and (B) only

46. Read the following Statements and find out the correct option.

Statement-I: Agarose gel electrophoresis is employed to check the progression of a restriction enzyme digestion.

Statement-II: DNA is a negatively charged molecule, hence it moves towards the positive electrode (anode).

(1) Both are correct Statements

(2) Both are wrong Statements

(3) Only Statement-I correct

(4) Only Statement-II correct

47. Go through the following statements and find out the correct option:

(A) A stirred-tank reactor is usually cylindrical or with a curved base to facilitate the mixing of the reactor contents.

(B) The stirrer facilitates even mixing and oxygen availability throughout the bioreactor.

(C) To produce in large quantities, the development of **bioreactors**, where large volumes (1 lac to 2 lac litres) of culture can be processed, was required.

(1) (A) and (B) only

(2) (B) and (C) only

(3) (A), (B), (C)

(4) (A) only

48. Find out the correct statements and choose correct option-

(A) The downstream processing include separation and purification only.

(B) The product has to be formulated with suitable preservatives.

(C) Such formulation has to undergo thorough clinical trials as in case of drugs.

(D) Strict quality control testing for each product is also required.

(1) (A) and (B) only

(2) (B) (A) (C) only

(3) (B) and (D) only

(4) All are correct

49. Consider the following Statements:

(A) Rice is an important food grain, the presence of which goes back 100 of years in Australia's agricultural history.

(B) There are an estimated 2 lac varieties of rice in India alone.

(C) The diversity of rice in India is one of the richest in the world.

(D) Basmati rice is distinct for its unique aroma and flavour and 27 documented varieties of Basmati are grown in India.

(E) There is reference to Basmati in ancient texts, folklore and poetry, as it has been grown for centuries.

(F) In 1997, an American company got patent rights on Basmati rice through the US Patent and Trademark Office.

Which of the above Statements are correct:

(1) (A) and (C) only

(2) (B), (C), (D), (E), (F)

(3) (B) and (D) only

(4) (A), (B), (C), (D), (E), (F)

50. Read the following statement:

(i) In gene therapy, lymphocytes from the blood of the patient are grown in a culture outside the body.

(ii) A functional ADA cDNA (using a retroviral vector) is then introduced into these lymphocytes, which are subsequently returned to the patient.

(iii) These cells are not immortal, the patient requires periodic infusion of such genetically engineered lymphocytes.

(iv) The gene isolate from marrow cells producing ADA is introduced into cells at early embryonic stages, it never be a permanent cure.

How many of them are incorrect:

(1) One

(2) Two

(3) Three

(4) Four

1. Consider the following Statements and find out the correct option:

(A) In some animals, the body is externally and internally divided into segments with a serial repetition of at least some organs called as Metameric segmentation.

(B) Metameric segmentation not found in Chordata.

(C) The body of arthropods is covered by chitinous exoskeleton.

(D) The body of arthropods consists of **head, Foot** and **abdomen**.

(E) Arthropods have **jointed appendages.**

Which of the above are incorrect:

(1) (A), (E), (C) only

(2) (B), (D) only

(3) (A), (C), (D), (E) only

(4) All are incorrect

2. Match the List-I and List-II:

	List-I	List-II
(i)	*Pila*	Apple snail
(ii)	*Limulus*	King crab
(iii)	*Petromyzon*	Lamprey
(iv)	*Carcharodon*	Great white shark

How many of them are correctly matched:

(1) One

(2) Two

(3) Three

(4) Four

3. Consider the following features:

(A) Circulatory system is of closed type.

(B) Respiration takes place through gills.

(C) Excretory organ is proboscis gland.

(D) Sexes are separate.

(E) Fertilisation is external.

(F) Development is indirect.

Which above features are/is not found in **Hemichordates:**

(1) Only (A)

(2) Only (E) and (C)

(3) Only (C) and (D)

(4) All are correct

4. Read the following statement carefully with respect to Cyclostomata:

(i) Their body is devoid of scales and paired fins.

(ii) Circulation is of closed type.

(iii) Cyclostomes are marine but migrate for spawning to fresh water.

(iv) After spawning, within a few days, they die.

(v) Their larvae, after metamorphosis, return to the ocean.

How many of them are correct:

(1) Three

(2) Four

(3) Five

(4) Two

5. Consider the following Statements and find out the correct option.

Statement-I: The **squamous epithelium** is made of a single thin layer of flattened cells with smooth boundaries.

Statement-II: They are found in the inner wall of ureter and Urinary bladder.

(1) Both are correct Statements

(2) Only Statement-I correct

(3) Both are wrong Statements

(4) Only Statement-II correct

6. Go through the following statements:

Assertion-A: The bone cells (osteocytes) are present in the spaces called lacunae.

Reason-R: Bones have a hard and pliable ground substance rich in calcium salts and collagen fibres which give bone its strength.

(1) **A** correct and **R** is correct explanation of **A**

(2) **A** correct and **R** is also correct but R is not correct explanation of **A**

(3) **A** correct but **R** incorrect

(4) **A** and **R** both are incorrect

7. Which statement is incorrect w.r.t. muscle fibers:

(1) Each muscle is made of many long, cylindrical fibres arranged in parallel arrays.

(2) These fibres are composed of numerous fine fibrils, called myofibrils.

(3) Muscle fibres contract (shorten) in response to stimulation, then relax (lengthen) and return to their uncontracted state in a coordinated fashion.

(4) All muscles are mesodermal in origin.

8. Consider the following Statements and find out the correct option:

Statement-I: Each restriction endonuclease recognizes a specific palindromic nucleotide sequences in the RNA.

Statement-II: Each restriction endonuclease functions by 'inspecting' the length of a DNA sequence.

(1) Both are wrong Statements

(2) Only Statement-I correct

(3) Both are correct Statements

(4) Only Statement-II correct

9. Consider the following Statements and find out the correct option:

Statement-I: Cnidarians, commonly known as sea walnuts.

Statement-II: The body of flatworm bears eight external rows of ciliated comb plates, which help in locomotion.

(1) Both are wrong Statements

(2) Only Statement-I correct

(3) Both are correct Statements

(4) Only Statement-II correct

10. Consider the following Statements and find out the correct option

Statement-I: Inspiration is initiated by the contraction of diaphragm which increases the volume of thoracic chamber in the antero-posterior axis.

Statement-II: Larynx is a cartilaginous box which helps in sound production and hence called the **sound box**.

(1) Both are wrong Statements

(2) Only Statement-I correct

(3) Both are correct Statements

(4) Only Statement-II correct

11. Read the following Statements very carefully and find out the incorrect:

(A) As the solubility of CO_2 is 20-25 times higher than that of O_2.

(B) The diffusion membrane contain thin squamous epithelium of alveoli, the endothelium of alveolar capillaries and the basement substance in between them.

(C) The total thickness of diffusion membrane is much more than a millimeter.

(D) All the factors in our body are favourable for diffusion of O_2 from alveoli to tissues and that of CO_2 from tissues to alveoli.

Which above statement is/are incorrect?

(1) (A) and (C) both   (2) (C) only

(3) (D) and (A) both   (4) (B) and (C) both

12. Go through the following statement:

Assertion-A: Basophils secrete histamine, serotonin and heparin.

Reason-R: Platelets are cell fragments produced from megakaryocytes (special cells in the bone marrow)

(1) **A** correct and **R** is correct explanation of **A**

(2) **A** correct and **R** is also correct but **R** is not correct explanation of **A**

(3) **A** correct but **R** incorrect

(4) **A** and **R** both are incorrect

13. Find out incorrect statement with respect to ECG of Heart:

(1) Each peak in the ECG is identified with a letter from P to T that corresponds to a specific electrical activity of the heart.

(2) The P-wave represents systole of ventricles.

(3) The QRS complex represents the **depolarisation of the ventricles**.

(4) The contraction starts shortly after Q wave and marks the beginning of the systole.

14. Read the following Statements and find out correct option:

(i) Glycine is the simplest amino acid.

(ii) Lecithin is a phospholipid.

(iii) Primary metabolites have identifiable functions and play known roles in normal physiologial processes,

(iv) We do not understand the role or functions of all the

'secondary metabolites' in host organisms.

How many of them are/is correct:

(1) Four   (2) One

(3) Two   (4) Three

15. Consider the following Statements and find out the correct option:

Statement-I: the long protein chain is also folded upon itself like a hollow wollen ball, giving rise to the **primary structure**

Statement-II: This gives us a 3-dimensional view of a protein and is absolutely necessary for the many biological activities of proteins.

(1) Both are wrong Statements

(2) Only Statement-I correct

(3) Both are correct Statements

(4) Only Statement-II correct

16. Consider the following Statements:

(A) Enzymes are divided into 6 classes each with 4-13 subclasses and named accordingly by a four-digit number.

(B) **Lyases:** Enzymes that catalyse removal of groups from substrates by mechanisms other than hydrolysis leaving double bonds.

(C) **Isomerases:** Includes all enzymes catalysing interconversion of optical, geometric or positional isomers.

(D) **Ligases:** Enzymes catalysing the linking together of 2 compounds, e.g., enzymes which catalyse joining of C-O, C-S, C-N, P-O etc. bonds.

Which above Statements are correct:

(1) (A), (C), (B)

(2) (A), (B), (C), (D)

(3) (A), (B), (D)

(4) (B), (C), (D)

17. Consider the following:

(A) A hairpin shaped **Henle's loop** is the next part of PCT.

(B) The ascending limb continues as another highly coiled tubular region called **distal convoluted tubule** (DCT).

(C) The DCTs of many nephrons open into a straight tube called *collecting duct*, many of which converge and open into the renal pelvis through medullary pyramids in the calyces.

(D) The Malpighi an corpuscle, PCT and DCT of the nephron are situated in the cortical region of the kidney whereas the loop of Henle dips into the medulla.

Which above statement are correct?

(1) (A) and (C) only

(2) (C) and (B) only

(3) (A), (B), (C), (D)

(4) (A), (B), (C) only

18. Match the List-I and List-II

	List-I		List-II
(A)	Each organised skeletal muscle in our body is made of a number of **muscle bundles** or **fascicles** held together by a common collagenous connective tissue layer called	(i)	fibrous cartilage
(B)	A characteristic feature of the muscle fibre is the presence of a large number of parallelly arranged filaments in the sarcoplasm called	(ii)	appendicular skeleton
(C)	The bones of the limbs alongwith their girdles constitute the	(iii)	fascia
(D)	The two halves of the pelvic girdle meet ventrally to form the pubic symphysis containing	(iv)	myofibrils

Find out the correct option:

(1) (A)-(ii), (B)-(i), (C)-(iii), (D)-(iv)

(2) (A)-(ii), (B)-(iii), (C)-(i), (D)-(iv)

(3) (A)-(iii), (B)-(iv), (C)-(ii), (D)-(i)

(4) (A)-(iii), (B)-(i), (C)-(iv), (D)-(ii)

19. Consider the following Statements and find out the incorrect one with respect to humans:

(1) JGA is a special sensitive region formed by cellular modifications in the distal convoluted tubule and the afferent arteriole at the location of their contact

(2) A fall in GFR can activate the JG cells to release renin which can stimulate the glomerular blood flow and thereby the GFR back to normal.

(3) A comparison of the volume of the filtrate formed per day (180 litres per day).

(4) The urine released (1.5 litres), suggest that nearly 9 per cent of the filtrate has to be reabsorbed by the renal tubules.

20. Read the following Statements:

(i) Pectoral and Pelvic girdle contain total 6 bones in adults.

(ii) Each girdle is formed of two halves.

(iii) Each half of pectoral girdle consists of a clavicle and a scapula.

(iv) Scapula is a large triangular flat bone situated in the dorsal part of the thorax between the second and the seventh ribs.

(v) The dorsal, flat, triangular body of scapula has a slightly elevated ridge called the spine which projects as a flat, expanded process called the acromion.

How many of them are correct Statements:

(1) Two   (2) Three

(3) Four   (4) Five

21. Consider the following Statements and find out the correct option for humans:

Statement-I: Acetylcholine is a neurotransmitters

Statement-II: The neurotransmitters bind to their specific **receptors**, present on the post-synaptic membrane.

(1) Both are wrong Statements

(2) Only Statement-I correct

(3) Both are correct Statements

(4) Only Statement-II correct

22. Go through the following statement and find out the correct option:

Assertion-A: The hypothalamus is part of forebrain.

Reason-R: It also contains several groups of neurosecretory cells, which secrete hormones called hypothalamic hormones.

(1) **A** correct and **R** is correct explanation of **A**

(2) **A** correct and **R** is also correct but **R** is not correct explanation of **A**

(3) **A** correct but **R** incorrect

(4) **A** and **R** both are incorrect

23. Consider the following statements:

(i) The exaggerated response of the immune system to certain antigens present in the environment is called allergy.

(ii) The substances to which such an immune response is produced are called allergens.

(iii) The antibodies produced to these are of IgE type.

(iv) Common examples of allergens are mites in dust, pollens, animal dander, etc.

How many of above are/is correct:

(1) Three

(2) Four

(3) Two

(4) One

24. Read the Statements given below:

(A) The thymus gland is a lobular structure located on the dorsal side of the kidney and the aorta.

(B) The thymus plays a major role in the development of the immune system.

(C) This gland secretes the peptide hormones called **thymosins**.

(D) Thymosins play a major role in the differentiation of **T-lymphocytes**, which provide **cell-mediated immunity**. Which above statement is/are correct?

(1) (A) and (C) only

(2) (A) only

(3) (D) and (E) only

(4) (B), (C), (D)

25. Which statement is incorrect one:

(1) Glucagon is a peptide hormone, and plays an important role in maintaining the normal blood glucose levels.

(2) Glucagon increases blood sugar (**hyperglycemia**).

(3) In addition, this hormone stimulates the process of gluconeogenesis which also contributes to hyperglycemia.

(4) Glucagon increases the cellular glucose uptake and utilisation.

26. Read the following statement:

(i) The spleen is a large bean shaped organ.

(ii) It mainly contains lymphocytes and phagocytes.

(iii) It acts as a filter of the blood by trapping blood-borne microorganisms.

(iv) Spleen is a Primary lymphoid organ.

How many of above are/is correct:

(1) Three

(2) Four

(3) Two

(4) One

27. Consider the following Statements:

(i) Open circulatory system is present fishes.

(ii) All Annelids and chordates have a closed circulatory system.

(iii) Closed circulatory system more advantageous as the flow of fluid can be more precisely regulated.

(iv) All vertebrates possess a muscular chambered heart.

(v) Fishes have a 3-chambered heart with two atrium and a ventricle.

How many of them are/is incorrect:

(1) Five

(2) Two

(3) Three

(4) Four

28. Read the following and out the incorrect:

(1) The wall of the uterus has three layers of tissue.

(2) The external thin membranous layer called **perimetrium.**

(3) **The** middle thick layer of smooth muscle called **myometrium.**

(4) **The** inner non-glandular layer called **endometrium** that lines the uterine cavity.

29. Consider the following statements and find out incorrect one:

(i) **Mons pubis** is a cushion of fatty tissue not covered by skin and pubic hair.

(ii) The **labia majora** are fleshy folds of tissue, which extend down from the mons pubis and surround the vaginal opening.

(iii) The **labia minora** are paired folds of tissue under the labia majora.

(iv) The opening of the vagina is often covered partially by a membrane called **hymen.**

(v) The **clitoris** is a tiny finger-like structure which lies at the upper junction of the two labia minora above the urethral opening.

How many of them are correct:

(1) Two

(2) Four

(3) Three

(4) Five

30. Read the following facts:

(i) The spermatids are transformed into **spermatozoa (sperms)** by the process called **spermiogenesis.**

(ii) After spermiogenesis, sperm heads become embedded in the **leyding cells,** and are finally released from the seminiferous tubules by the process called **spermiation.**

(iii) Spermatogenesis starts at the age of puberty due to significant increase in the secretion of gonadotropin releasing hormone (GnRH).

(iv) The increased levels of GnRH then acts at the anterior pituitary gland and stimulates secretion of two gonadotropins-luteinising hormone (LH) and follicle stimulating hormone (FSH).

(v) FSH acts at the Leydig cells and stimulates synthesis and secretion of androgens.

How many of them are incorrect:

(1) Four

(2) Two

(3) Three

(4) Five

31. Read the following Statements and find out the correct option:

Statement-I: The blastomeres in the blastocyst are arranged into an outer layer called **trophoblast.**

Statement-II: The trophoblast layer then gets attached to the perimetrium and the inner cell mass gets differentiated as the embryo.

(1) Both are wrong Statements

(2) Both are correct Statements

(3) Only Statement-I correct

(4) Only Statement-II correct

32. Go through the following statement and find out the correct option:

Assertion-A: The primary follicles get surrounded by more layers of granulosa cells and a new theca and called **secondary follicles.**

Reason-R: The primary follicle soon transforms into a tertiary follicle which is characterised by a fluid filled cavity called **antrum.**

(1) **A** correct and **R** is correct explanation of **A**

(2) **A** correct and **R** is also correct but R is not correct explanation of **A**

(3) **A** correct but **R** incorrect

(4) **A** and **R** both are incorrect

33. Find out the incorrect statement:

(1) **Condoms** are barriers made of thin rubber/ latex sheath.

(2) The 'Nirodh' is a popular brand of condom for the male.

(3) Use of condoms has increased in recent years due to its additional benefit of protecting the user from contracting STDs and AIDS.

(4) Both the male and the female condoms are reusable, can be self-inserted and thereby gives privacy to the user.

34. Read the following events with respect to ART:

(1) **Intra cytoplasmic sperm injection** (ICSI) is another specialised procedure to form an embryo in the laboratory in which a sperm is directly injected into the vagina.

(2) Infertility cases either due to inability of the male partner to inseminate the female or due to very low sperm counts in the ejaculates, could be corrected by **artificial insemination** (AI) technique.

(3) In this technique, the semen collected either from the husband or a healthy donor is artificially introduced either into the vagina or into the uterus (IUI-**intra-uterine insemination**) of the female.

(4) All of above techniques require extremely high precision handling by specialised professionals and expensive instrumentation.

35. Which of the following is incorrect with respect to origin of life:

(1) The geological history of earth closely correlates with the biological history of earth.

(2) A common permissible conclusion is that earth is very old, not thousands of years as was thought earlier but billions of years old.

(3) The first cellular form of life did not possibly originate till about 2000 billion years ago.

(4) All life forms were in water environment only.

36. Consider the following statements:

(i) The **Big Bang** theory attempts to explain to us the origin of universe.

(ii) Big Bang talks of a singular huge explosion unimaginable in physical terms.

(iii) The universe expanded and hence, the temperature came down.

(iv) Hydrogen and Helium formed sometime later.

Which above Statements are correct w.r.t. Big Bang:

(1) (i), (ii) only

(2) (i), (iii), (iv) only

(3) (i), (ii), (iii) only

(4) All are correct

37. Read the following Statements:

(i) *Homo sapiens* arose in Australia and moved across continents and developed into distinct races.

(ii) During ice age between 75,000-10,000 billion years ago modern *Homo sapiens* arose.

(iii) Pre-historic cave art developed about 18,000 years ago. (iv) Agriculture came around 10, 0000 years back and human settlements started.

(v) The skull of baby chimpanzee is more like adult human skull than adult chimpanzee skull.

Which of the above statements is/are incorrect:

(1) (v) and (ii) only

(2) (iii) and (ii) only

(3) (iv) only

(4) (i) (ii) only

38. Consider the following:

(A) When migration of a section of population to another place and population occurs, gene frequencies change in the original as well as in the new population.

(B) New genes/alleles are added to the new population and these are lost from the old population.

(C) The above phenomenon known as gene migration. (D) If the change in allele occurs by chance, it is called genetic drift.

(1) (A) and (B) only

(2) (B) only

(3) (A), (B), (C), (D)

(4) (A), (B), (C) only

39. Read the following Statements and find out the correct option:

Statement-I: The pathogens can enter our body by various means, multiply and interfere with normal vital activities, resulting in morphological and functional damage.

Statement-II: Maintenance of personal and public hygiene is very important for prevention and control of many infectious diseases.

(1) Both are wrong Statements

(2) Both are correct Statements

(3) Only Statement-I correct

(4) Only Statement-II correct

40. Read the following Statements:

(A) *Physical barriers*: Skin on our body is the main barrier which prevents entry of the micro-organisms.

(B) *Physiological barriers*: Acid in the stomach, saliva in the mouth, tears from eyes–all prevent microbial growth.

(C) *Cellular barriers*: Certain types of leukocytes (WBC) of our body like polymorpho-nuclear leukocytes and monocytes and natural killer.

(D) *Cytokine barriers*: Virus-infected cells secrete proteins called **interferons** which protect non-infected cells from further viral infection.

Which of the above statements are correct?

(1) (A) and (B) only

(2) (B) and (C) only

(3) (C) and (D)only

(4) (A), (B), (C) (D)

41. Go through the following statement and find out the correct option:

Assertion-A: The chemical carcinogens present in tobacco smoke have been identified as a major cause of lung cancer.

Reason-R: Cancer causing viruses called **oncogenic viruses** have genes called **viral oncogenes**.

(1) **A** correct and **R** is correct explanation of **A**

(2) **A** correct and **R** is also correct but R is not correct explanation of **A**

(3) **A** correct but **R** incorrect

(4) **A** and **R** both are incorrect

42. Find out the incorrect statement for HIV:

(1) It is important to note that HIV/AIDS is not spread by mere touch or physical contact; it spreads only through body fluids.

(2) It is, hence, imperative, for the physical and psychological well-being, that the HIV/AIDS infected persons are not isolated from family and society.

(3) There is always a time-lag between the infection and appearance of AIDS symptoms.

(4) After getting into the body of the person, the virus enters into Killer T-cells directly.

43. Consider the following Statements:

(i) Yeast (*Saccharomyces cerevisiae)* is used for commercial production of ethanol.

(ii) Lipases are used in detergent formulations and are helpful in removing oily stains from the laundry.

(iii) The bottled fruit juices bought from the market are clearer as compared to those made at home.

(iv) The bottled juices are clarified by the use of pectinases and proteases.

(v) Streptokinase produced by the bacterium *Streptococcus* and modified by genetic engineering is used as a 'clot buster'.

How many of them are correct:

(1) One

(2) Three

(3) Four

(4) Five

44. Read the following Statements and find out the correct option with respect to sewage treatment:

Statement-I: Once the BOD of sewage or waste water is reduced significantly, the effluent is then passed into a settling tank where the bacterial 'flocs' are allowed to sediment. This sediment is called **activated sludge**.

Statement-II: A small part of the activated sludge is pumped back into the aeration tank to serve as the inoculum. The remaining major part of the sludge is pumped into large tanks called **anaerobic sludge digesters**.

(1) Both are correct Statements

(2) Both are wrong Statements

(3) Only Statement-I correct

(4) Only Statement-II correct

45. Consider the following Statements and find out the correct option:

(A) WBCs shows amoeboid movement.

(B) Cilia found in fallopian tube.

(C) In trachea cilia present.

(D) Human beings can move limbs, jaws, eyelids, tongue with the help of muscles.

Which of the above are correct with respect to humans:

(1) (A), (B), (C)   (2) (B), (C)

(3) (D), (C), (A)   (4) (A), (B), (C), (D)

46. Read the following Statements and find out the correct option:

Statement-I: pBR 322 is an example of a vector.

Statement-II: Ti plasmid obtained from a Fungus.

(1) Both are correct Statements

(2) Both are wrong Statements

(3) Only Statement-I correct

(4) Only Statement-II correct

47. Match the List-I and List-II:

	List-I		List-II
(A)	*Monascus purpureus*	(i)	Bread making
(B)	*Saccharomyces cerevisiae*	(ii)	Statin
(C)	*Aspergillus niger*	(iii)	Citric acid
(D)	*Trichoderma polysporum*	(iv)	*Immuno suppressive*

Find out the correct option:

(1) (A)-(ii), (B)-(i), (C)-(iii), (D)-(iv)

(2) (A)-(ii), (B)-(iii), (C)-(i), (D)-(iv)

(3) (A)-(iii), (B)-(i), (C)-(ii), (D)-(iv)

(4) (A)-(iii), (B)-(i), (C)-(iv), (D)-(ii)

48. Read the following Statements:

(i)   If any protein encoding gene is expressed in a heterologous host, is called a **recombinant protein.**

(ii) The cells harbouring cloned genes of interest may be grown on a small scale in the laboratory.

(iii) A stirred-tank reactor is usually cylindrical or with a curved base to facilitate the mixing of the reactor contents.

(iv) The processes include separation and purification, which are collectively referred to as downstream processing.

(v)   Each restriction endonuclease recognises a specific **palindromic nucleotide sequences** in the DNA.

How many of them are correct:

(1) One   (2) Three

(3) Four   (4) Five

	List-I		List-II
(A)	Bt –cotton	(i)	C peptide
(B)	Proinsulin	(ii)	RNAi
(C)	Insulin used for diabetes was earlier extracted from pancreas of slaughtered	(iii)	cry
(D)	A novel strategy was adopted to prevent this infestation which was based on the process of	(iv)	cattle and pigs

49 Match the List-I and List-II:

Find out the correct option:

(1) (A)-(ii), (B)-(i), (C)-(iii), (D)-(iv)

(2) (A)-(ii), (B)-(iii), (C)-(i), (D)-(iv)

(3) (A)-(iii), (B)-(iv), (C)-(ii), (D)-(i)

(4) (A)-(iii), (B)-(i), (C)-(iv), (D)-(ii)

50. Read the following with respect to GMO:

The Indian Government has set up organisations such as X, which will make decisions regarding the validity of Y and the safety of introducing GM-organisms for public services.

Here X and Y respectively:

(1) GEAC, GM research (2) CDRI, GM research

(3) NBRI, GM research (4) IIPR, GM research

1. **Consider the following matching with respect to Arthropoda and find out the correct option:**

   (A) Economically important insect-*Laccifer*

   (B) Vector-*Anopheles*

   (C) Gregarious pest-*Locusta*

   (D) Living fossil-*Limulus*

   Which of the above are correct:

   (1) (A), (C)

   (2) (B), (D)

   (3) (D), (A)

   (4) (A), (B), (C), (D)

2. **Match the List-I and List-II:**

	List-I		List-II
(A)	*Culex*	(i)	Cnidoblasts
(B)	*Dentalium*	(ii)	jointed appendages
(C)	*Hydra*	(iii)	visceral hump
(D)	*Antedon*	(iv)	water vascular system

   Find out the correct option:

   (1) (A)-(ii), (B)-(i), (C)-(iii), (D)-(iv)

   (2) (A)-(ii), (B)-(iii), (C)-(i), (D)-(iv)

   (3) (A)-(iii), (B)-(i), (C)-(ii), (D)-(iv)

   (4) (A)-(iii), (B)-(i), (C)-(iv), (D)-(ii)

3. **Consider the following features:**

   (A) The most distinctive feature of echinoderms is the presence of **water vascular system.**

   (B) Usually external fertilization present.

   (C) The anterior head region has sensory tentacles.

   (D) The mouth contains a file-like rasping organ for feeding, called **radula.**

   (E) Larva absent.

Which above features are found in phylum **Echinodermata**:

(1) (A), (B)
(2) Only (A)

(3) Only (C) and (D)
(4) (A), (B), (C), (D), (E)

4. Read the following statement carefully with respect to Reptilia:

(i)   They do not have external ear openings.

(ii) Tympanum represents ear.

(iii) Heart is usually three-chambered, but four-chambered in crocodiles.

(iv) Snakes and lizards shed their scales as skin cast.

(v)   Bisexual.

How many of them are correct:

(1) Three
(2) Four

(3) Five
(4) two

5. Consider the following Statements and find out the correct option:

STATEMENT-I: Frog shows sexual dimorphism.

STATEMENT-II: Male Frog has vocal sac.

(1) Both are wrong Statements

(2) Only Statement-I correct

(3) Both are correct Statements

(4) Only Statement-II correct

6. Go through the following statements:

Assertion-A: Neurons, the unit of neural system are excitable cells

Reason-R: Neuroglia make up more than one half the volume of neural tissue in our body.

(1) **A** correct and **R** is correct explanation of **A**

(2) **A** correct and **R** is also correct but **R** is not correct explanation of **A**

(3) **A** correct but **R** incorrect

(4) **A** and **R** both are incorrect

7. Find out the incorrect statement:

(1) Smooth muscles are 'involuntary' as their functioning cannot be directly controlled.

(2) **Cardiac muscle tissue** is a contractile tissue present only in the heart and Liver.

(3) Cell junctions fuse the plasma membranes of cardiac muscle cells and make them stick together.

(4) Communication junctions (intercalated discs) at some fusion points allow the cells to contract as a unit.

8. Consider the following:

Corvus (Crow), Columba (Pigeon), Psittacula (Parrot), Struthio (Ostrich), Pavo (Peacock), Aptenodytes (Penguin), Neophron (Vulture), Macaca (Monkey), Rattus (Rat), Canis (Dog), Felis (Cat), Frog (Rana)

How many of them has four chambered heart:

(1) 9

(2) 1

(3) 7

(4) 11

9. Consider the following Statements and find out the correct option:

Statement-I: Gap junctions facilitate the cells to communicate with each other.

Statement-II: Tight junctions help to stop substances from leaking across a tissue

(1) Both are correct Statements

(2) Only Statement-I correct

(3) Both are wrong Statements

(4) Only Statement-II correct

10. Consider the following Statements and find out the correct option:

Statement-I: Volume of air that will remain in the lungs after a normal expiration termed as FRC.

Statement-II: FRC includes ERV + RV.

(1) Both are wrong Statements

(2) Only Statement-I correct

(3) Both are correct Statements

(4) Only Statement-II correct

11. Read the following Statements very carefully and find out the incorrect:

(1) A sigmoid curve is obtained when percentage saturation of haemoglobin with O_2 is plotted against the pO_2.

(2) This curve is called the Oxygen dissociation curve and is highly useful in studying the effect of factors like pCO_2, H^+ concentration, etc., on binding of O_2 with haemoglobin.

(3) In the alveoli, where there is high pO_2, low pCO_2, lesser H^+ concentration and lower temperature, the factors are all favourable for the formation of oxyhaemoglobin, whereas in the tissues, where low pO_2, high pCO_2, high H^+ concentration and higher temperature exist, the conditions are favourable for dissociation of oxygen from the oxyhaemoglobin.

(4) This curve never indicates that O_2 gets bound to haemoglobin in the lung surface and gets dissociated at the tissues.

12. Go through the following statement:

Assertion-A: Lymph is a colourless fluid containing specialised lymphocytes which are responsible for the immune responses of the body.

Reason-R: Fats are absorbed through lymph in the lacteals present in the intestinal villi.

(1) **A** correct and **R** is correct explanation of **A**

(2) **A** correct and **R** is also correct but **R** is not correct explanation of **A**

(3) **A** correct but **R** incorrect

(4) **A** and **R** both are incorrect

13. Go through the following Statements:

(A) Heart is protected by a double walled membranous bag, **pericardium,** enclosing the pericardial fluid.

(B) Our heart has four chambers, two relatively small upper chambers called **atria** and two larger lower chambers called **ventricles.**

(C) A thin, muscular wall called the interatrial septum separates the right and the left atria, whereas a thick-walled, the inter-ventricular septum, separates the left and the right ventricles.

(D) The atrium and the ventricle of the same side are also separated by a thick neural tissue called the atrio-ventricular septum.

Find out the correct Statements and choose the suitable option for Humans:

(1) (A), (B) only

(2) (A), (B), (C)

(3) (B), (C), (A) only

(4) All are correct

14. Read the following Statements and find out correct option:

(i) In a polypeptide or a protein, amino acids are linked by a **peptide bond** which is formed when the carboxyl (-COOH) group of one amino acid reacts with the amino (-NH2) group of the next amino acid with the elimination of a water moiety (the process is called dehydration).

(ii) In a polysaccharide the individual monosaccharides are linked by a **glycosidic bond**.

(iii) **Glycosidic bond** formed by dehydration method.

(iv) **Glycosidic bond** is formed between two carbon atoms of two adjacent monosaccharides.

How many of them is/are correct:

(1) Three

(2) Four

(3) Two

(4) One

15. Consider the following Statements and find out the correct option

Statement-I: Paper made from plant pulp is cellulose.

Statement-II: Cellulose is made by amino acid monomers.

(1) Both are wrong Statements

(2) Only Statement-I correct

(3) Both are correct Statements

(4) Only Statement-II correct

16. Find out the incorrect statement:

(1) A nucleotide has three chemically distinct components.

(2) One is a heterocyclic compound, the second is a protein and the third a phosphoric acid or phosphate.

(3) The heterocyclic compounds in nucleic acids are the nitrogenous bases named adenine, guanine, uracil, cytosine, and thymine.

(4) Adenine and Guanine are substituted purines while the uracil is substituted pyrimidines.

17. Consider the following:

(A) A comparison of the volume of the filtrate formed per day (180 litres per day) with that of the urine released (1.5 litres), suggest that nearly 99 per cent of the filtrate has to be reabsorbed by the renal tubules. This process is called **reabsorption.**

(B) The tubular epithelial cells in different segments of nephron perform **reabsorption** either by active or passive mechanisms.

(C) For example, substances like glucose, amino acids, Na+, etc., in the filtrate are reabsorbed actively whereas the nitrogenous wastes are absorbed by passive transport.

(D) Reabsorption of water not occurs passively in the initial segments of the nephron. Which above statement are correct?

(1) (A) and (C) only   (2) (B) and (C) only

(3) (A), (B), (C), (D),   (4) (A), (B) and (C) only

18. Match the List-I and List-II:

	List-I	List-II
(A)	GFR	125 ml/minute
(B)	*Vasa recta*	counter current
(C)	Glomerulus and Bowman's capsule	malpighian body

Find out the correct option:

(1) Only (A)   (2) Only (A), (B)

(3) Only (C), (B)   (4) (A), (B), (C)

19. Consider the following Statements and find out the incorrect one:

(1) The macrophages and leucocytes in blood exhibit amoeboid movement.

(2) It is effected by pseudopodia formed by the streaming of protoplasm (as in *Amoeba*).

(3) Cytoskeletal elements like microfilaments are involved in amoeboid movement.

(4) Ciliary movement occurs in most of our internal tubular organs which are not lined by ciliated epithelium.

20. Find out the odd one out:

(i) Ball and socket joint-between humerus and pectoral girdle

(ii) Hinge joint - knee joint

(iii) Pivot joint - between humerus and axis

(iv) Gliding joint - between the carpals

How many of them are correct:

(1) One   (2) Two

(3) Three   (4) Four

21. **Consider the following Statements and find out the correct option.**

   Statement-I: The electrical potential difference across the resting plasma membrane is called as the **Action potential.**

   Statement-II: A nerve impulse is transmitted from one neuron to another through junctions called synapses.

   (1) Both are wrong Statements

   (2) Only Statement-I correct

   (3) Both are correct Statements

   (4) Only Statement-II correct

22. **Go through the following Statements:**

   (i) Trachea is a primary site of exchange of gases.

   (ii) Exchange of gases also occur between blood and tissues.

   (iii) O_2 and CO_2 are exchanged in these sites by simple diffusion mainly based on pressure/concentration gradient.

   (iv) Solubility of the gases as well as the thickness of the membranes involved in diffusion are also some important factors that can affect the rate of diffusion.

   How many of them are correct:

   (1) Two   (2) Three

   (3) Four   (4) One

23. **Consider the following:**

   (A) Renette cells are the tubular excretory structures of earthworms and other annelids.

   (B) Nephridia help to remove nitrogenous wastes and maintain a fluid and ionic balance.

   (C) Kidneys are the excretory structures of most of the annelids including cockroaches.

   (D) Green glands perform the excretory function in crustaceans like cockroach.

   Which above statement are/is correct?

   (1) (A) only   (2) (A), (C) and (D) only

   (3) (D) and (B) only   (4) (A), (B), (C)

24. **Melatonin plays a very important role in the regulation of:**

   (A) Maintaining the normal rhythms of sleep-wake cycle

   (B) Body temperature

   (C) Metabolism and pigmentation

   (D) The menstrual cycle

   (E) Defense capability

   Which above statement are correct?

   (1) (B), (C), (D) only   (2) (A) and (C) only

   (3) (D) and (E) only   (4) All are correct

25. Which statement is incorrect for Hormone releasing form adrenal medulla:

(1) The adrenal medulla secretes two hormones called **adrenaline** or **epinephrine** and **noradrenaline** or **norepinephrine.**

(2) These are commonly called as **catecholamines.**

(3) Adrenaline and noradrenaline are rapidly secreted in response to stress of any kind and during emergency situations and are called **emergency hormones** or **hormones of Fight or Flight.**

(4) These hormones decreases alertness, pupilary dilation, piloerection (raising of hairs), sweating etc.

26. Consider the following Statements:

(i) Earthworms, sponge, tapeworm and leech, typical examples of bisexual animals.

(ii) Cockroach is an example of a unisexual species.

(iii) The cows, sheep, rats, deers, dogs, tiger, etc. are non-primate mammals.

(iv) In rotifers, honeybees and even some lizards and birds turkey etc. **parthenogenesis found.**

How many of them is/are correct:

(1) One   (2) Two

(3) Three   (4) Four

27. Match the List-I and List-II:

	List-I		List-II
(A)	A cushion of fatty tissue covered by skin and pubic hair	(i)	Labia majora
(B)	Are fleshy folds of tissue, which extend down from the mons pubis and surround the vaginal opening	(ii)	Hymen
(C)	A tiny finger-like structure which lies at the upper junction of the two labia minora above the urethral opening	(iii)	Mons pubis
(D)	The opening of the vagina is often covered partially by a membrane called	(iv)	Clitoris

Find out the correct option:

(1) (A)-(ii), (B)-(i), (C)-(iii), (D)-(iv)

(2) (A)-(ii), (B)-(iii), (C)-(i), (D)-(iv)

(3) (A)-(iii), (B)-(iv), (C)-(ii), (D)-(i)

(4) (A)-(iii), (B)-(i), (C)-(iv), (D)-(ii)

28. Consider the following Statements with respect to mammary glands:

(i) The cells of alveoli secrete milk, which is stored in the cavities (lumens) of alveoli.

(ii) The alveoli open into mammary tubules.

(iii) The tubules of each lobe join to form a **mammary duct.**

(iv) Several mammary ducts join to form a wider mammary ampulla which is connected to **lactiferous duct** through which milk is sucked out. How many of them is/are correct:

(1) One	(2) Two
(3) Three	(4) Four

29. Find out the incorrect one:

(1) The human male ejaculates about 200 to 300 billion sperms during a coitus of which, for normal fertility, at least 80 per cent sperms must have normal shape and size and for at least 40 per cent of them must show vigorous motility.

(2) The acrosome is filled with enzymes that help fertilisation of the ovum.

(3) The middle piece possesses numerous mitochondria, which produce energy for the movement of tail that facilitate sperm motility essential for fertilisation.

(4) The sperm head contains an elongated haploid nucleus, the anterior portion of which is covered by a cap-like structure, **acrosome**.

30. Read the following Statements:

(i) The corpus luteum secretes large amounts of progesterone which is essential for maintenance of the endometrium.

(ii) Such an endometrium is necessary for implantation of the fertilized ovum and other events of pregnancy.

(iii) During pregnanacy all events of the menstrual cycle stop and there is no menstruation.

(iv) In the absence of fertilisation, the corpus luteum degenerates.

(v) In human beings, menstrual cycles ceases around 50 years of age; that is termed as **menarche**.

How many of them are correct for Human female:

(1) Five	(2) Two
(3) Three	(4) Four

31. Read the following Statements and find out the correct option:

Statement-I: The signals for parturition originate from the partially developed foetus and the placenta which induce mild uterine contractions called **foetal ejection reflex.**

Statement-II: Parturition is induced by a simple neuroendocrine mechanism.

(1) Both are wrong Statements

(2) Both are correct Statements

(3) Only Statement-I correct

(4) Only Statement-II correct

32. Go through the following statement and find out the correct option:

Assertion-A: An ideal contraceptive should be user-friendly, easily available, effective and reversible with no or least side-effects.

Reason-R: Use of condoms has increased in recent years due to its additional benefit of protecting the user from contracting STDs and AIDS.

(1) **A** correct and **R** is correct explanation of **A**

(2) **A** correct and **R** is also correct but R is not correct explanation of **A**

(3) **A** correct but **R** incorrect

(4) **A** and **R** both are incorrect

33. Consider the following statements and find out the correct option for humans-

STATEMENT 1. Natural methods work on the principle of avoiding chances of ovum and sperms meeting.

STATEMENT 2. Periodic abstinence is one such method in which the couples avoid or abstain from coitus from day 10 to 17 of the menstrual cycle when ovulation could be expected.

1. Both are wrong statements

2. Only Statement 1 correct

3. Both are correct statements

4. Only statement 2 correct

34. Read the following events with respect to evolution:

(i) The universe is very old-almost 20 billion years old.

(ii) Galaxies contain stars and clouds of gas and dust.

(iii) The **Big Bang** theory attempts to explain to us the origin of universe.

(iv) The universe expanded and hence, the temperature came down.

(v) Hydrogen and Helium formed sometime later.

How many of above are correct:

(1) Three   (2) Four

(3) Five   (4) Two

35. Which of the following is incorrect:

(1) A study of fossils in different sedimentary layers indicates the geological period in which they existed.

(2) The study showed that life-forms varied over time and certain life forms are restricted to certain geological timespans.

(3) Deepest the fossil indicates fossil is more newer.

(4) Rocks form sediments and a cross-section of earth's crust indicates the arrangement of sediments one over the other during the long history of earth.

36. Which of the following is incorrect statement:

(1) *Tyrannosaurus rex* was about 20 feet in height and had huge fearsome dagger like teeth.

(2) About 65 mya, the dinosaurs suddenly disappeared from the earth.

(3) Natural selection is a process in which heritable variations enabling better survival are enabled to reproduce and leave greater number of progeny.

(4) About 15 bya, primates called *Dryopithecus* and *Ramapithecus* were existing.

37. Read the following Statements:

(i) **Branching descent** and **natural selection** are the two key concepts of Lamarckian Theory of Evolution

(ii) Sweet potato (root modification) and potato (stem modification) is an example of analogy.

(iii) The biochemical similarities point to the same shared ancestry as structural similarities among diverse organisms.

(iv) Man never domesticated wild animals and crops.

Which above Statements are correct:

(1) (i) and (ii) only

(2) (iii) And (ii) only

(3) (iv) and (iii) only

(4) All are correct

38. Which statement is/are true for ringworms:

(A) Many fungi belonging to the genera *Microsporum*, *Trichophyton* and *Epidermophyton* are responsible for **ringworms** which is one of the most common infectious diseases in man.

(B) Appearance of dry, scaly lesions on various parts of the body such as skin, nails and scalp are the main symptoms of the disease.

(C) These lesions are accompanied by intense itching.

(D) Heat and moisture help these fungi to grow, which makes them thrive in skin folds such as those in the groin or between the toes.

(E) Ringworms are generally acquired from soil or by using towels, clothes or even the comb of infected individuals.

(1) (A) and (B) only

(2) (B) and (C) only

(3) (A), (B), (C), (D), (E)

(4) (D) only

39. Find out the correct Statements:

(A) Acquired immunity, on the other hand, is pathogen specific. It is characterised by memory.

(B) Our body when encounters a pathogen for the first time produces a response called **primary response** which is of low intensity.

(C) Subsequent encounter with the same pathogen elicits a highly intensified secondary or anamnestic response.

(D) This is ascribed to the fact that our body appears to have memory of the first encounter.

(E) The primary and secondary immune responses are carried out with the help of two special types of lymphocytes present in our blood, i.e., **B**-lymphocytes and **T**-lymphocytes.

Which of the following are correct:

(1) (A) and (D) only

(2) (A), (B) and (E) only

(3) (B) and (D) only

(4) All are correct

40. Read the following Statements:

(A) Coca alkaloid or **cocaine** is obtained from coca plant.

(B) *Erythroxylum coca*, native of South America.

(C) It interferes with the transport of the neuro-transmitter dopamine.

(D) Cocaine, commonly called **coke** or **crack** is usually snorted.

(E) It has a potent stimulating action on central nervous system, producing a sense of euphoria and increased energy. Which of the above are/is correct?

(1) (A) and (B) only

(2) (B) and (C) only

(3) (C) and (D) only

(4) All are correct

41. Read the following events for HIV and find out the incorrect one:

(1) The word AIDS stands for **Acquired Immuno Deficiency Syndrome**.

(2) This means deficiency of immune system, acquired during the lifetime of an individual indicating that it is not a congenital disease. 'Syndrome' means a group of symptoms.

(3) AIDS was first reported in 1981 and in the last twenty five years or so, it has spread all over the world killing more than 25 million persons.

(4) AIDS is caused by the Human Immuno deficiency Virus (HIV), a member of a group of viruses called **retrovirus**, which have an envelope enclosing the DNA genome.

42. Match the List-I and List-II:

	List-I	List-II
(A)	*Pila*	Devil fish
(B)	*Euspongia*	King crab
(C)	*Petromyzon*	Dog fish
(D)	*Carcharodon*	Great white shark

How many of them is/are correctly matched:

(1) One

(2) Two

(3) Three

(4) Four

43. Consider the following Statements and find out the correct option:

Statement-I: Palmitic acid is an example of MUFA.

Statement-II: MUFA are good for health.

(1) Both are wrong Statements

(2) Only Statement-I correct

(3) Both are correct Statements

(4) Only Statement-II correct

44. Find out the incorrect:

(1) Alexander Fleming was worked on *Staphylococci* bacteria.

(2) Alexander Fleming discovered Penicillin from *Penicillium notatum*.

(3) This antibiotic was extensively used to treat American soldiers wounded in World War I.

(4) Fleming, Chain and Florey were awarded the Nobel Prize in 1945.

45. Consider the following and find out the incorrect one:

(1) The Ministry of Environment and Forests has initiated **Ganga Action Plan** and **Yamuna Action Plan.**

(2) Under these plans, it is proposed to build a large number of sewage treatment plants so that only treated sewage may be discharged in the rivers.

(3) Baculoviruses are pathogens that attack insects and other arthropods.

(4) Many members of the genus *Rhizobium* form antibiotics.

46. Read the following Statements and find out the correct option:

Statement-I: The DNA fragment seprated on an agarose gel can be seen after staining with ethidium bromide.

Statement-II: Retroviruses have also been disarmed and are now used to deliver desirable genes into animal cells.

(1) Both are correct Statements

(2) Both are wrong Statements

(3) Only Statement-I correct

(4) Only Statement-II correct

47. Go through the following statement and find out the correct option:

Assertion-A: The cutting of DNA by Ligase results in the fragments of DNA.

Reason-R: These fragments can be separated by a technique known as **PCR.**

(1) **A** correct and **R** is correct explanation of **A**

(2) **A** correct and **R** is also correct but **R** is not correct explanation of **A**

(3) **A** correct but **R** incorrect

(4) **A** and **R** both are incorrect

48. Find out the incorrect Statement:

(i) PCR not used to detect HIV in suspected AIDS patients.

(ii) PCR is being used to detect mutations in genes in suspected cancer patients too.

(iii) Transgenic animals that produce useful biological products can be created by the introduction of the portion of DNA (or genes) which codes for a particular product such as human protein (alpha-1-antitrypsin) used to treat emphysema.

(iv) In 2007, the first transgenic cow, Rosie, produced human protein-enriched milk (2.4 grams per litre).

How many of above are incorrect:

(1) Three

(2) Four

(3) One

(4) Two

49. Consider the following Statenmts:

(A) Insulin used for diabetes was earlier extracted from pancreas of slaughtered cattle and pigs.

(B) At present, about 30 recombinant therapeutics have been approved for human-use the world over.

(C) In India, 27 of recombinant therapeutics are presently being marketed.

(D) The main challenge for production of insulin using r-DNA techniques was getting insulin assembled into a mature form.

(E) In 1900, Eli Lilly an American company prepared two DNA sequences corresponding to A and B, chains of human insulin and introduced them in plasmids of *E.coli* to produce insulin chains.

Which above Statements are incorrect:

(1) (E) and (C) only

(2) (A), (B), (D) only

(3) (B) and (D) only

(4) All are correct

50. Consider the following Statements and find out the incorrect:

(1) **Biopiracy** is the term used to refer to the use of bioresources by multinational companies and other organisations without proper authorisation from the countries and people concerned without compensatory payment.

(2) Most of the industrialised nations are rich financially and also rich in biodiversity and traditional knowledge.

(3) Traditional knowledge related to bio-resources can be exploited to develop modern applications and can also be used to save time, effort and expenditure during their commercialisation.

(4) There has been growing realisation of the injustice, inadequate compensation and benefit sharing between developed and developing countries.

Answer Keys

Chapter-01 ANIMAL KINGDOM (Answer key)

1	2	3	4	5	6	7	8	9	10
3	2	3	4	3	1	3	4	2	2
11	12	13	14	15	16	17	18	19	20
4	2	4	2	2	2	4	4	1	4
21	22	23	24	25	26	27	28	29	30
2	2	3	4	1	1	4	3	2	1
31	32	33	34	35	36	37	38	39	40
2	2	2	3	1	4	4	3	4	1
41	42	43	44	45	46	47	48	49	50
1	4	4	4	4	1	3	2	4	4

Chapter-02 STURCTURAL ORGANISATION OF ANIMALS (Answer key)

1	2	3	4	5	6	7	8	9	10
4	3	4	2	4	2	1	3	3	4
11	12	13	14	15	16	17	18	19	20
3	4	2	1	3	3	4	4	1	3
21	22	23	24	25	26	27	28	29	30
3	2	4	2	4	2	4	4	2	1
31	32	33	34	35	36	37	38	39	40
2	2	3	2	2	4	3	3	2	4
41	42	43	44	45	46	47	48	49	50
2	2	1	1	2	4	1	4	4	4
51	52	53	54	55	56	57	58	59	60
4	1	4	1	1	3	3	4	4	3

Chapter-03 BIOMOLECULES (Answer key)

1	2	3	4	5	6	7	8	9	10
4	1	4	2	3	1	4	3	3	3
11	12	13	14	15	16	17	18	19	20
4	2	3	3	2	4	3	2	4	2
21	22	23	24	25	26	27	28	29	30
3	2	4	4	4	2	4	2	3	4
31	32	33	34	35	36	37	38	39	40
2	3	3	4	4	2	4	4	4	4
41	42	43	44	45	46	47	48	49	50
4	2	2	4	4	1	2	2	4	4

Chapter-04 BREATHING AND EXCHANGE OF GASES (Answer key)

1	2	3	4	5	6	7	8	9	10
4	3	4	3	1	3	4	3	3	2
11	12	13	14	15	16	17	18	19	20
3	2	2	1	2	4	4	4	3	3
21	22	23	24	25	26	27	28	29	30
3	1	4	2	4	3	4	4	4	1
31	32	33	34	35	36	37	38	39	40
2	2	4	2	2	4	4	1	2	4
41	42	43	44	45	46	47	48	49	50
2	2	3	1	3	1	2	4	4	4

Chapter-05 BODY FLUIDS AND CIRCULATION (Answer key)

1	2	3	4	5	6	7	8	9	10
4	1	2	2	1	2	2	3	3	3
11	12	13	14	15	16	17	18	19	20
3	2	2	2	3	4	4	2	2	3
21	22	23	24	25	26	27	28	29	30
3	1	4	4	4	1	3	4	2	1
31	32	33	34	35	36	37	38	39	40
2	1	4	4	4	4	3	4	2	4
41	42	43	44	45	46	47	48	49	50
2	2	3	1	4	1	2	4	3	3

Chapter-06 EXCRETORY PRODUCTS AND THEIR ELIMINATION (Answer key)

1	2	3	4	5	6	7	8	9	10
3	3	4	3	1	2	4	4	3	3
11	12	13	14	15	16	17	18	19	20
3	1	4	1	3	4	4	4	4	3
21	22	23	24	25	26	27	28	29	30
3	2	4	4	3	4	4	4	1	2
31	32	33	34	35	36	37	38	39	40
2	2	4	3	1	4	4	2	2	4
41	42	43	44	45	46	47	48	49	50
2	3	1	1	4	1	2	1	4	4

Chapter-07 LOCOMOTION AND MOVEMENT (Answer key)

1	2	3	4	5	6	7	8	9	10
4	2	4	3	1	2	4	4	3	3
11	12	13	14	15	16	17	18	19	20
3	2	4	4	2	4	3	4	3	3
21	22	23	24	25	26	27	28	29	30
3	1	4	4	4	4	4	4	1	1
31	32	33	34	35	36	37	38	39	40
2	2	1	4	3	4	4	2	2	3
41	42	43	44	45	46	47	48	49	50
2	4	4	1	4	3	3	3	4	4

Chapter-08 NEURAL CONTROL AND COORDINATION (Answer key)

1	2	3	4	5	6	7	8	9	10
3	4	4	2	1	1	2	3	3	3
11	12	13	14	15	16	17	18	19	20
4	2	4	1	3	4	4	4	3	3
21	22	23	24	25	26	27	28	29	30
3	3	3	4	4	4	4	4	4	1
31	32	33	34	35	36	37	38	39	40
2	2	1	2	3	4	4	2	2	4
41	42	43	44	45	46	47	48	49	50
3	4	4	3	3	1	3	2	4	4

Chapter-09 CHEMICAL COORDINATION AND INTEGRATION (Answer key)

1	2	3	4	5	6	7	8	9	10
4	4	4	2	1	2	4	1	3	3
11	12	13	14	15	16	17	18	19	20
2	1	3	1	2	4	4	3	3	3
21	22	23	24	25	26	27	28	29	30
3	1	2	2	4	1	3	4	2	3
31	32	33	34	35	36	37	38	39	40
2	3	1	4	4	3	4	4	2	4
41	42	43	44	45	46	47	48	49	50
1	3	4	1	3	3	4	2	4	4

Chapter-10 HUMAN REPRODUCTION (Answer key)

1	2	3	4	5	6	7	8	9	10
4	3	2	4	4	3	1	3	2	2
11	12	13	14	15	16	17	18	19	20
3	2	4	2	3	4	4	4	4	3
21	22	23	24	25	26	27	28	29	30
3	2	4	1	4	4	2	2	2	3
31	32	33	34	35	36	37	38	39	40
3	2	2	4	4	4	2	2	2	4
41	42	43	44	45	46	47	48	49	50
3	4	3	1	4	1	2	4	4	4

Chapter-11 REPRODUCTIVE HEALTH (Answer key)

1	2	3	4	5	6	7	8	9	10
3	2	4	4	4	4	4	4	2	4
11	12	13	14	15	16	17	18	19	20
3	2	2	3	2	2	4	1	1	4
21	22	23	24	25	26	27	28	29	30
2	3	2	3	1	3	1	4	2	2
31	32	33	34	35	36	37	38	39	40
4	4	1	1	1	1	2	2	3	4
41	42	43	44	45	46	47	48	49	50
3	2	4	1	2	2	2	1	1	1

Chapter-12 EVOLUTION (Answer key)

1	2	3	4	5	6	7	8	9	10
4	3	2	1	1	2	4	3	3	3
11	12	13	14	15	16	17	18	19	20
3	2	2	2	3	4	4	4	4	3
21	22	23	24	25	26	27	28	29	30
3	2	4	2	2	1	4	4	4	4
31	32	33	34	35	36	37	38	39	40
3	2	4	3	2	4	4	4	2	4
41	42	43	44	45	46	47	48	49	50
1	4	1	1	1	1	2	3	4	3

Chapter-13 HUMAN HEALTH AND DISEASE (Answer key)

1	2	3	4	5	6	7	8	9	10
4	3	4	4	1	2	1	4	4	4
11	12	13	14	15	16	17	18	19	20
3	3	1	2	3	3	4	4	4	3
21	22	23	24	25	26	27	28	29	30
3	3	4	2	4	1	3	2	3	1
31	32	33	34	35	36	37	38	39	40
2	1	4	4	2	2	4	4	2	4
41	42	43	44	45	46	47	48	49	50
2	2	3	1	1	1	2	4	4	4

Chapter-14 MICROBES IN HUMAN WELFARE (Answer key)

1	2	3	4	5	6	7	8	9	10
4	3	4	1	1	3	4	4	4	3
11	12	13	14	15	16	17	18	19	20
3	3	2	2	3	3	4	4	4	3
21	22	23	24	25	26	27	28	29	30
3	1	4	2	4	4	3	4	4	1
31	32	33	34	35	36	37	38	39	40
3	2	4	4	3	4	4	4	3	3

Chapter-15 BIOTECHNOLOGY - PRINCIPLES AND PROCESSES (Answer key)

1	2	3	4	5	6	7	8	9	10
4	1	4	4	1	3	1	3	3	3
11	12	13	14	15	16	17	18	19	20
3	2	4	4	3	4	4	4	4	3
21	22	23	24	25	26	27	28	29	30
3	2	4	2	4	4	3	4	1	4
31	32	33	34	35	36	37	38	39	40
2	2	4	4	1	4	4	1	2	4

Chapter-16 BIOTECHNOLOGY AND ITS APPLICATIONS (Answer key)

1	2	3	4	5	6	7	8	9	10
4	1	4	1	1	1	3	3	3	3
11	12	13	14	15	16	17	18	19	20
4	3	4	4	3	4	4	4	4	3
21	22	23	24	25	26	27	28	29	30
3	2	4	2	4	4	3	4	3	4
31	32	33	34	35	36	37	38	39	40
2	2	1	4	4	4	2	2	2	4

Answer key - Mock test-01

1	2	3	4	5	6	7	8	9	10
2	1	2	2	2	4	4	2	4	4
11	12	13	14	15	16	17	18	19	20
3	3	3	1	3	4	4	2	2	2
21	22	23	24	25	26	27	28	29	30
1	4	3	1	4	3	2	4	3	2
31	32	33	34	35	36	37	38	39	40
2	4	4	3	4	4	3	1	2	2
41	42	43	44	45	46	47	48	49	50
2	3	2	3	3	3	1	3	4	2

Answer key - Mock test-02

1	2	3	4	5	6	7	8	9	10
1	3	4	3	3	2	4	3	4	4
11	12	13	14	15	16	17	18	19	20

4	2	3	3	4	4	3	3	3	3
21	22	23	24	25	26	27	28	29	30
4	4	1	4	4	2	2	1	3	1
31	32	33	34	35	36	37	38	39	40
4	4	4	1	1	1	3	3	4	4
41	42	43	44	45	46	47	48	49	50
3	4	1	2	3	1	1	2	2	1

Answer key - Mock test-03

1	2	3	4	5	6	7	8	9	10
2	4	1	3	3	3	4	4	1	3
11	12	13	14	15	16	17	18	19	20
2	2	2	1	1	2	3	3	4	4
21	22	23	24	25	26	27	28	29	30
3	2	2	2	4	1	3	4	2	2
31	32	33	34	35	36	37	38	39	40
2	3	4	1	3	4	4	3	2	4
41	42	43	44	45	46	47	48	49	50
2	4	4	1	4	3	1	3	4	1

Answer key - Mock test-04

1	2	3	4	5	6	7	8	9	10
4	2	1	2	3	2	2	4	1	3
11	12	13	14	15	16	17	18	19	20
4	2	2	2	2	2	3	4	4	3
21	22	23	24	25	26	27	28	29	30
4	2	1	4	4	4	4	4	1	4
31	32	33	34	35	36	37	38	39	40
1	2	3	3	3	4	2	3	4	4
41	42	43	44	45	46	47	48	49	50
4	1	1	3	4	4	4	4	1	2

Next book coming soon.....
which contain
1500+ statement based,
Assertion and reason type,
list 1 and list 2 type
NCERT based high quality questions for
NEET
so stay tuned.